Explainable Artificial Intelligence in Medical Imaging

Artificial intelligence (AI) in medicine is rising, and it holds tremendous potential for more accurate findings and novel solutions to complicated medical issues. Biomedical AI has potential, especially in the context of precision medicine, in the healthcare industry's next phase of development and advancement. Integration of AI research into precision medicine is the future; however, the human component must always be considered.

Explainable Artificial Intelligence in Medical Imaging: Fundamentals and Applications focuses on the most recent developments in applying artificial intelligence and data science to health care and medical imaging. Explainable artificial intelligence is a well-structured, adaptable technology that generates impartial, optimistic results. New healthcare applications for explicable artificial intelligence include clinical trial matching, continuous healthcare monitoring, probabilistic evolutions, and evidence-based mechanisms. This book overviews the principles, methods, issues, challenges, opportunities, and the most recent research findings. It makes the emerging topics of digital health and explainable AI in health care and medical imaging accessible to a wide audience by presenting various practical applications.

Presenting a thorough review of state-of-the-art techniques for precise analysis and diagnosis, the book emphasizes explainable artificial intelligence and its applications in healthcare. The book also discusses computational vision processing methods that manage complicated data, including physiological data, electronic medical records, and medical imaging data, enabling early prediction. Researchers, academics, business professionals, health practitioners, and students all can benefit from this book's insights and coverage.

Amjad Rehman Khan (Senior Member, IEEE) earned a Ph.D. from the Faculty of Computing, Universiti Teknologi Malaysia (UTM), Malaysia, specializing in information security using image processing techniques in 2010. He received a Rector Award for the 2010 Best Student from UTM Malaysia. He is currently associate professor at CCIS Prince Sultan University Riyadh, Saudi Arabia. He is also a principal investigator in several projects and completed projects funded by MoHE Malaysia, Saudi Arabia. His research interests are bioinformatics, IoT, information security, and pattern recognition.

Tanzila Saba (Senior Member, IEEE) received his Ph.D. degree in document information security and management from the Faculty of Computing, Universiti Teknologi Malaysia (UTM), Malaysia, in 2012. She is currently a full professor with the College of Computer and Information Sciences, Prince Sultan University (PSU), Riyadh, Saudi Arabia, and also the leader of the AIDA Laboratory. She has published over 300 publications in high-ranked journals. Her primary research interests include bioinformatics, data mining, and classification using AI models. She received the Best Student Award from the Faculty of Computing, UTM, in 2012 and also received the best researcher award from PSU, from 2013 to 2016. She is the editor of several reputed journals and on a panel of TPC of international conferences.

Advances in Computational Collective Intelligence
Edited by
Dr. Subhendu Kumar Pani
Principal, Krupajal Group of Institutions, India

Deep Learning for Smart Healthcare: Trends, Challenges and Applications
K. Murugeswari, B.Sundaravadivazhagan, S. Poonkuntran, and Thendral Puyalnithi
ISBN: 978-1-032-455815

Edge Computational Intelligence for AI-Enabled IoT Systems
By Shrikaant Kulkarni, Jaiprakash Narain Dwivedi, Dinda Pramanta, and Yuichiro Tanaka
ISBN: 978-1-032-207667

Explainable AI and Cybersecurity
By Mohammad Tabrez Quasim, Abdullah Alharthi, Ali Alqazzaz, Mohammed Mujib Alshahrani, Ali Falh Alshahrani, and Mohammad Ayoub Khan
ISBN: 978-1-032-422213

Machine Learning in Applied Sciences
By M. A. Jabbar, Shankru Guggari, Kingsley Okoye, and Houneida Sakly
ISBN: 978-1-032-251721

Social Media and Crowdsourcing
By Sujoy Chatterjee, Thipendra P Singh, Sunghoon Lim, and Anirban Mukhopadhyay
ISBN: 978-1-032-386874

AI and IoT Technology and Applications for Smart Healthcare
By Alex Khang
ISBN: 978-1-032-684901

Innovations and Applications of Technology in Language Education
By Hung Phu Bui, Raghvendra Kumar, and Nilayam Kamila
ISBN: 978-1-032-560731

Data-Driven Modelling and Predictive Analytics in Business and Finance
By Alex Khang, Rashmi Gujrati, Hayri Uygun, RK Tailor and Sanjaya Singh Gaur
ISBN: 978-1-032-60191-5

Explainable Artificial Intelligence in Medical Imaging
Fundamentals and Applications

Edited by
Amjad Rehman Khan
and Tanzila Saba

CRC Press
Taylor & Francis Group
Boca Raton London New York

CRC Press is an imprint of the
Taylor & Francis Group, an **informa** business

Cover: Shutterstock

First edition published 2025
2385 NW Executive Center Drive, Suite 320, Boca Raton FL 33431
and by CRC Press

4 Park Square, Milton Park, Abingdon, Oxon, OX14 4RN

CRC Press is an imprint of Taylor & Francis Group, LLC

ISBN: 9781032598987 (hbk)
ISBN: 9781032626338 (pbk)
ISBN: 9781032626345 (ebk)

DOI: 10.1201/9781032626345

Typeset in Garamond
by KnowledgeWorks Global Ltd.

Contents

Preface

This book focuses on the most recent developments in applying artificial intelligence and data science to healthcare and medical imaging. Explainable artificial intelligence is a well-structured, adaptable technology that generates impartial, optimistic results. New healthcare applications for explicable artificial intelligence include clinical trial matching, continuous healthcare monitoring, probabilistic evolutions, and evidence-based mechanisms. This book overviews the principles, methods, issues, challenges, opportunities, and the most recent research findings. It makes the emerging topics of digital health and explainable AI in healthcare and medical imaging accessible to a wide audience by presenting various practical applications.

Principles and Methods of *Explainable Artificial Intelligence in Medical Imaging* presents a thorough review of state-of-the-art techniques for precise analysis and diagnosis with an emphasis on explainable artificial intelligence and its applications in healthcare. The book also discusses computational vision processing methods that handle complicated data, including physiological data, electronic medical records, and medical imaging data, enabling early prediction. Researchers, academics, business professionals, health practitioners, and students will all benefit from the knowledge in this book.

Contributors

Naveed Abbas received his Ph.D. degree in image processing (medical imaging) and machine learning from Universiti Teknologi Malaysia, Malaysia, in 2016. During his Ph.D., he proposed novel techniques for occlusion splitting of red blood cells in medical imaging and segmentation and classification of malaria parasites for proper quantification of malaria parasitemia. He is currently conducting research under his supervision for four Ph.D. students while co-supervising 2 Ph.D. students abroad. He is the author of many papers published in international journals and conferences of high repute. He is currently working as assistant professor in the Department of Computer Sciences Islamia College Peshawar. His research interests include DIP,VP, CV, XAI, ML, and DL for various tasks in images, videos, and data science.

Aiesha Ahmad earned her Ph.D. in Computer Science with major in AI from NCBA&E Lahore and M.Phil. in Computer Science with Major in SE &AI from COMSATS University Islamabad, Lahore Campus. Currently, she is working as assistant professor at the Institute of Computer Science & Information Technology, The Women University Multan, Pakistan. Her area of research is artificial intelligence, machine learning, deep learning, machine consciousness, deliberative and non-deliberative rationality evaluation, fuzzy modeling, and knowledge base systems.

Qurat ul Ain is a lecturer at Riphah International University's Faisalabad campus, where she has been serving since March 2023. She holds an MS in Computer Science from Riphah International University, Faisalabad.

Shahzad Akbar is associate professor at Riphah College of Computing, Riphah International University, Faisalabad Campus, Pakistan. His area of research is image processing, machine & deep learning, biometrics, medical image analysis, and pattern recognition. He is a recipient of different national awards. He has more than 20 years of teaching and industry experience and supervised many undergraduate and postgraduate students. He is the head of Riphah Artificial Intelligence

(RAIR) Lab, Riphah International University, Faisalabad Campus, Pakistan. He is an approved supervisor by the Higher Education Commission (HEC), Pakistan, and is also a reviewer of some reputed journals and conferences.

Theeb Rabie Alafan did his Ph.D. at the University Technology Malaysia in 2024. He was an active member of the ViCube Research Lab, UTM, JB, Malaysia. He is certified data management professional (CDMP) with professional skills and experiences in Data Governance, Data Privacy & Protection, Data Strategy, Data analytics, Business Intelligence, Business Analysis, and Information Systems of over 10 years. Leading multiple projects and professional teams in various information technology projects, data management projects, and business strategy.

Abdullah Alaulamie is currently assistant professor with the Department of Information Systems, King Faisal University. His research interests include computer in human behavior, human–computer interaction, IS theories, the Internet of Things (IoT), and immersion.

Bandar Ali Al-Rami Al-Ghamdi, holds a Ph.D. from Universite de Reims Champagne-Ardenne in 2015, Reims, France; the M.Sc. degree in Information Technology from De Montfort University, Leicester, UK, in 2008; and the B.Cs. degree in Computer Sciences from the University of King Abdul-Aziz University, Jeddah, Saudi Arabia, in 2003. Currently, he is assistant professor at Arab Open University, Riyadh, KSA. His research interests are Sensor Networks, Distributed Systems, eHealth Systems, Networking, Testing, Verification, Software Engineering, and Real-Time Systems. He has multiple publications in national and international sources.

Anees Ara (Member, IEEE) received her B.Sc. degree in computer science and the M.Sc. degree in mathematics with computer science from Osmania University, Hyderabad, India. She has a Ph.D. in computer science with network security as her specialization from King Saud University, Riyadh, Saudi Arabia. She is currently working as assistant professor at Prince Sultan University. She also an active researcher at AIDA Lab, PSU. She published her research work in various national and international journals, conferences and as book chapters. Her research interest includes network security, wireless sensor networks, cyber physical systems, Internet of things, cloud computing, and ubiquitous computing.

Fetoun Alzahrani specializes in machine learning and deep learning. She holds master's degree in Information Technology from King Saud University, where her thesis focused on artificial intelligence and deep learning fields. She deeply understands core programming languages and statistical analytics, showcasing her superior technical aptitude. Her expertise extends beyond theoretical knowledge, as she has demonstrated a strong practical understanding of managing complex tasks and other technical projects. Her contributions to the academic community are evident through her four published works in various fields, including natural language processing, artificial intelligence, cloud computing, and information technology projects such as IoT and mobile development using web technologies. Fetoun is affiliated with the AIDA Lab at Prince Sultan University, where she serves as a research assistant, further enriching her portfolio with hands-on experience and cutting-edge research in the field.

Rida Arif holds an MS in Computer Science from Riphah International University. Her area of research is machine learning.

Hareem Ayesha completed her M.Sc. in Computer Science from the Department of Computer Science, Bahauddin Zakariya University, Multan, Pakistan, in 2020. Currently, she is working as lecturer of Computer Science at the Institute of Computer Science & Information Technology, The Women University Multan, Pakistan. Her research interests include artificial intelligence, machine learning, deep learning, explainable artificial intelligence, computer vision and medical image analysis.

Noor Ayesha completed her medical degree from School of Clinical Medicine, Zhengzhou University, Zhengzhou, China. She has interest in medical imaging, cancer diagnosis, and artificial intelligence techniques. She is also a competent researcher in the domain of medical images analysis and cancer diagnosis.

Ayesha Azam is working as research officer at the Bioinformatics Research Laboratory (BRL), Al-Khawarizmi Institute of Computer Science (KICS), UET, Lahore. Her research interests include medical image processing, augmented reality in healthcare and education, computer vision, and deep learning. Azam received her bachelor's degree in computer science from the University of Engineering and Technology (UET) in Lahore, Pakistan, in 2022. Currently, she is pursuing a master's degree in computer science at the same university.

Mahsa Bahadori is an undergraduate student at the Department of Industrial Engineering, Islamic Azad University of Mashhad, Iran. She has research interest in machine learning, healthcare optimization, and data analysis.

Mina Bahadori, M.Sc. Systems Engineering, Bachelor of Industrial Engineering, Ph.D. candidate at the Department of Industrial Engineering of Clemson University, USA. She has research interest in machine learning, reinforcement leaning, stochastic optimization, and data analysis.

Chintan Bhatt is working as an assistant professor in the Department of Computer Science and Engineering (CSE), School of Technology, Pandit Deendayal Energy

University (PDEU), Gujarat, India. Before joining PDEU, Dr. Bhatt served as assistant professor in CE Department (CSPIT, CHARUSAT) for 11 years. Dr. Bhatt is the author and coauthor of 80+ publications in the areas of computer vision, Internet of Things, and fog computing. Dr. Bhatt has won several awards, including "CSI Award" and "Best Paper Award" for his CSI articles and conference publications. Dr. Bhatt was involved in successful organization of few Special Issues in SCI/Scopus Journals.

Mehdi Davari received his master's degree in Financial Management and graduated from the Department of Management, Isfahan Branch, Islamic Azad University, Isfahan, Iran. He is interested in human factor ergonomics for understanding the interaction between humans and their environment, including the tools, tasks, and systems they use to achieve organizational goals.

Alex Elyassih (Senior Member, Australian Computer Society) earned his PhD in computer science and information technology from USA with a focus on straight line motion of robot manipulations in Cartesian space. His research was based in the development and implementations of the straight-line motion algorithms processing techniques. He was honored with certification Award as Certified Professional from the Australian Computer Society in association with IPP accreditation (International professional Practice Programme). Currently, he is assistant professor at the College of Computer and Information Sciences, Prince Sultan University, Riyadh, Saudi Arabia. His research interests include Cybersecurity, IoT, information security, GRC (Governance, Risk & compliance and pattern recognition.

Ahmad Bilal Farooq is a lecturer at Riphah International University's Faisalabad campus, where he has been serving since October 2023. He holds an MS in Computer Science from Riphah International University, Faisalabad.

Umer Farooq received his bachelor's degree in information technology in 2017 and master's degree in information technology from the Department of Information Sciences, University of Education, Lahore, in July 2023. His research interests include Biomedical Image Processing, Machine Learning, Deep Learning, Transfer Learning, and CNN.

Amit Ganatra served as a provost in Parul University, Waghodia, Gujarat, India. His record of excellence has allowed him to establish his mark in academics through developing policies, designing curriculums, and furthering research. Additionally, he holds memberships across multiple academic bodies where he has been instrumental toward shaping the trajectory of technical education. Also, to note, Dr. Ganatra is a member of IEEE, ACM, and CSI professional society chapters. He has also been known for his contributions to the academic knowledge bank through his authorship of 130+ research publications and his supervision of over 100 industry projects, 100+ dissertations, and 12 Ph.D. research scholars.

Sahar Gull holds an MS in Computer Science from Riphah International University. Her area of research is machine learning, image processing, and deep learning.

Abdul Hai is a computer vision researcher at the Intelligent Information Processing (IIP) lab. He earned his B.Sc. in Software Engineering from Islamia College University in 2023.

Sajid Iqbal has completed his Ph.D. from the Department of Computer Science, University of Engineering and Technology, Lahore, Pakistan. Currently, he is working as assistant professor in the Department of Information Systems, College of Computer Science and Information Technology, King Faisal University, Saudi Arabia. His research areas include medical image analysis, computer vision, and natural language processing. He has published more than 40 articles on national and international platforms.

Karrar A. Kadhim received his B.Sc. degree in computer science from Kufa University, Iraq, in 2010 and M.Sc. degree from the School of Computing, Faculty of Engineering, UTM, in 2013. where he is currently pursuing a Ph.D. degree. Currently, he is a lecturer in the Computer Techniques Engineering Department, Faculty of Information Technology, Imam Ja'afar Al-Sadiq University, Baghdad, Iraq. His research interests include computer vision, digital image processing, medical image processing, deep learning, and machine learning.

Muhammad Usman Ghani Khan has over 18 years of research experience specifically in the areas of image processing, computer vision, bioinformatics, medical imaging, computational linguistics, and machine learning. He is director of Intelligent Criminology Lab under the Center of Artificial Intelligence. He is also director and founder of five research labs, including Computer Vision & ML Lab, Bioinformatics Lab, Virtual Reality & Gaming Lab, Data Science Lab, and Software Systems Research Lab. He is a well-groomed teacher and mentor for subjects related to artificial intelligence, ML, and deep learning. He has recorded freely available video lectures on YouTube for courses of Bioinformatics, Image Processing, Data Mining & Data Science, and Computer Programming. Khan received his Ph.D. degree from Sheffield University, Sheffield, UK, in 2012. During his Ph.D. degree, he worked on statistical modeling for machine vision signals, specifically generating language descriptions of video streams. He is currently working as chairperson of the Department of Computer Science, University of Engineering and Technology, Lahore, Pakistan.

Fatima Nayer Khan is a member of Artificial Intelligence and Research Analysts (AIDA) lab and her research interests include data science, artificial intelligence, machine learning, and software engineering. She has published in well-recognized prestigious scientific journals. She is the co-ambassador for Women in Data Science (WiDS) conference and is associate director for Evaluation and Academic Accreditation Center at Prince Sultan University, Riyadh, Saudi Arabia.

Amjad R. Khan (Senior Member, IEEE) earned a Ph.D. from the Faculty of Computing, Universiti Teknologi Malaysia (UTM), Malaysia, specializing in information security using image processing techniques in 2010. He received a Rector Award for the 2010 Best Student from UTM Malaysia. He is currently associate professor at CCIS Prince Sultan University Riyadh, Saudi Arabia. He is also PI in several projects and has completed projects funded by MoHE Malaysia, Saudi Arabia. His research interests are Bioinformatics, IoT, Information Security and Pattern Recognition.

Tanzila S. Khan (Senior Member, IEEE) received a Ph.D. degree in document information security and management from the Faculty of Computing, Universiti Teknologi Malaysia (UTM), Malaysia, in 2012. She is associate chair in the Information Systems Department, College of Computer and Information Sciences, Prince Sultan University, Riyadh, Saudi Arabia, where she is an Artificial Intelligence and Data Analytics Research Laboratory leader. Her primary research interests include medical imaging, pattern recognition, data mining, MRI analysis, and soft computing. She is Active Professional Member of ACM, AIS, and IAENG organizations. She is PSU Women in Data Science (WiDS) ambassador at Stanford University and the Global Women Tech Conference. She was a recipient of the Best Student Award from the Faculty of Computing, UTM, in 2012

Ahmad Kokhahi, M.Sc. and Bachelor of Industrial Engineering, PhD candidate at the Department of Industrial Engineering of Clemson University, USA. He has research interest in machine learning, metaheuristic, and scheduling.

Deep Kothadiya received his bachelor's and master's degrees in computer science and engineering from Gujarat Technological University. He is currently pursuing Ph.D. at Charotar University of Science and Technology (CHARUSAT). He is also assistant professor with the U & P U Patel Department of Computer Engineering, Chandubhai S. Patel Institute of Technology, CHARUSAT. He is also a research scholar with CHARUSAT and Prince Sultan University, Riyadh, Saudi Arabia. He has already published many research papers, including one SCI-indexed paper. He is also Technical Reviewer of *International Journal of Computing and Digital Systems*.

Hannan Bin Liaqat received his B.S. degree in information technology from the COMSATS Institute of Information Technology, Lahore, Pakistan, in 2006, M.S. degree in computer networks from the COMSATS Institute of Information Technology in 2009, and Ph.D. degree from the Dalian University of Technology, Dalian, China, in 2016. From 2009 to 2011, he was lecturer in the Computer Science Department, University of Gujrat, Gujrat, Pakistan. He is currently associate professor and M.Phil. supervisor in the Department of Information Sciences, University of Education, Lahore. Dr. Hannan has a number of publications to his credits in international journals and conferences. He is the reviewer of several international journals.

Shiza Maham received her bachelor's degree in Computer Science from the University of Engineering & Technology and recently completed her master's degree in Computer Science from the University of Engineering & Technology. She is designated as research officer in the Intelligent Criminology Research Laboratory under the National Center of Artificial Intelligence. Her research interests lie in the fields of Natural Language Processing, Machine Learning, and Deep Learning.

Krunal Maheriya has received his bachelor degree from Silver Oak College of Engineering and Technology (GTU), Ahmedabad, Gujarat, India, in 2021, Master's degree in Computer Engineering from CHARUSAT University, Gujarat, India, in 2023. Currently, he is working as assistant professor at CHARUSAT. His major area of research includes computer vision and deep learning.

Tariq Mahmood is assistant professor at the Faculty of Information Sciences, University of Education, Vehari Campus, Vehari, Pakistan. He has completed his doctoral degree in Software Engineering from the Beijing University of Technology, China, and his master's degree in Computer Science from the University of Lahore, Pakistan. He is a renowned expert in Image Processing, Healthcare Informatics and Social Media Analysis, Adhoc Networks, and WSN. He has contributed various research articles in well-reputed international journals and conferences. He is the editorial member and reviewer of various journals, including *PLoS One, Journal of Supercomputer, Journal of Digital Imaging, International Journal of Sensors, Wireless Communications and Control*, etc. His research interests include Image Processing, Social Media Analysis, Medical Image Diagnosis, Machine Learning, and Data Mining. He aims to contribute to interdisciplinary research of computer science and human-related disciplines.

Abeer Rashad Mirdad is associate professor in the college of Computer and Information Sciences, Department of Information Systems, Prince Sultan University, Riyadh, Saudi Arabia. She is also a member of Artificial Intelligence & Data Analytics (AIDA) Lab. Her key research interests are in blockchain technology, data analytics, artificial intelligence, machine learning, and deep learning.

Farhan Mohamed (Senior Member, IEEE) received his B.Sc. and M.Sc. degrees from Universiti Teknologi Malaysia (UTM), and the Ph.D. degree in computer science from Swansea University, in 2014. He is currently senior lecturer in the School of Computing, Faculty of Engineering, UTM, Malaysia. He is also research fellow with the Media and Games Innovation Centre of Excellence (MaGICX), Institute of Human Centered Engineering, UTM. He led a study with SME Corp-Huawei in analyzing SME digitalization, in 2018. His current research interests include visual analytics, virtual environment, and procedural computer graphics. He received the Leaders in Innovation Fellowship from Newton Fund, Royal Academy of Engineering, UK, in 2017. He is on the Executive Committee of the IEEE Computer Society Malaysia.

Muhammad Mujahid received master's degree of Computer Science from the Islamia University of Bahawalpur, Pakistan. Currently, he is pursuing Ph.D. degree. He is a reviewer of the *Journal of Super Computing* and *PLoS One*. He is also engaged with IEEE Journals, Springer, and some other journals. His main research interests include text mining, machine learning, data science, artificial intelligence, bioinformatics, Internet of Things, and sentiment analysis.

Zunaira Naqvi is a lecturer at Riphah International University's Faisalabad campus, where she has been serving since October 2023. She holds an MS in Computer Science from Riphah International University, Faisalabad.

Shahid Naseem is working as assistant professor (IT) in the Department of Information Sciences, University of Education, Lahore, Pakistan. He did his Ph.D. in Computer Science from National College of Business Administration and Economics, Lahore, Pakistan. His research of interest is Artificial Intelligence, Machine Learning, and Explainable Artificial Intelligence.

Zubaira Naz has worked at Bioinformatics Research Lab as senior research officer. She has authored few articles in international refereed journals. Her research interests include medical image processing, bioinformatics, augmented reality, virtual reality, metaverse, image processing, and deep learning. Naz received her bachelor's and master's degrees in computer science from the University of Engineering and Technology (UET) Lahore, Pakistan, in 2018 and 2022, respectively. She is currently working as lecturer in the Department of Computer Science, Information and Technology University, Lahore, Pakistan.

Martin Parmar received his diploma degree from SSPC, Visnagar, Gujarat, India, in 2003, Bachelor's Degree in Computer Engineering from CITC, Gujarat, India, in 2007, and Master's Degree in Computer Science and Engineering from L.D. College of Engineering, Ahmedabad, Gujarat, India, in 2014. Currently, he is pursuing doctoral course in Computer Engineering at CHARUSAT. He is working as assistant professor at CHARUSAT. His major area of research includes information security, blockchain and cryptocurrency.

Atul Patel is a seasoned professional with a Ph.D. in Wireless Communications from Sardar Patel University (2012), complemented by master's Degree in Computer Applications from D.D.I.T., Nadiad, Gujarat University, India (1993). With over 30 years of progressive experience in industry, academia, and research, he has held various leadership roles, including Registrar at CHARUSAT University and professor and dean at CMPICA, Faculty of Computer Science, CHARUSAT. Dr. Patel's expertise spans across artificial intelligence, deep learning, machine learning, cloud computing, big data analytics, and network technologies, making him a versatile and accomplished individual in the field.

Mrugendrasinh Rahevar is assistant professor in U & P U Patel Department of Computer Engineering, CHARUSAT University, Gujarat, India. He completed his B.E.C.E. from Gujarat University in 2006 and M.E.C.S.E. from Gujarat Technological University in 2014. He completed his Ph.D. in action recognition in computer vision in 2023 from CHARUSAT University. His research interest includes computer vision and deep learning.

Ghalib Ahmed Salman received his bachelor's degree in statistics and computer science from Baghdad University, Iraq, in 1993 and M.Sc. degree from ALRASHEED College, University of Technology, Iraq, in 2002. He received his Ph.D. in computer science from the Faculty of Computing at University of Technology, Malaysia. Currently, he is a lecturer in the Cyber Security Department, Middle Technical University. His research interests include computer vision, digital image processing, medical image processing, data and image security, and computer networking.

Masoumeh Soleimani holds a Ph.D. in Mathematics, specializing in graph theory and algebra. Currently pursuing a Ph.D. in Industrial Engineering at the Department of Industrial Engineering, Clemson University, USA, her research focus centers on optimization, machine learning, and data analysis.

Morteza Soltani, M.Sc. Industrial Engineering, Bachelor of Industrial Engineering, Ph.D. candidate at the Department of Industrial Engineering of Clemson University, USA. He has research interest in machine learning, reinforcement leaning, and stochastic optimization.

Abdullah Tariq is a seasoned researcher in the field of machine learning and deep learning. Currently, he completed his Master's degree in Computer Science with a specialization in Deep Learning and Machine Learning. He completed his Bachelor's degree from the University of Engineering and Technology Lahore in 2020. He has been working at the National Center of Artificial Intelligence in Lahore, where he has been contributing to cutting-edge research in the field of artificial intelligence. With four years of research experience in machine learning and deep learning, he has been an active participant in various research projects and has published several research papers in top-tier conferences and journals.

Mehreen Tariq, an accomplished computer scientist, completed her M.Sc. in Computer Science from Bahauddin Zakariya University, Multan, Pakistan, in 2020. Her proficiency encompasses artificial intelligence, machine learning, deep learning, explainable AI, computer vision, and medical image analysis. Committed to ethical and transparent AI, Mehreen's academic journey showcases a blend of theoretical expertise and practical application. Her diverse skill set and unwavering dedication to innovation position her as a valuable contributor to the dynamic field of computer science.

Talha Tasleem is a computer vision researcher at the Digital Image Processing (DIP) lab. He earned his B.Sc. in Software Engineering from Islamia College University in 2023.

Farwa Urooj holds an MS in Computer Science from Riphah International University. Her area of research is machine learning.

Chapter 1

Explainable Artificial Intelligence in Medicine: Social and Ethical Issues

Shahid Naseem[1], Tariq Mahmood[2,3], Hannan Bin Liaqat[1], Amjad R. Khan[2], and Umer Farooq[1]

[1]*Department of Information Sciences, Division (S&T), University of Education, Lahore, Pakistan*

[2]*Artificial Intelligence and Data Analytics (AIDA) Lab, CCIS Prince Sultan University Riyadh, Kingdom of Saudi Arabia*

[3]*Faculty of Information Sciences, University of Education, Vehari Campus, Vehari, Pakistan*

1.1 Introduction

Computer programs that can recognize images, comprehend speech, make judgments, and translate languages are referred to as artificial intelligence (AI) systems. AI has diverse applications across various domains, including economics, biometrics, online commerce, and the automotive sector. Healthcare systems are facing mounting challenges due to increasing patient demands, a rise in chronic diseases, and resource limitations (Gupta, Anpalagan, Guan, & Khwaja, 2021). Concurrently, the adoption of digital health technologies is on the upswing, leading to a proliferation of data in healthcare settings. If properly applied, these technologies could free up healthcare professionals to concentrate on figuring out the underlying causes of illnesses and keeping track of how well treatments and preventative measures are working. Therefore, it is important for lawmakers, politicians, and other decision-makers

DOI: 10.1201/9781032626345-1

to be aware of this tendency. Many computer scientists, data scientists, and clinical entrepreneurs contend that integrating AI should be one of the key components of healthcare reform (Amann et al., 2020; Rehman et al., 2023).

Globally, healthcare expenses are rising as a result of variables like rising chronic illness rates, longer life expectancy, and the continual discovery of pricey new treatments. Several researchers forecast a difficult future for the global sustainability of healthcare systems. AI holds the promise of mitigating the power of these trends by enhancing healthcare quality and cost-effectiveness (Khan et al., 2022; Larabi-Marie-Sainte et al., 2019). AI is frequently employed in healthcare to aid in treatment decisions and assists clinical experts in diagnosing chronic diseases. However, despite their undeniable potential, AI-based models, which are trained on individual patient data to match their unique characteristics, do not offer a one-size-fits-all solution (Sadad et al., 2021). Several challenges are associated with AI-based systems, encompassing technical aspects as well as legal, medical, and patient perspectives, necessitating a multidisciplinary approach. While AI-based systems support humans in performing various analytical tasks, their explainability remains a subject of criticism (Mahmood et al., 2021). In these systems, explainability is not merely a technical concern but also raises numerous medical, legal, ethical, and social issues that require investigation. This study delves into assessing the role of explainable AI in the medical field and conducts an ethical assessment of explainability for the integration of AI-based systems into clinical practice (Mahmood et al., 2020).

1.1.1 Ethical Issues in Healthcare

The realm of ethics in AI is a burgeoning field of research, arising in response to the challenges posed by AI in the healthcare sector (Vainio-Pekka et al., 2023). One of the central challenges in implementing ethical considerations in AI is transparency. In any medical treatment scenario, ethical issues invariably come into play. These encompass concerns related to waiting lists, equitable access to medical resources, and making ethically sound decisions regarding the appropriate course of treatment (Mahmood et al., 2023). While the integration of AI into clinical practice holds immense potential for enhancing healthcare, it also brings forth ethical dilemmas that demand attention. Establishing ethical standards is imperative to assess the benefits and complexities of medical procedures in healthcare, focusing on the moral decision-making applied to medical practices and policies, as outlined below:

Determine a patient's wishes in order to respect their autonomy.

- *Justice:* Adhere to the proper procedures to set healthcare spending caps and treat all patients fairly.
- *Beneficence:* Look out for the patient's best interests and determine what constitutes desirable outcomes.
- *Non-maleficence:* Decide what harms need to be avoided.

These principles serve as valuable tools for healthcare professionals in recognizing ethical dilemmas and engaging in meaningful conversations with patients to understand their needs and preferences.

    i. Informed consent for data usage
   ii. Safety and clearness
  iii. Algorithmic impartiality and bias
   iv. Data secrecy

The main objective is to assist policymakers in taking a proactive approach to address the ethical challenges posed by the implementation of AI in healthcare settings. The growing prominence of AI in high-stakes situations has heightened the need for responsible, fair, and transparent AI design and governance. Transparency, encompassing accessibility and comprehensibility of information, is of utmost importance. Often, information regarding the functioning of machine learning algorithms is intentionally obscured. The integration of AI may result in situations where accountability for any potential harm becomes elusive (Borda, Molnar, Neesham, & Kostkova, 2022; Yousaf et al., 2019).

1.1.2 Ethical Issues in Medicine

As the integration of AI-powered systems in healthcare remains to expand, it becomes imperative to delve into the ethical considerations accompanying this impending paradigm shift. A widely adopted and well-suited ethical framework for measuring biomedical ethical challenges is crucial in this context. It is worth noting that moral and ethical values in the field of medicine often exhibit variations based on the country and cultural norms. Many ethical issues in medical practice revolve around matters of life and death. These issues encompass concerns related to patient rights, informed consent, confidentiality, competence, advance directives, negligence, and more.

1.1.3 Social Issues

AI models have the capacity to incorporate and propagate human and societal biases within the healthcare domain. However, it is crucial to understand that the responsibility often lies more with the underlying data than with the algorithms themselves. These models can be trained on datasets that contain human decisions or data reflecting the indirect consequences of historical or societal inequalities. Additionally, the process of data collection and utilization can also contribute to bias, with user-generated data acting as a feedback loop that perpetuates such biases.

Within the healthcare context, social issues, often referred to as social determinants of health, pertain to the conditions in which individuals reside, work, learn, and engage in recreational activities. These conditions are a direct result of the distribution of financial resources and power on both international and national scales, as

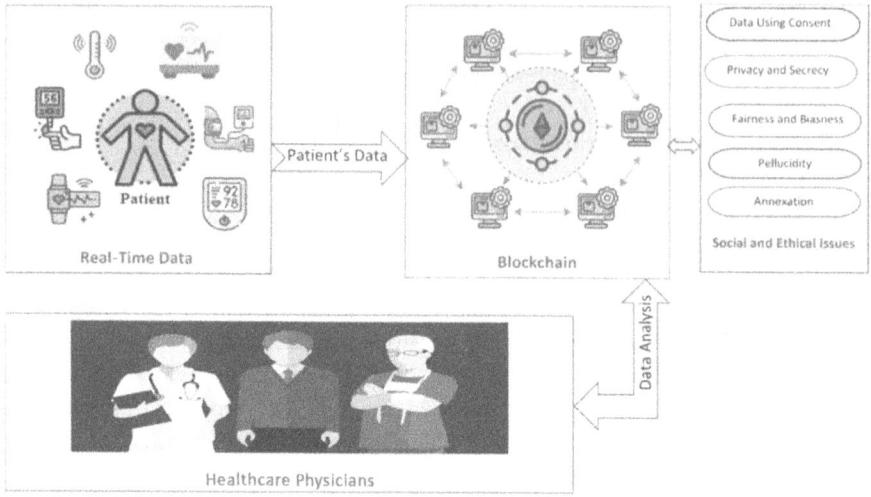

Figure 1.1   AI model for healthcare.

well as at regional levels. Frequently, systematic health disparities can be attributed to these underlying social issues (Webster, Taylor, Thomas, & Weller, 2022).

As our reliance on AI for decision-making continues to expand, it becomes paramount to ensure that these systems are developed ethically and free from unjust biases. AI systems are increasingly being employed to enhance patient care pathways and surgical outcomes, surpassing human capabilities in certain domains, as illustrated in Figure 1.1. This trend is likely to persist, with AI either complementing or potentially replacing existing systems, ushering in an era of AI in healthcare. In this context, abstaining from the utilization of AI could be seen as unscientific and ethically questionable (Stuckler, 2008).

Table 1.1 illustrates that having access to healthcare means that an individual can avail healthcare services from a healthcare provider, aiming to optimize their personal health. The impact of this access is visually represented in Figure 1.2. This access necessitates that an individual can enter the healthcare system, and any barriers to this entry can hinder a person's ability to reach healthcare services. As per

Table 1.1   Social Factor Impact in Healthcare

Sr. No.	Social Factors	Impact in Healthcare (%)
1.	Uninsured of healthcare industry workers	30
2.	Uninsured of disabled persons	9
3.	Uninsured and Latinx	38
4.	Insured and don't have bachelor degree	86

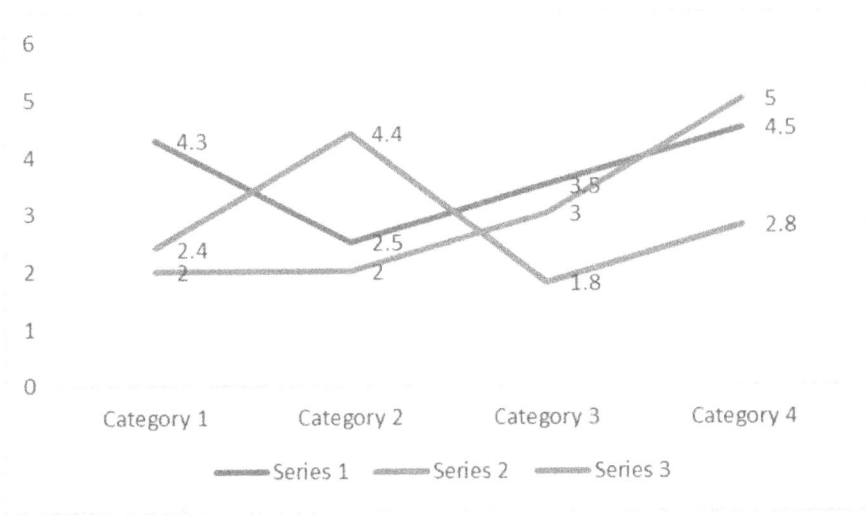

Figure 1.2   Impact of social factors in healthcare.

the Patient Protection and Affordable Care Act of 2019, a significant portion of the population, approximately 27.9 million individuals, remained without health insurance, primarily comprising low-income workers. Likewise, the Kaiser Family Foundation has reported that cost serves as a substantial impediment to health-care access for economically disadvantaged individuals in Europe. Additionally, Medicaid is available to people with disabilities who are unable to work and get support like Social Security Disability Insurance (Naik et al., 2022).

As indicated in Table 1.2, a notable 55% of business leaders within the healthcare industry express apprehension regarding the potential threats to security and privacy associated with the implementation of AI in healthcare. Additionally, 45% of these

Table 1.2   AI-Based Ethical Concerns in Healthcare

Sr. No.	AI-Based Ethical Concerns in Healthcare	Effects in Healthcare (%)
1.	Security and privacy threats	55
2.	Safety issues	45
3.	Machine learning issues	35
4.	Effects of malicious entities	35
5.	Personal interaction	30
6.	Concentration of wealth	28
7.	Loss of job for healthcare employees	15

leader's harbor concerns related to safety issues linked to AI, while 35% specifically worry about machine learning–related issues, along with similar concerns pertaining to malicious entities. Moreover, 30% of these leaders have reservations regarding the personal interaction aspect with AI-based healthcare systems, and another 28% are concerned about the prominent role of wealth within AI-based healthcare systems. Lastly, 15% of respondents are troubled by the possibility that AI-based healthcare systems could result in job displacement for healthcare employees.

1.2 Materials and Methods

In recent years, AI has made major inroads into the field of healthcare, aiding doctors in making more informed clinical decisions. AI has demonstrated its ability in a variety of applications, including the detection of malignancies in magnetic resonance images and the evaluation of reports written by radiologists and pathologists. Nevertheless, AI comes with a significant risk: It can sometimes be supposed as a "black box," eroding reliance in its trustworthiness. This issue is particularly critical in a domain where a single decision can literally be a matter of life or death. The introduction of new technology raises concerns about the potential for inaccuracies and data breaches, particularly in the high-stakes realm of healthcare (Singh & Garg, 2014). Errors in this field can have grave consequences for patients who may become victims of such inaccuracies. It is crucial to keep in mind that patients often interact with healthcare professionals at times when they are most vulnerable. However, if utilized wisely, the partnership between AI and physicians can be quite fruitful. AI can be used to provide doctors with evidence-based advice and serve as a medical decision support tool (AI-Health). Its contributions to healthcare can be seen in a variety of areas, such as diagnosis, medication discovery, epidemiology, individualized care, and improving operational effectiveness (Tang et al., 2022).

1.2.1 Explainable AI

The idea of explainable artificial intelligence (XAI) has been gaining significant traction, primarily focused on ensuring that AI algorithms are comprehensible to humans. This research aims to explore whether XAI can genuinely propel advancements in healthcare, particularly by enhancing understanding and trust. XAI strives to transition from the concept of a "black box" to that of a transparent "white box." In a white-box model, complete transparency is achieved. However, in numerous scenarios, such as deep learning models, the level of explainability may fall within a range, akin to a "translucent white box," with opacity varying from 0% to 100%.

Higher opacity in the translucent white box can contribute to a more profound understanding of the model, potentially fostering greater trust. Within the realm of healthcare, various stakeholders have distinct requirements for explanations. For instance, while users like healthcare professionals and patients mainly have to do

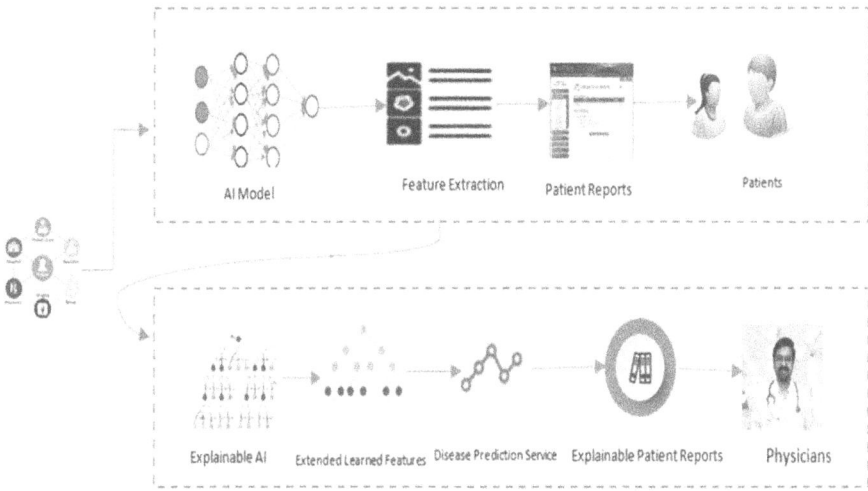

Figure 1.3   Explainable AI for healthcare.

with having confidence in the predictions made by the model, data scientists are mostly interested in understanding the model itself (as shown in Figure 1.3). As a result, while trust for patients and healthcare providers generally relates to the model, trust for data researchers generally relates to what the model predicts. By offering numerous predictions and supporting explanations, it is possible to address the issue of model trust (Yang, Ye, & Xia, 2022).

1.2.2 Explainable AI for Healthcare

As AI continues to advance within the healthcare sector, the need for transparency and trustworthiness in AI-driven clinical decision-making becomes increasingly critical. In response to this challenge, XAI has emerged as a promising solution, offering clear and interpretable explanations for the predictions and recommendations generated by AI algorithms. XAI plays a vital role in facilitating informed decision support for clinical practitioners and aligning with evidence-based medical practices. In the realm of XAI, ongoing efforts are dedicated to developing effective evaluation methods. While one straightforward approach involves user feedback for evaluation, this method requires substantial effort and may still be susceptible to various biases. Additionally, computational evaluations are being explored to assess the ethics and unsupervised learning behavior of XAI systems, as illustrated in Figure 1.4 (Li et al., 2020).

This chapter delves into the application of XAI techniques within the healthcare domain, with a particular focus on their potential to enhance patient outcomes, foster trust among clinicians, and ensure compliance with regulatory standards. The study examines a range of XAI methods, including rule-based models, decision

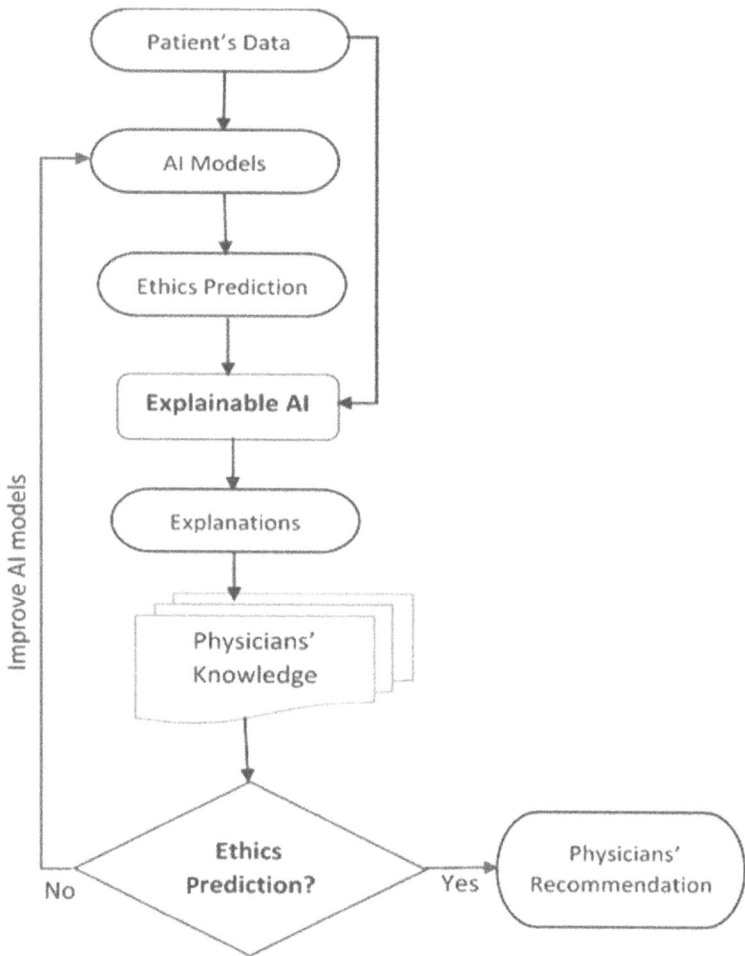

Figure 1.4 XAI for explanation of AI ethics.

trees, and model-agnostic techniques, within the context of healthcare research. The chapter thoroughly explores the advantages and limitations associated with these methods. Furthermore, the research addresses ethical considerations as well as challenges and outlines future directions for the integration of XAI into health-care systems. XAI is deemed crucial for providing clinical users with insightful decision support from AI and aligning with evidence-based medical practices. In the field of XAI, the development of effective evaluation methods is an ongoing endeavor. While one straightforward approach involves assessing XAI through user feedback, this method has its complexities and potential biases. To tackle this challenge, the chapter proposes a computational evaluation method tailored for medical experts and physicians. The output of XAI models (local feature importance) is used as a feature in this method, while the labels from prediction tasks are used as labels. Real-time medical records are consulted during the review process. In the end, the work aims to answer the research query of how to statistically analyze XAI models for particular prediction models and datasets (Meethongjan et al., 2013; Nazar, Alam, Yafi, & Su'ud, 2021).

Within the realm of healthcare, XAI plays a crucial role in addressing and analyzing various social and ethical issues. It provides a valuable tool for enhancing the understanding of technological, medical, and patient-centric perspectives efficiently. This is achieved through the utilization of XAI algorithms, as illustrated in the algorithm described by Bell, Nov, and Stoyanovich (2023).

Algorithm 1.1: XAI for AI Ethics Evaluation

```
1. Function EMC (D, L, FI)      //EMC  → Electronic Medicine
   Compendium
2. Input: D (observations), L (classes) and FI (local
   feature imp.)
3. Output: AU ROC       //Area Under the Receiver Operating
   Characteristic
4. DFI ← D x FI;        //DFI: Development financing
   institutions
5. Train X, text X, train Y, text Y ←     train.test.
   split (D, L);
6. RF_EMC model ←    train. Classifier (train X, train Y);
                     //X: Ethics issues, Y: Social issues
7. Pred.classes ← RF_EMC model. Predict (text X);
                  //RF: Radio Frequency
8. Return AUROC (Pred_classes, test Y).    //Pred: Prediction
9. Function EMR (D, P, FI)
10. Input: D (Observations), P (Predicted proba). And FI
    (local feature imp.)
11. Output: RMSE              //RMSE: Root Mean Square Error
12. DFI ← D x FI;
13. train X, test X, train Y, test Y ←     train_test_split
    (D,P);
14. RF_EMC model    train_regressor (train X, train Y);
15. Pred. proba     RF_EMC model.predict (text X);
16. return RMSE (Pred_Proba, test Y);
```

At its core, explainability can be defined as a quality of AI-based systems that enables individuals to comprehend the rationale behind a particular AI-generated prediction. In the medical field, the absence of explainability in these technologies can lead to ethical and professional concerns, neglect important issues, and potentially result in significant harm. To contribute to the ongoing discussion regarding AI in medicine, this chapter aims to emphasize the critical role of explainable AI in shaping the future of healthcare.

Despite numerous studies showing that AI algorithms may outperform humans in particular analytical tasks like pattern recognition, the medical industry has come under fire for its lack of explainability. Uncertainties in social and ethical matters may obstruct progress and prevent breakthrough technologies from reaching their full potential for improving patient and public health. In this study, we do a thorough conceptual review of the literature that is currently available about explainable AI within these domains (Norouzi et al., 2014).

A major goal of our analysis was to identify the pertinent elements that are essential for establishing the value and requirement of explainability within each individual area. We then come to conclusions that summarize the ethical ramifications of adopting explainability for the future of AI in healthcare based on these identified elements. As stated by Sheu and Pardeshi (2022) in their 2022 study, we also want to assess explainability in the context of four core ethical principles—independence, kindness, impartiality, and integrity.

Within the framework of the XAI model, we incorporate a class activation mapping approach. This approach serves the purpose of highlighting the affected areas, enhancing visual interpretability, and generating local features and maps (M_1, M_2, …M_k) for healthcare images, each associated with corresponding weights (w_1, w_2, …w_k). The weighted sum is subsequently input into a backbone ResNet model. In this process, a specific cross section of the Kth map Mk, with A × B representing its shape, is condensed, where wk belongs to Rk × c. Here, K signifies the map count. The score S_c for a specific class *c* is calculated using Equation (1.1):

$$S_c = \sum_{i=1}^{k} w_{k,c}^{fc} \left(\frac{1}{AB} \sum_{i=1}^{A} \sum_{j=1}^{B} F_{i,j}^{k} \right) \tag{1.1}$$

For the S_c score for *c* class, we define the activation map M_c^{fc} for the *k*th feature map for share $A \times B$, as presented in Equation (1.2).

$$\left(M_c^{fc} \right)(i, j) = \sum_{i=1}^{k} w_{k,c}^{fc} \, F_{i,j}^{k} \tag{1.2}$$

The processing burden is increased by using this strategy. When it comes to healthcare, some photos are labeled as having huge lesions, even if the majority of positive cases only catch a small amount. A categorization module is offered to handle the issue. A joint pattern of distribution of an image and the mode viral infection probability is taken into account by the classification module. We take into account a sample set and a multiple-instance learning module. Equation (1.3) illustrates how the classification module's total sections are separated into |S| disjoint parts.

$$|S| = \max\left(1, \left[\frac{n}{S_i} \right] \right) \tag{1.3}$$

Here S_i is the length of one section of the classification module. The join probability can be expressed using Equation (1.4):

$$P(C|P) = P(C \,|\, \{C_i\}_{i=1}^{|S|}) = \frac{1}{1 + \Pi_{i=1}^{|S|}(1 \,/\, P(c \,|\, P_i - 1)} \qquad (1.4)$$

Here $P(c|P_i)$ is the probability of section i in C.

In certain instances, the pursuit of explainability can potentially lead to a trade-off with reduced performance in the XAI model. To make a model fully explainable, it may necessitate simplification or the introduction of additional, simpler steps to enhance transparency, potentially resulting in a performance decrease. Hulsen (2023) observed that, when system accuracy is taken into account, the level of explainability in AI systems within the healthcare domain tends to be lower than in non-healthcare domains.

In the development of policies pertaining to the explainability of health AI, active consultation with patients is essential, as their perspectives may differ from those made up by healthcare professionals. Depending on the ramifications of an incorrect decision based on the AI algorithm, the trade-off among transparency and precision may change depending on the scenario. According to Iqbal et al. (2023), the usage of machine learning and deep learning applications in healthcare can lead to outcomes related to liability, trust, and interpretability. The black-box nature of many deep learning models presents an obstacle to clinical utilization, necessitating the establishment of trust with clinicians and patients through explanation of model decisions (Mughal et al., 2018).

Furthermore, Arshad et al. (2023) emphasize the need to keep a moral framework that benefits both end users and XAI while gaining the trust of medical professionals and patients through clarifications for black-box models. These explanations should encompass complete information and refrain from misleading the end user. They should also elucidate the reasons behind errors in results to enhance justice and consistency. Unfortunately, the absence of criteria for evaluating the accuracy and extensiveness of clarifications poses challenges. This dearth of measures could potentially have adverse effects on the application of XAI in clinical settings. Additionally, it is ethically necessary to comprehend how explanations affect patients' dignity and well-being because the reconstructed information from justifications could be negatively abused (Muhsin et al., 2014; Mujeeb et al., 2019).

As highlighted by Jayatilake and Ganegoda (2021), the increasing adoption of AI methods in various industries, including medicine, underscores the critical importance of explaining machine decisions. This need is particularly significant for healthcare applications such as medication recommendations, disease prognosis or prediction (Mahmood et al., 2022), and mortality prediction, where explainable decisions are essential for ethical reasons and to garner societal acceptance (Iqbal et al., 2022).

1.3 Results and Discussion

We used a multidisciplinary approach in our intelligence-based clinical decision support system to investigate the importance of explainability in medical AI from multiple angles, covering technological, legal, healthcare, and patient viewpoints. The originality of this study resides in its thorough analysis of explainability's function in clinical practice as well as its moral analysis of the use of AI-driven instruments in the healthcare industry.

Understanding the function of explainability in clinical practice requires an understanding of specific core considerations and values, which are illuminated by each of these areas. Explainable AI must be taken into account from a technological standpoint, in terms of both how it can be accomplished and its developmental advantages. We have identified crucial touch points for explainability when assessing the legal perspective within clinical practice, such as informed consent, certification and approval of medical devices, and liability. These elements highlight the complex interaction between human actors and medical AI. Additionally, it is critical to comprehend the dynamic interactions between human beings and medical AI systems, according to both the medical and patient perspectives. In conclusion, we stress that ignoring explainability in clinical decision support systems poses a serious challenge to fundamental medical ethical principles and may have negative effects on both individual and societal health (Taha, Alsaqour, Uddin, Abdelhaq, & Saba, 2017). An algorithm's ability to explain things can either be a built-in property or it can be estimated using techniques like black-box models and artificial neural network models. However, compared to current approaches, which merely provide approximations of explainability, innate explainability is typically more accurate.

1.4 Conclusion

To unlock the full potential of medical AI, it is crucial to increase awareness among developers, healthcare professionals, and lawmakers regarding the challenges and limitations associated with opaque algorithms within this field. Furthermore, fostering interdisciplinary collaboration is paramount in effectively addressing these issues. This chapter delves into the significance of explainable AI within clinical decision support systems, incorporating insights from technological experts, legal authorities, medical practitioners, and patient perspectives. To ensure that explainable AI delivers on its promises for healthcare professionals and legislators, and to tackle the challenges and restrictions posed by algorithms in medical AI, it is vital to sensitize all stakeholders and encourage cross-disciplinary cooperation. The integration of medical AI introduces challenges that demand a reevaluation of the roles and responsibilities of healthcare professionals. Through our comprehensive analysis, we contend that explainability stands as an indispensable requirement for effectively managing these challenges while adhering to established professional norms and values. Within the context of this chapter, we posit that explainable AI can play a pivotal role in upholding patients as the central focus of healthcare decision-making. Collaboratively, patients and clinicians can make informed and autonomous decisions about their health with the support of explainable AI. Furthermore, explainable AI has the potential to promote the fair allocation of available healthcare resources. In conclusion, we emphasize that the absence of explainability within clinical decision support systems poses a significant threat to fundamental ethical principles in medicine and may result in adverse consequences for both individuals and public health.

Acknowledgment

This chapter is published with support of Artificial Intelligence & Data Analytics Lab (AIDA), CCIS, Prince Sultan University, Riyadh, Saudi Arabia.

References

Amann, J., Blasimme, A., Vayena, E., Frey, D., Madai, V. I., & Consortium, P. Q. (2020). Explainability for artificial intelligence in healthcare: A multidisciplinary perspective. BMC Medical Informatics and Decision Making, 20, 1–9.

Arshad, W., Masood, T., Mahmood, T., et al. (2023). Cancer unveiled: A deep dive into breast tumor detection using cutting-edge deep learning models. IEEE Access, 11, 133804–133824.

Bell, A., Nov, O., & Stoyanovich, J. (2023). Think about the stakeholders first! Toward an algorithmic transparency playbook for regulatory compliance. Data & Policy, 5, e12.

Borda, A., Molnar, A., Neesham, C., & Kostkova, P. (2022). Ethical issues in AI-enabled disease surveillance: Perspectives from global health. Applied Sciences, 12(8), 3890.

Gupta, A., Anpalagan, A., Guan, L., & Khwaja, A. S. (2021). Deep learning for object detection and scene perception in self-driving cars: Survey, challenges, and open issues. Array, 10, 100057.

Hulsen, T. (2023). Explainable artificial intelligence (XAI): Concepts and challenges in healthcare. AI, 4(3), 652–666.

Iqbal, S., Qureshi, A. N., Li, J., Choudhry, I. A., & Mahmood, T. (2023). Dynamic learning for imbalance data in learning chest X-ray and CT images. Heliyon, 9(6), e16807.

Iqbal, S., Qureshi, A. N., Ullah, A., Li, J., & Mahmood, T. (2022). Improving the robustness and quality of biomedical CNN models through adaptive hyperparameter tuning. Applied Sciences, 12(22), 11870.

Jayatilake, S. M. D. A. C., & Ganegoda, G. U. (2021). Involvement of machine learning tools in healthcare decision making. Journal of Healthcare Engineering, 2021, 6679512.

Khan, M. A., Sharif, M. I., Raza, M., Anjum, A., Saba, T., & Shad, S. A. (2022). Skin lesion segmentation and classification: A unified framework of deep neural network features fusion and selection. Expert Systems, 39(7), e12497.

Larabi-Marie-Sainte, S., Aburahmah, L., Almohaini, R., et al. (2019). Current techniques for diabetes prediction: Review and case study. Applied Sciences, 9(21), 4604.

Li, X.-H., Cao, C. C., Shi, Y., et al. (2020). A survey of data-driven and knowledge-aware explainable AI. IEEE Transactions on Knowledge and Data Engineering, 34(1), 29–49.

Mahmood, T., Li, J., Pei, Y., & Akhtar, F. (2021). An automated in-depth feature learning algorithm for breast abnormality prognosis and robust characterization from mammography images using deep transfer learning. Biology, 10(9), 859.

Mahmood, T., Li, J., Pei, Y., Akhtar, F., Imran, A., & Rehman, K. U. (2020). A brief survey on breast cancer diagnostic with deep learning schemes using multi-image modalities. IEEE Access, 8, 165779–165809.

Mahmood, T., Li, J., Pei, Y., Akhtar, F., Rehman, M. U., & Wasti, S. H. (2022). Breast lesions classifications of mammographic images using a deep convolutional neural network-based approach. PLoS One, 17(1), e0263126.

Mahmood, T., Rehman, A., Saba, T., Nadeem, L., & Bahaj, S. A. O. (2023). Recent advancements and future prospects in active deep learning for medical image segmentation and classification. IEEE Access, 11, 113623–113652.

Meethongjan, K., Dzulkifli, M., Rehman, A., et al. (2013). An intelligent fused approach for face recognition. Journal of Intelligent Systems, 22(2), 197–212.

Mughal, B., Sharif, M., Muhammad, N., et al. (2018). A novel classification scheme to decline the mortality rate among women due to breast tumor. Microscopy Research and Technique, 81(2), 171–180.

Muhsin, Z. F., Rehman, A., Altameem, A., Saba, T., & Uddin, M. (2014). Improved quadtree image segmentation approach to region information. The Imaging Science Journal, 62(1), 56–62.

Mujeeb, S., Alghamdi, T. A., Ullah, S., et al. (2019). Exploiting deep learning for wind power forecasting based on big data analytics. Applied Sciences, 9(20), 4417.

Naik, N., Hameed, B., Shetty, D. K., et al. (2022). Legal and ethical consideration in artificial intelligence in healthcare: Who takes responsibility? Frontiers in Surgery, 9, 266.

Nazar, M., Alam, M. M., Yafi, E., & Su'ud, M. M. (2021). A systematic review of human–computer interaction and explainable artificial intelligence in healthcare with artificial intelligence techniques. IEEE Access, 9, 153316–153348.

Norouzi, A., Rahim, M. S. M., Altameem, A., et al. (2014). Medical image segmentation methods, algorithms, and applications. IETE Technical Review, 31(3), 199–213.

Rehman, A. (2023). Brain stroke prediction through deep learning techniques with ADASYN strategy. 2023 16th International Conference on Developments in eSystems Engineering (DeSE), Istanbul, Turkiye, pp. 679–684.

Sadad, T., Rehman, A., Munir, A., et al. (2021). Brain tumor detection and multi-classification using advanced deep learning techniques. Microscopy Research and Technique, 84(6), 1296–1308.

Sheu, R.-K., & Pardeshi, M. S. (2022). A survey on medical explainable AI (XAI): Recent progress, explainability approach, human interaction and scoring system. Sensors, 22(20), 8068.

Singh, M. M., & Garg, U. S. (2014). Laws applicable to medical practice and hospitals in India. International Journal of Research Foundation of Hospital and Healthcare Administration, 1(1), 19–24.

Stuckler, D. (2008). Population causes and consequences of leading chronic diseases: A comparative analysis of prevailing explanations. The Milbank Quarterly, 86(2), 273–326.

Taha, A., Alsaqour, R., Uddin, M., et al. (2017). Energy efficient multipath routing protocol for mobile ad-hoc network using the fitness function. IEEE Access, 5(2019), 10369–1038.

Tang, H., Huang, H., Liu, J., Zhu, J., Gou, F., & Wu, J. (2022). AI-assisted diagnosis and decision-making method in developing countries for osteosarcoma. Healthcare, 10(11), 2313.

Vainio-Pekka, H., Agbese, M. O.-O., Jantunen, M., et al. (2023). The role of explainable AI in the research field of AI ethics. ACM Transactions on Interactive Intelligent Systems, 13(4), 1–39.

Webster, C. S., Taylor, S., Thomas, C., & Weller, J. M. (2022). Social bias, discrimination and inequity in healthcare: Mechanisms, implications and recommendations. BJA Education, 22(4), 131.

Yang, G., Ye, Q., & Xia, J. (2022). Unbox the black-box for the medical explainable AI via multi-modal and multi-centre data fusion: A mini-review, two showcases and beyond. Information Fusion, 77, 29–52.

Yousaf, K., Mehmood, Z., Saba, T., et al. (2019). Mobile-health applications for the efficient delivery of health care facility to people with dementia (PWD) and support to their carers: A survey. BioMed Research International, 2019, 7151475.

Chapter 2

Explainable AI for Diagnosis of Pneumonia Using Chest X-ray Images: Current Achievements and Analysis on Benchmark Datasets

Muhammad Mujahid, Tanzila S. Khan, Fetoun Alzahrani, Alex Elyassih, and Abeer Rashad Mirdad

Artificial Intelligence and Data Analytics (AIDA) Lab, CCIS Prince Sultan University, Riyadh, Kingdom of Saudi Arabia

2.1 Introduction

Pneumonia is a life-threatening condition characterized by inflammation of the lungs, derived from the Greek word "pneuma" meaning "breath." Pneumonia is a very lethal illness that claims the lives of almost 4 million individuals annually, particularly affecting newborns and the elderly. The condition might be caused by a virus, bacterium, or fungus, depending on the specific infectious pathogen that impacts the delicate air sacs (alveoli) in the lung. The symptoms encompass a forceful or parched cough, an elevated temperature accompanied by spasms, rapid respiration, and difficulty breathing; chest uneasiness when coughing; an accelerated

DOI: 10.1201/9781032626345-2

pulse; profound exhaustion or weakness. Patients exhibiting severe symptoms may have anorexia, general malaise, or hemoptysis. Pneumonia may be transferred by several means. When a young individual inhales, microorganisms present in their nasal passages or throat have the potential to invade their respiratory system. Airborne droplets can transmit while coughing or sneezing. Pneumonia may be classified into three primary categories: (a) community-acquired pneumonia with poor transmission, (b) viral pneumonia, and (c) bacterial pneumonia.

2.1.1 Pneumonia Transmission

Furthermore, pneumonia can be transmitted through the blood, particularly during or soon after birth. More research is needed on the several bacteria that cause pneumonia, including how they should be transmitted, as they are crucial for control and diagnosis. Even though those most healthy children's natural defenses can resist infection, children with lower immune systems tend to be more prone to pneumonia. Starvation can harm a baby's immune system, especially in non-breastfed infants. Symptoms of HIV infection, as well as infections such as measles, enhance a child's risk of pneumonia. Cooking, "heating with biomass" (such as wood or compost), and living in crowded dwellings with smoking parents are all variables that raise the risk of pneumonia in children. Symptoms, physical examination, clinical examination, and medical examination all are commonly used to reach a diagnosis. Despite the existence of advanced CNN-based categorization algorithms that provide similar network structures to the trial-and-error methodology, CNN-motivated deep learning models continue to be the preferred choice for medical image classification. Identifying pneumonia using chest X-ray (CXR) images is a challenging and time-consuming operation in image processing, as the illness mostly impacts the lung boundaries (Mughal et al., 2018a,b). CNN-inspired deep learning (DL) models have been the dominant preference for enhancing performance. According to the data, the proposed approach performed better than the current technique, with the logistic regression (LR) classifier getting a slightly higher precision of 95.63% and the multilayer perceptron achieving 95.39% (Bhandary et al., 2020). Pneumonia symptoms, types, risk factors, treatment, and its diagnosis are illustrated in Figure 2.1.

Certain researchers employ digital imaging techniques to autonomously identify pneumonia. The objective of picture analysis is to get valuable data through the process of extracting and disseminating applications (Parveen & Khan, 2020). The act of dividing a digital picture into distinct sections is referred to as segmentation, whereas the act of conveying information depending on local frequency is known as modulation. Parveen and Khan employed several wavelet transforms, including discrete wavelet transform (DWT), repetition wavelet transform (WFT), particle packet transform (WPT), and ambiguous classification applications, to detect pneumonia. The concept of obscure C entails assigning a weight to each pixel in order to accurately determine its value.

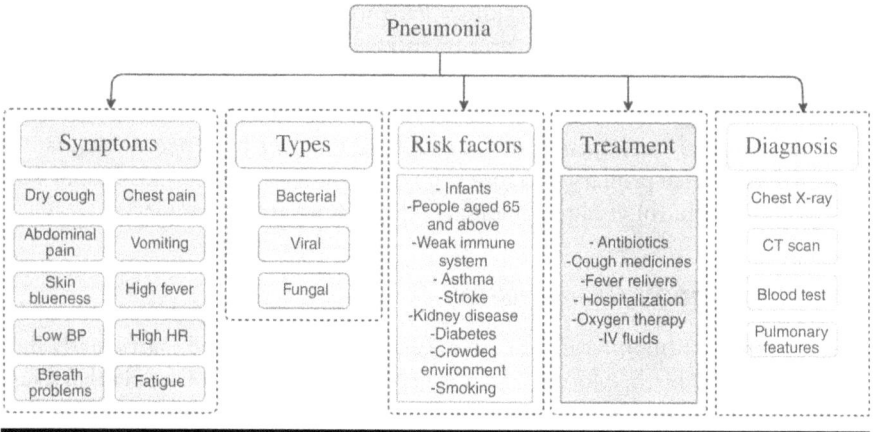

Figure 2.1 Pneumonia symptoms, types, risk factors, treatment, and its diagnosis.

Abdullah et al. (2011) proposed a method for identifying pneumonia symptoms by employing a cellular neural network. Cellular neural networks employ a 3×3 spatial model that is linear and remains unaltered. This model is built upon state equations, output equations, boundary equations, and essential values. The proposed architecture will enable rapid identification of pneumonia symptoms. The integration of these techniques yields an effective algorithm for identifying the signs of pneumonia in an image. Candy-software is employed as a CNN simulator in certain regions to detect indications of pneumonia. The distinction between the grayscale CT images is fundamental in differentiating the normal region from the area of pneumonia, yielding superior outcomes (Fahad et al., 2018).

2.1.2 Pneumonia Deaths

Pneumonia is responsible for one-third of all deaths globally, as reported by the World Health Organization (WHO). World Pneumonia Day is observed globally on November 12th every year. Each year, pneumonia impacts millions of individuals globally. In 2010, the number of children under the age of 5 who died from pneumonia was 1,123,375. Annually, pneumonia claims the lives of 90,000 children in Pakistan. Pneumonia has a significant impact on families and children worldwide, with the biggest number of cases occurring in South Asia and Sub-Saharan Africa. In Pakistan, it remains the second highest prevalent cause of mortality within children in their age grouping. Before any treatments, the estimated yearly mortality rate from pneumonia among children under the age of 5 in Abbottabad, Pakistan, was 14 fatalities per 1,000 children. Between 1988 and 1991, pneumonia accounted for 44% of the overall deaths in infants below the age of 5 in a small village located in Pakistan's North Areas, as determined through verbal forensic methods. According to the verbal analysis carried out by the "Aga Khan Health Services," Pakistan (AKHSP) in the North Areas, pneumonia is the primary cause of death among babies and young children aged 1–4 years (McAllister et al., 2019; Pneumonia, 2021; WHO, 2021).

Nigeria is among the top five nations responsible for 50% of global pneumonia deaths and has the third-highest mortality rate. This suggests that Nigeria is facing a severe pneumonia issue. In Nigeria, pneumonia is the predominant cause of disease among children. In 2016, a total of 140,520 children below the age of 5 succumbed to pneumonia, which translates to almost 16 fatalities occurring per hour. In 2017, a total of 153,068 children under the age of 5 died as a result of pneumonia. Nigeria has the greatest case fatality rate and the largest differential in internal death rates internationally, as indicated by current statistics on lower respiratory tract infections. Unfortunately, Nigeria has not seen the same level of success as many other countries in reducing death rates from pediatrics pneumonia. While the global rate has reduced by 51% over the MDG years, Nigeria has only seen an 8% decline (Wonodi et al., 2020).

As a result, there has been a substantial decrease in the mortality rate of pneumonia in children under the age of 5, with the number of cases dropping from 1.7 million in 2000 to 1.3 million in 2011. Nevertheless, pneumonia remains the leading source of mortality for human beings above the age of 1. This is alarming since most fatalities caused by pneumonia may be avoided. Pneumonia is the primary reason for adult hospital admissions in Sub-Saharan Africa, resulting in around 4 million cases and 200,000 fatalities each year. The specific kind of pneumonia and the extent of the sickness determine the therapeutic approach. The diagnosis of pneumonia is essential for therapy as it allows a clinician to determine if a patient with many symptoms truly has pneumonia or not. In cases when the patient has acquired hospital-acquired pneumonia (HAP) or ventilator-associated pneumonia (VAP), the work of diagnosis becomes more complex since the symptoms may not manifest until after a period of 48 hours. The sample CXR images are shown in Figure 2.2.

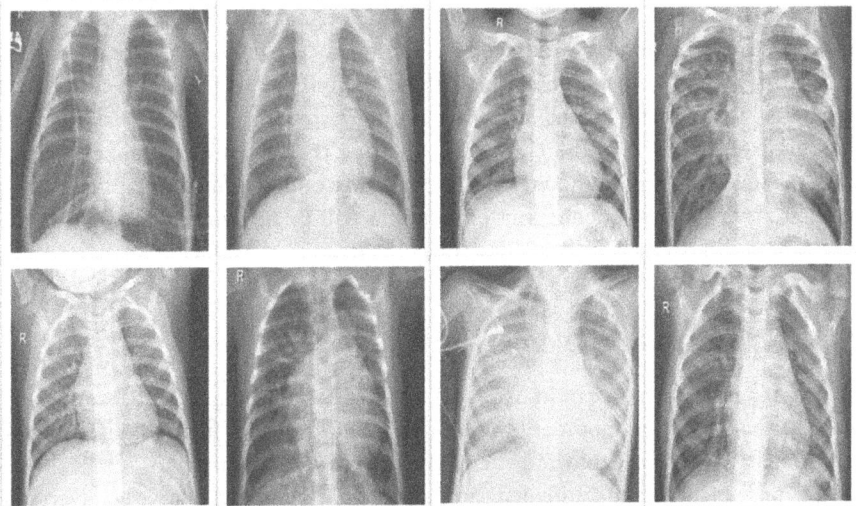

Figure 2.2   Sample of CXR images.

2.1.3 CXR

X-ray, sometimes referred to as X-radiation, is a kind of electromagnetic radiation that can penetrate objects. These beams penetrate specific areas of the human body, allowing for viewing of its innermost structures. An X-ray picture is a monochromatic depiction of the body's innermost anatomical structures (Bhatt & Shah, 2023). The X-ray is a highly established and extensively utilized diagnostic procedure in therapeutic settings. A CXR is employed for the detection of chest-related ailments, such as pneumonia and other pulmonary diseases, since it offers an image of the thoracic cavity, including the chest and spinal bones, as well as delicate organs such as the lungs, blood vessels, and airways. X-ray imaging offers various advantages as a substitute for dialysis. X-ray imaging technology offers substantial benefits over conventional testing approaches as an alternative analytic tool for pneumonia. The advantages of X-ray imaging are its affordability, widespread accessibility, noninvasiveness, time efficiency, and adjustable settings. Considering the ongoing worldwide healthcare crisis, X-ray imaging presents itself as a more effective approach for the widespread, convenient, and rapid identification of pandemics (Reshi et al., 2021).

Pneumonia is often detected by proficient experts utilizing a CXR. On X-rays, it often manifests as one or more areas of heightened opacity, and the diagnosis may be verified by a medical history, significant symptoms, and laboratory tests. Additional conditions, such as pulmonary edema, hemorrhage, atelectasis, lung malignancy, and post-radiation or post-surgical alterations, might complicate the identification of pneumonia on a CXR. To maximize benefits, ensure that all four components are readily available whenever possible. Several factors, such as the patient's position and depth of breathing, might modify the appearance of the X-ray, thereby complicating its interpretation. In recent years, there has been an increase in the use of computer-controlled systems for detecting pneumonia. These systems aim to improve the efficacy and accuracy of healthcare providers. DL algorithms surpass conventional machine learning (ML) techniques in the realm of medical image analysis, namely, in the areas of tracking, categorization, and classification (Rajpurkar et al., 2017). The chest radiograph is the globally recognized benchmark for investigating pulmonary disorders. Consequently, the development of an automated method for identifying pneumonia will be advantageous in promptly treating the illness, especially in rural areas (Varshni et al., 2019).

2.1.4 Scope and Problems

Pneumonia is more prevalent in economically disadvantaged and destitute nations, characterized by high population density, pollution, and filthy environmental conditions. This has exacerbated the issue, and there is a scarcity of medical supplies. Consequently, timely identification and treatment can effectively avert the illness from reaching a lethal stage. Magnetic resonance imaging and computed

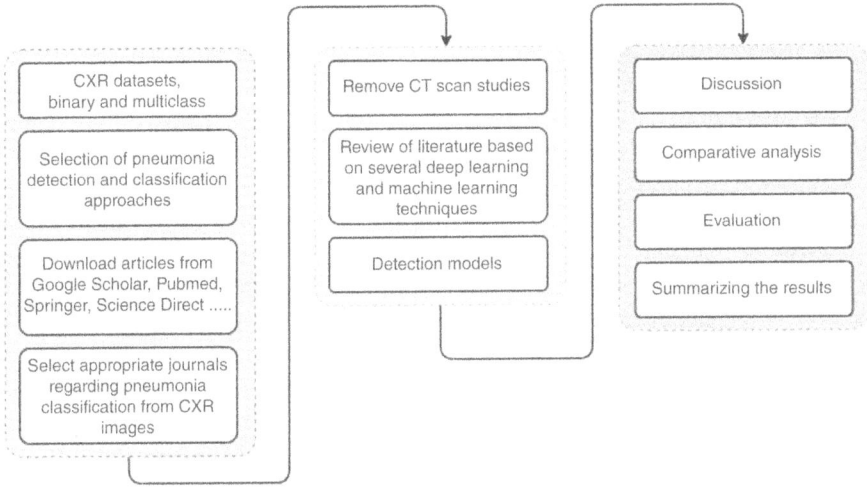

Figure 2.3   Review diagram based on literature.

tomography, sometimes known as radiography, are commonly used diagnostic techniques to check the lungs. X-ray imaging is a noninvasive and often inexpensive method used to assess the condition of the lungs. The regions of consolidation on the pneumonic X-ray that distinguish a pneumonic condition from a healthy one is known as infiltrates. Nevertheless, CXR diagnostics for pneumonia identification are prone to subjective variability. Hence, it is crucial to devise an automated approach for detecting pneumonia (Sirazitdinov et al., 2019).

Medical images are more intricate and diverse compared to normal images, making it demanding to create an active model due to limited data collection. The effective ML model can solely be trained utilizing the datasets obtained in a research setting. The complexity of medical images makes it more challenging to train the ML model using lab-based datasets. Researchers struggle to decipher the patterns present in medical images. Utilizing real-time data can enhance the refinement of the model. Data sharing poses a challenging hurdle for hospitals and other medical facilities. Review diagram based on literature is presented in Figure 2.3.

2.2 Background

The principal aim of this chapter is to propose a remedy for the concern through the implementation of a novel deep neural network architecture. Incorporating dropout into the convolutional component of the network was the proposed innovation. The proposed method was trained and assessed utilizing a dataset comprising 5,856 annotated images acquired from a Kaggle-hosted medical imaging challenge. From a retrospective study of pediatrics patients aged 1–5 years at the Guangzhou Women and Children's Medical Centre in Guangzhou, China, the anterior–posterior CXR images were selected. With the following remarkable metrics, their network outperformed the competition in the Kaggle competition: 97.2% accuracy, 97.3% recall, 97.4% precision, and an AUC of 0.982. These outcomes exhibit parity with the most cutting-edge systems presently accessible (Szepesi & Szilágyi, 2022).

This work employs a DL model, namely, VGG16, to accurately diagnose and categorize pneumonia using two datasets of CXR images. The study's results demonstrate that VGG16 with NN achieves superior performance compared to VGG16 with SVM, KNN, RF, and NB for both datasets. Furthermore, the proposed method enhances the performance of prior models on both datasets 1 and 2 (Sharma & Guleria, 2023).

In developing nations, 15% of children under 5 dies from preventable acute lung cell inflammation. The hybrid technique extracted features using DL models. Three steps were used to evaluate the model's performance: pretrained transfer learning on individual models, DL ensemble implementation. The hybrid DL model identified multiclass with 98.19% accuracy and 97.29% F1 score. For binary classification, the model was 99.21% accurate. The recommended model outperforms advanced DL algorithms in binary and multiclass classification, according to assessment criteria. This shows that CXRs can detect pneumonia early. Heat and saliency maps are easier to read for identification using the hybrid XAI model (Ukwuoma et al., 2023).

The goal of another study was to show that CXRs can be used in a simpler way to find pneumonia (Yi et al., 2023). To do this, authors look at how well 15 different convolutional neural network (CNN) models work after being trained on the same dataset. After looking at the results, they picked the best model that meets one of the greatest performance standards, was easy to understand, and can be trained with fewer computer resources and time. These measurements were about the same for the chosen architecture as they are for cutting-edge designs taught on CXRs. This shows that CNN designs need to be made simpler so that they are easier to understand without lowering accuracy or performance. Based on the results of this study, authors recommend doing more research to improve designs that aren't as complicated so that we can get even higher levels of accuracy. A set of 5,856 images was used with the image enhancement method. The CNN model was 90% accurate and had an AUC of 96% (Gourisaria et al., 2021).

The biological course of pneumonia and its detection via X-ray imaging was investigated in research (Saul et al., 2019). It describes the methods and results of an automated system for diagnosing the disease in its early stages, as well as a review of past studies aiming at enhancing diagnostic accuracy. The research provides a DL architecture for classification tasks that was learned using changed images and several preprocessing stages. CNNs and residual network architecture was used in the classification approach. The results show an accuracy of 78.73%, which was higher than the previous record accuracy of 76.8%.

Authors implemented automated systems for classifying pneumonia and normal CXR images utilizing nine advanced DL architectures: CNN, VGG16, VGG19, DenseNet201, Inception_ResNet_V2, Inception_V3, Xception, Resnet50, and MobileNet_V2. The primary objective was to address the following research inquiry: Can DL techniques surpass DCNN approaches in terms of performance? A total of 5,856 CXR and CT pictures were utilized, consisting of 4,273 cases of pneumonia and 1,583 cases of normal conditions. The tests were conducted and assessed based on several performance criteria. Furthermore, the Resnet50, MobileNet_V2, and Inception_Resnet_V2 designs outperformed other architectures in this study, with an accuracy of 84% (El Asnaoui et al., 2021).

The study (Rahman et al., 2020) trained and compared four popular DL approaches based on CNN for classifying CXR images into normal and pneumonia patients. Classification accuracy, precision, and recall were respectively 98%, 97%, and 99% for normal and pneumonia images, 95%, 95%, and 96% for bacterial and viral pneumonia images, and 93.3%, 93.7%, and 93.2% for normal, bacterial, and viral pneumonia images. Millions of children are killed by this disease every year. Many people may be saved if medical professionals act quickly with a treatment plan based on an accurate diagnosis. In developing countries, where there is a greater need for doctors to treat patients in the field, access to medical professionals is limited. Therefore, computer-aided diagnostic (CAD) systems can play a crucial role in preventing unnecessary deaths. Furthermore, the input images from the X-ray equipment exhibit significant diversity as a result of variances in the skill of the radiologists (Mordani, 2019).

This study experiment employed a comparable methodology, wherein X-ray images were utilized for the purpose of diagnosing pneumonia. The dataset has undergone preprocessing to make it suitable for tasks using transfer learning. Pretrained variants of CNNs such as VGG16, Inception-v3, and ResNet50 were utilized. The three networks commonly used to create ensembles are CNN, Inception-V3, VGG-16, and ResNet50. Cohen's kappa and AUC were employed as assessment metrics for assessing the performance of pretrained and ensemble DL models, in addition to the conventional metrics. These metrics were utilized to assess the performance of the models. The experimental results indicate that Inception-V3 with CNN earned the best possible accuracy and recall scores, reaching 99.29% and 99.73%, respectively (Mujahid et al., 2022).

Barakat et al. present a novel ML approach to precisely detect pediatric pneumonia based on CXR images. This approach involves equalizing the distribution of classes in the dataset by using data augmentation techniques, improving the method used to extract features, and evaluating the performance of various ML models. The Quadratic SVM model achieved an accuracy of 97.58% with this method, surpassing the accuracy reported in the current ML literature. Moreover, this method is more cost-effective in terms of processing resources and more feasible because it has a significantly lower classification time compared to the TL benchmark

(Barakat et al., 2023). Hence, the results indicate that the proposed technique is appropriate and has potential for detecting pediatrics pneumonia in CXRs.

In reality (Madhuri et al., 2023), physicians employ chest radiography to detect pneumonia. In the realm of computer science, a hybrid CNN and ML classifiers have a common objective. Incorporating DL and ML technology into CAD systems can enhance their performance. This can assist radiologists and physicians in making medical determinations. CNNs excel in image classification and segmentation, making them a popular choice for constructing DL-based CAD systems. The results indicate that the most effective predictor was an ensemble model that combines radial basis function (RBF), support vector machine (SVM), and LR, with a success rate of 97%. This concept was employed to develop a cloud-based CAD system that significantly simplifies the process for doctors to detect pneumonia. Several scholars worked on infectious diseases (Chakraborty et al., 2019; Ge et al., 2020; Rehman, 2023; Rustam et al., 2020; Yee & Raymond, 2020).

In order to eliminate the need for single-image investigations and drastically reduce overall expenditures, this chapter proposes a novel method for identifying the residency of pneumonia by integrating computational algorithms to CXRs. Although recent developments in DL have shown impressive results in picture classification across several domains, there is currently limited applicability of this technology for the diagnosis of pneumonia. Therefore, the primary goal was to conduct an analysis that will advance this field of study, offering a novel approach to the use of pretrained CNNs in the feature extraction stage of the disease detection process. Authors suggest combining SVM with ResNet which extract the hierarchical features from the individual X-rays using the boosting approach to choose the relevant features. They have shown, by performance analysis of the available dataset, that the new scheme in pneumonia classification has a higher level of precision than most contemporary techniques, leading to a significant increase in clinical outcomes.

The dataset comprised CXR images that were processed using the locally adaptable regression kernel (LARK) descriptors proposed by the developer. The method employed was a calculation-based approach that was integrated with the novel SVM classifier. The research is mostly limited to a paired arrangement, utilizing ANN and ResNet as the experimental models. According to the developer, this technique has the potential to distinguish between bacterial and viral pneumonia in the future by improving contrast, color space, and artificially illuminating the images. Authors used pulmonary radiography categorization to explore the site of pneumonia. CNN was used as the analytical approach. According to the developer, this technique was the best strategy for X-ray characterization. Given that X-ray images are used to detect pneumonia, climate pneumonia must be classified to establish whether it is caused by a virus or bacteria. This study shows that the proposed approach correctly diagnoses pneumonia. Furthermore, it provides significant advice for other researchers to improve accuracy and efficiency by using high-performance processors (Naz et al., 2023). The authors conducted research where they examined CXRs to identify the specific locations where pneumonia was detected. The collection consists of 5,856 CXR images captured from different perspectives. The CNN utilized these datasets to develop their work, employing the Adam optimization approach, which offers superior computing efficiency and reduced time compared to other techniques. This study aimed to provide state-of-the-art results for pneumonia detection using CXRs. They employed a CNN architecture to identify and classify CXRs as either prone to pneumonia or not (Mujahid et al., 2022).

The disease known as pneumonia mostly affects small, constricted areas. The inadequate alignment of the CXR was caused by a breakdown in network performance. A three-branch AG-CNN design was presented in the study, and it is essential for improving alignment and reducing noise in the various disease-affected regions. Moreover, it integrates global divisions to help mitigate the existence of discriminatory markers in local chapters. ChestX-ray-14 datasets have made it easier for us to understand various parts of CNN. This method's value, when applied to this dataset, is 0.87. However, the flexibility of this method to handle changes in parameters is restricted. The model's inability to adapt to parameter changes might make it more difficult for it to predict a wide variety of facts with accuracy. The CheXNet technique, including 121 layers of CNN, was employed in the experiment. The technique was used to detect and determine if a pneumonia infection was present in CXR images (Table 2.1) (Muhsin et al., 2014).

2.3 Materials and Methods

2.3.1 X-ray Imaging Dataset for Pneumonia Detection

The main objective of a classifier is to successfully accomplish its intended purpose by utilizing the information it is provided with. A dataset of X-ray images is necessary for the classification of pneumonia. A CNN is employed to develop the classification algorithm for distinguishing the characteristics in X-ray images. Although DL networks have demonstrated superior efficacy in detecting and classifying cataracts, the initial training of these networks is a time-consuming endeavor. Furthermore, their performance is greatly dependent on larger datasets of pneumonia. Figure 2.4 shows the workflow diagram for pneumonia detection and classification.

2.3.2 Kaggle Dataset

Kaggle provided the CXR image dataset for pneumonia utilized in this investigation. The dataset consists of 7,750 images in total, of which 6,200 are designated for training purposes and 1,550 are for the test set. Resizing is performed on the X-ray images as part of the preprocessing phase. Diverse dimensions of the original images are captured, including 1,344 by 600, 1,272 by 1,144, and so forth.

Table 2.1 Summary of Literature Review

Reference	Techniques/Approach	Dataset Employed	Results (%)	Limitations	Year
Szepesi and Szilágyi (2022)	CNN+Dropout	X-ray images	97.2	Only 5,856 labeled images can produce valid results, yet the dataset is skewed	2022
Alshmrani et al. (2023)	VGG-19+CNN	X-ray images	96.4	Achieved results are poor	2023
Sharif et al. (2019)	NN+VGG16	X-ray images	95.4	The authors used VGG-19 and ML; however, they were unable to get correct results	2023
Ukwuoma et al. (2023)	XAI model	X-ray images	98.1	The hybrid model requires a lot of time to train and yield results	2023
Gourisaria et al. (2021)	CNN	X-ray images	90.0	Only 90% accuracy was achieved by the CNN model on a small number of pneumonia samples	2021
Ozsoz et al. (2020)	DCNN	X-ray images	94.4	The dataset was categorized into multiple classes by the authors, and no optimal processing technique was used	2020
Saul et al. (2019)	CNN	X-ray images	78.7	The dataset is constrained, and the achieved results are unsatisfactory	2019

(Continued)

Table 2.1 (Continued)

Reference	Techniques/ Approach	Dataset Employed	Results (%)	Limitations	Year
El Asnaoui et al. (2021)	Inception_Resnet_V2	X-ray images	84.0	A total of 5,856 images are employed in the experiments, with an imbalance between the normal and pneumonia classes	2021
Mamlook et al. (2020)	CNN	X-ray images	98.4	The authors exclusively utilized CNN and other ML models, while failing to mention the computational time	2020
Rahman et al. (2020)	Inception-V3 with CNN	X-ray images	99.9	The authors utilized preprocessing and augmentation techniques to expand the dataset, although its size remained limited	2022
Barakat et al. (2023)	SVM	X-ray images	97.5	After assessing the impact of modifying the number of feature extraction regions of interest (ROIs) on both the classification time and accuracy, it has been determined that the ROI feature extraction approach is the most unfavorable option	2022

(Continued)

Table 2.1 (Continued)

Reference	Techniques/ Approach	Dataset Employed	Results (%)	Limitations	Year
Madhuri et al. (2023)	RBF	X-ray images	97.0	The authors employ multiple models, which results in a time-consuming process	2023
Bhandary, Prabhu, Rajinikanth, Thanaraj, Satapathy, Robbins, et al. (2020)	NN	X-ray images	84.1	The neural network was able to achieve a lower level of accuracy	2020
Mujeeb et al. (2019)	CNN	X-ray images	93.4	Adam may also be utilized to analyze the data of several participants and different X-rays	2020
Naz et al. (2019)	SVM	X-ray images	98	The use of GPU and other ML classifiers can enhance accuracy	2020
Mujahid et al. (2022)	CNN	X-ray images	97	The processing was inadequate, and the image input was also limited	2019
Yousaf et al. (2019)	VGG16	X-ray images	96.2	There were problems with the way the data were trained	2019
Muhsin et al. (2014)	DCNN	X-ray images	76	There is a shortage of radiographs	2020

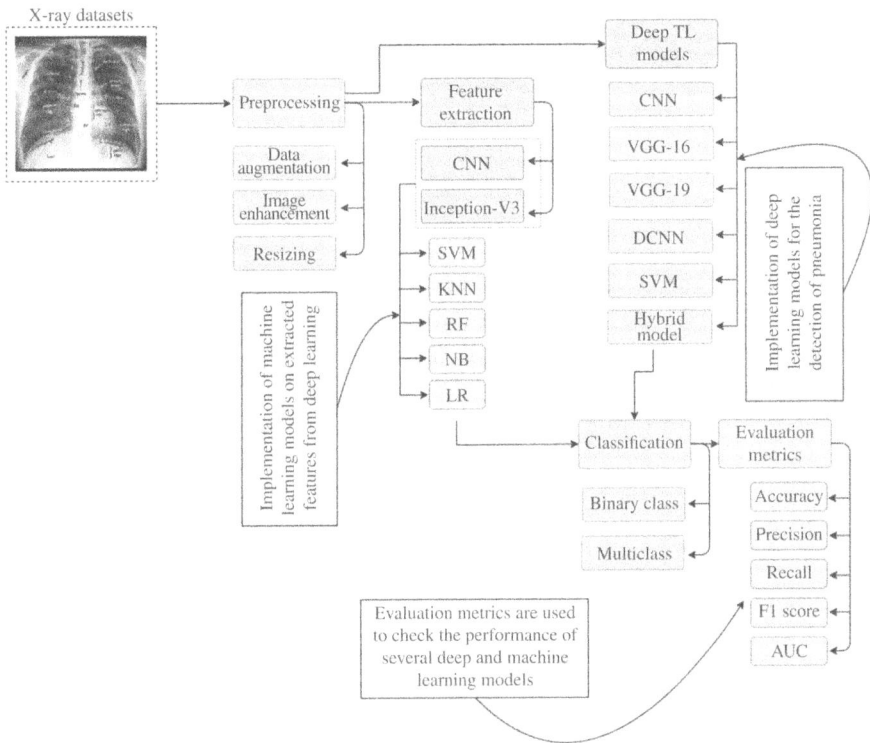

Figure 2.4   Workflow diagram for pneumonia detection and classification.

Therefore, regarding the computational and model implementation aspects, the X-ray images are reshaped to a standardized dimension. All image dimensions are adjusted to fixed size which corresponds to the height, width, and quantity of channels, correspondingly. Three channels are present: green, red, and blue.

2.3.3 ChestX-ray14 Dataset

The ChestX-ray14 dataset consists of 112,120 frontal-view X-ray images taken between 1992 and 2015. These images were collected from 30,805 different patients. The dataset includes text-mined reports from radiologists, which were analyzed using natural language processing techniques to identify 14 common diseases. It enhances the ChestX-ray8 dataset by incorporating six extra thorax diseases: edema, emphysema, fibrosis, pleural thickening, and hernia.

2.3.4 Viral Pneumonia Dataset

A total of 5,247 CXR images, with resolutions ranging from 400p to 2000p, were obtained from the Kaggle Chest X-ray Pneumonia Database for this study. Out of the total 5,247 CXR images, 1,341 depict normal subjects, while 3,906 show subjects affected by pneumonia. Among the pneumonia cases, 2,561 images are of bacterial pneumonia and 1,345 images are of viral pneumonia. Pneumonia cases may involve a coexistence of viral and bacterial infections. The dataset was partitioned into a training set and a test set.

2.3.5 Data Augmentation

Data augmentation is a post-resizing procedure utilized to enlarge the dataset. Data augmentation is performed using the image augmentor Python library to ensure that the number of images in the normal and pneumonia classes are equivalent (Eid & Elawady, 2021; Khan et al., 2022). The methodology for augmenting data is delineated in Algorithm 1.1. Data augmentation is a procedure that consists of a series of consecutive steps, which begins with rotation. Following this, the functions flip-left-right, flip-top-bottom, and zoom are executed. The random alteration function and sample ratio are ultimately utilized. Data augmentation is implemented solely on the normal images in the original dataset, as a significant number of pneumonia X-ray images were already present. The purpose of generating images is to normalize the dataset, which serves to prevent the model from being overfit to the majority class data (Larabi-Marie-Sainte et al., 2019; Sudheesh et al., 2023).

2.4 Comparative Analysis and Discussion

The objective and automated classification and detection of pneumonia is currently a significant research topic. Automatic pneumonia detection can reduce the workload of radiologists and clinicians. Furthermore, it offers an approach that is both impartial and prompt in evaluating the magnitude of the epidemic resulting from viral dissemination. This chapter discusses recent progress in machine learning–based pneumonia classification and detection using CXR imaging. The study centers on two domains of investigation: DL and ML methodologies. Conversely, DL methods have made substantial progress in classifying pneumonia. Nevertheless, there is still considerable opportunity for expansion and enhancement. Figure 2.5 shows the most utilized models in the literature for pneumonia detection and classification.

To begin with, it is necessary to have CXR images. These images will aid in the development of DL baseline methods. Furthermore, the field of automatic image annotation has been relatively neglected despite its potential for significant advancements. Furthermore, the advancement of precise and unbiased DL methods for pneumonia diagnosis is a cost-effective and efficient means to aid a larger population in enhancing their diagnostic accuracies (Sharif et al., 2019). Enhancing the intelligibility of DL is of utmost importance as it has the potential to facilitate its extensive utilization in pneumonia diagnosis. Furthermore, prior studies have

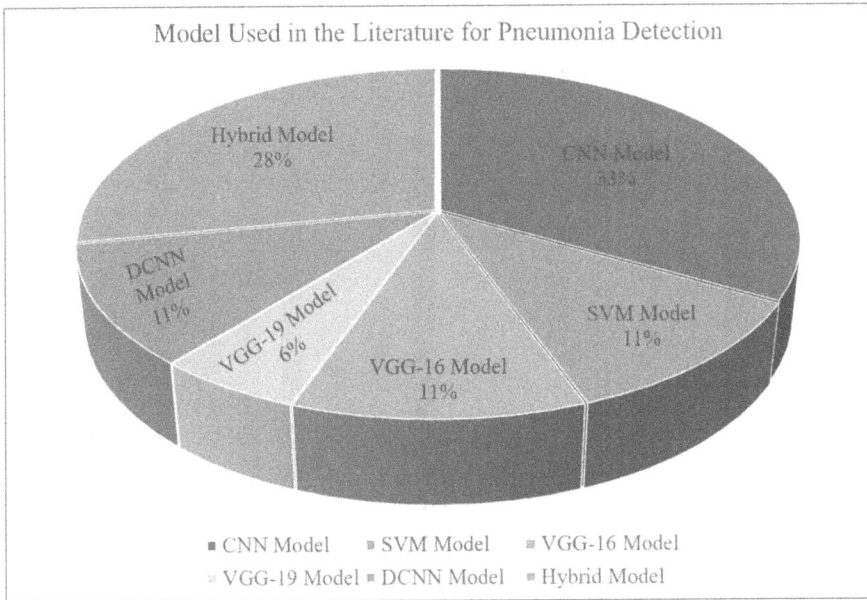

Figure 2.5 **Most utilized models in the literature for pneumonia detection and classification.**

employed blood or urine tests, which offer a more effective approach to developing lightweight ML methods that address the problem of pneumonia screening in developing countries with limited access to costly devices. This is due to the limited access that developing nations have to expensive devices. This idea is highly commendable for implementing efficient DL methods that specifically target the issue faced by developing countries, where there is a limited availability of costly radiology equipment. These methodologies can be employed to acquire knowledge in radiology while reducing the reliance on costly equipment. Figure 2.6 illustrate the comparative analysis of several recent studies.

It is of the utmost importance to work toward the development of an all-encompassing system for the identification and classification of cases of pneumonia utilizing X-ray images. The review of the relevant literature that was carried out as part of this study revealed that there has been a paucity of previous research on the diagnosis of pneumonia through the utilization of X-ray images. The diagnosis of pneumonia can be made in a straightforward manner and at a reduced financial outlay by making use of X-ray images. This method can speed up the process of timely identification of pneumonia cases, which makes it especially useful in remote areas of the country where access to healthcare resources is limited. They have the potential to be beneficial in areas where access to medical care is restricted because of their ability to detect early signs of disease.

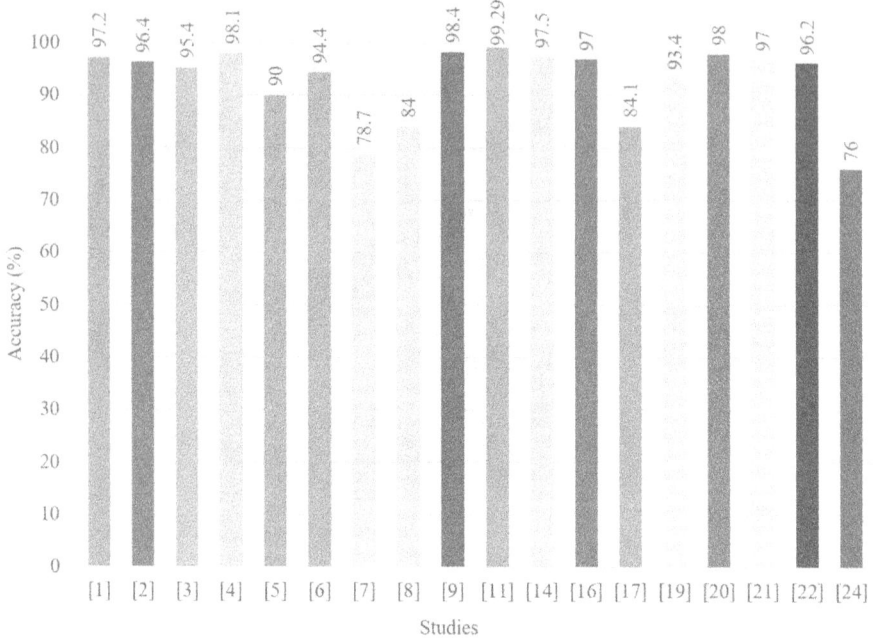

Figure 2.6 Comparative analysis of several recent studies.

This chapter presents an extensive overview of the findings that were obtained from earlier efforts at research. To provide a brief summary, the researchers and pioneers are working together to develop automated methods for identifying cases of pneumonia.

2.5 Conclusion

The automated detection and classification of pneumonia is alleviating the burden on radiologists and physicians. Furthermore, it provides an unbiased approach for evaluating the severity and aids in the prevention of pneumonia by facilitating a timely and precise diagnosis. This chapter provides a concise overview of different methodologies and techniques that have been devised for the detection and classification of pneumonia. Our research primarily focused on the automated diagnosis of pneumonia. We examined the different methodologies employed by other researchers, as well as the challenges and constraints encountered in previous studies, and potential novel directions for further study. Ultimately, it has been ascertained that further research is necessary to explore the potential for diagnostic classification, evaluate the cost-effectiveness of different DL and ML methods in medical application, and enhance the precision of detection.

Acknowledgment

This chapter is published with support of Artificial Intelligence & Data Analytics Lab (AIDA) CCIS Prince Sultan University, Riyadh, Saudi Arabia.

References

Abdullah, A. A., Posdzi, N. M., & Nishio, Y. (2011, June). Preliminary study of pneumonia symptoms detection method using cellular neural network. International Conference on Electrical, Control and Computer Engineering 2011 (InECCE).

Alshmrani, G. M. M., Ni, Q., Jiang, R., Pervaiz, H., & Elshennawy, N. M. (2023). A deep learning architecture for multi-class lung diseases classification using chest X-ray (CXR) images. Alexandria Engineering Journal, 64, 923–935.

Barakat, N., Awad, M., & Abu-Nabah, B. A. (2023). A machine learning approach on chest X-rays for pediatric pneumonia detection. Digital Health, 9, 20552076231180008.

Bhandary, A., Prabhu, G. A., Rajinikanth, V., Thanaraj, K. P., Satapathy, S. C., & Robbins, D. E. (2020). Deep-learning framework to detect lung abnormality: A study with chest X-ray and lung CT scan images. Pattern Recognition Letters, 129, 271–278.

Bhatt, H., & Shah, M. (2023). A convolutional neural network ensemble model for pneumonia detection using chest X-ray images. Healthcare Analytics, 3, 100176.

Chakraborty, S., Aich, S., Sim, J. S., & Kim, H. C. (2019). Detection of pneumonia from chest X-rays using a convolutional neural network architecture. International Conference on Future Information & Communication Engineering, 11, 98–102.

Eid, M. M., & Elawady, Y. H. (2021). Efficient pneumonia detection for chest radiography using ResNet-based SVM. European Journal of Electrical Engineering and Computer Science, 5(1), 1–8.

El Asnaoui, K., Chawki, Y., & Idri, A. (2021). Automated methods for detection and classification pneumonia based on X-ray images using deep learning. In Studies in Big Data (pp. 257–284). Springer International Publishing.

Fahad, H. M., Ghani Khan, M. U., Saba, T., et al. (2018). Microscopic abnormality classification of cardiac murmurs using ANFIS and HMM. Microscopy Research and Technique, 81(5), 449–457.

Ge, Z., Mahapatra, D., Chang, X., Chen, Z., Chi, L., & Lu, H. (2020). Improving multi-label chest X-ray disease diagnosis by exploiting disease and health labels dependencies. Multimedia Tools and Applications, 79, 14889–14902.

Gourisaria, H., Rautaray, M. K., & Pandey, S. S. (2021). Pneumonia detection using CNN through chest X-ray. Journal of Engineering Science and Technology (JESTEC), 16(1), 861–876.

Khan, M. A., Sharif, M. I., Raza, M., et al. (2022). Skin lesion segmentation and classification: A unified framework of deep neural network features fusion and selection. Expert Systems, 39(7), e12497.

Larabi-Marie-Sainte, S., Aburahmah, L., Almohaini, R., et al. (2019). Current techniques for diabetes prediction: Review and case study. Applied Sciences, 9(21), 4604.

Madhuri, A., Sk, R., Priya, Y., Sk, S., & Kumar, L. S. (2023, February). Pneumonia detection and classification using hybrid convolution neural network and machine learning classifiers. 2023 Third International Conference on Artificial Intelligence and Smart Energy (ICAIS).

Mamlook, A., Chen, R. E., & Bzizi, S. (2020). Investigation of the performance of machine learning classifiers for pneumonia detection in chest X-ray images. 2020 IEEE International Conference on Electro Information Technology (EIT), pp. 98–104. IEEE.

McAllister, D. A., Liu, L., Shi, T., et al. (2019). Global, regional, and national estimates of pneumonia morbidity and mortality in children younger than 5 years between 2000 and 2015: A systematic analysis. Lancet Global Health, 7(1), e47–e57.

Mordani, S. (2019). Pneumonia biggest killer infection in India, pollution worsening crisis, says report. In News18. https://www.news18.com/news/india/pneumonia-biggest-killer-infection-in-india-pollution-worsening-crisis-says-report-2384299.html

Mughal, B., Muhammad, N., Sharif, M., et al. (2018a). Removal of pectoral muscle based on topographic map and shape-shifting silhouette. BMC Cancer, 18(1), 1–14.

Mughal, B., Sharif, M., Muhammad, N., et al. (2018b). A novel classification scheme to decline the mortality rate among women due to breast tumor. Microscopy Research and Technique, 81(2), 171–180.

Muhsin, Z. F., Rehman, A., Altameem, A., et al. (2014). Improved quadtree image segmentation approach to region information. The Imaging Science Journal, 62(1), 56–62.

Mujahid, M., Rustam, F., Álvarez, R., Luis Vidal Mazón, J., Díez, I. D. L. T., & Ashraf, I. (2022). Pneumonia classification from X-ray images with inception-V3 and convolutional neural network. Diagnostics (Basel), 12(5), 1280.

Mujeeb, S., Alghamdi, T. A., Ullah, S., et al. (2019). Exploiting deep learning for wind power forecasting based on big data analytics. Applied Sciences, 9(20), 4417.

Naz, Z., Khan, M. U. G., et al. (2023). An explainable AI-enabled framework for interpreting pulmonary diseases from chest radiographs. Cancers, 15(1), 314.

Ozsoz, M., Ibrahim, A. U., Serte, S., Al-Turjman, F., & Yakoi, P. S. (2020). Viral and bacterial pneumonia detection using artificial intelligence in the era of COVID-19. https://www.researchsquare.com/article/rs-70158/v1

Parveen, S., & Khan, K. B. (2020, November). Detection and classification of pneumonia in chest X-ray images by supervised learning. 2020 IEEE 23rd International Multitopic Conference (INMIC).

Rahman, T., Chowdhury, M. E. H., Khandakar, A., et al. (2020). Transfer learning with deep convolutional neural network (CNN) for pneumonia detection using chest X-ray. Applied Sciences (Basel), 10(9), 3233.

Rajpurkar, P., Irvin, J., Zhu, K., et al. (2017). Chexnet: Radiologist-level pneumonia detection on chest x-rays with deep learning. arXiv:1711.05225.

Rehman, A. (2023). Brain stroke prediction through deep learning techniques with ADASYN strategy. 2023 16th International Conference on Developments in eSystems Engineering (DeSE), Istanbul, Turkiye, pp. 679–684.

Reshi, A. A., Rustam, F., Mehmood, A., et al. (2021). An efficient CNN model for COVID-19 disease detection based on X-ray image classification. Complexity, 2021(1), 12.

Rustam, Z., Yuda, R. P., Alatas, H., & Aroef, C. (2020). Pulmonary rontgen classification to detect pneumonia disease using convolutional neural networks. TELKOMNIKA, 18(3), 1522.

Saul, C. J., Urey, D. Y., & Taktakoglu, C. D. (2019). Early diagnosis of pneumonia with deep learning. https://doi.org/10.48550/arXiv.1904.00937

Sharif, A., Khan, M. A., Javed, K et al. (2019). Intelligent human action recognition: A framework of optimal features selection based on Euclidean distance and strong correlation. Journal of Control Engineering and Applied Informatics, 21(3), 3–11.

Sharma, S., & Guleria, K. (2023). A deep learning based model for the detection of pneumonia from chest X-ray images using VGG-16 and neural networks. Procedia Computer Science, 218, 357–366.

Sirazitdinov, I., Kholiavchenko, M., Mustafaev, T., Yixuan, Y., Kuleev, R., & Ibragimov, B. (2019). Deep neural network ensemble for pneumonia localization from a large-scale chest X-ray database. Computers & Electrical Engineering, 78, 388–399.

Sudheesh, R., Mujahid, M., Rustam, F., et al. (2023). Bidirectional encoder representations from transformers and deep learning model for analyzing smartphone-related tweets. PeerJ Computer Science, 9, e1432.

Szepesi, P., & Szilágyi, L. (2022). Detection of pneumonia using convolutional neural networks and deep learning. Biocybernetics and Biomedical Engineering, 42(3), 1012–1022.

Ukwuoma, C. C., Qin, Z., Belal Bin Heyat, M., et al. (2023). A hybrid explainable ensemble transformer encoder for pneumonia identification from chest X-ray images. Journal of Advanced Research, 48, 191–211.

Varshni, D., Thakral, K., Agarwal, L., Nijhawan, R., & Mittal, A. (2019, February). Pneumonia detection using CNN based feature extraction. 2019 IEEE International Conference on Electrical, Computer and Communication Technologies (ICECCT).

Wonodi, C., Obi-Jeff, C., Falade, A., Watkins, K., & Omokore, O. A. (2020). Pneumonia in Nigeria: The way forward. Pediatric Pulmonology, 55(S1), S5–S9.

Yee, S. L. K., & Raymond, W. J. K. (2020, September). Pneumonia diagnosis using chest X-ray images and machine learning. Proceedings of the 2020 10th International Conference on Biomedical Engineering and Technology.

Yi, R., Tang, L., Tian, Y., Liu, J., & Wu, Z. (2023). Identification and classification of pneumonia disease using a deep learning-based intelligent computational framework. Neural Computational and Applied, 35(20), 14473–14486.

Yousaf, K., Mehmood, Z., Saba, T., et al. (2019). Mobile-health applications for the efficient delivery of health care facility to people with dementia (PwD) and support to their carers: A survey. BioMed Research International, 2019, 7151475.

Chapter 3

Explainable AI for Medical Science: A Comprehensive Survey, Current Challenges, and Possible Directions

Deep Kothadiya[1,3], Chintan Bhatt[2], Amjad R. Khan[3], Anees Ara[3], and Fatima Nayer Khan[3]

[1]*U & P U Patel Department of Computer Engineering, Faculty of Technology (FTE), Chandubhai S. Patel Institute of Technology (CSPIT), Charotar University of Science and Technology (CHARUSAT), Changa, India*

[2]*Department of Computer Science and Engineering, School of Technology, Pandit Deendayal Energy University, Gandhinagar, 382007, Gujarat, India*

[3]*Artificial Intelligence and Data Analytics Laboratory (AIDA), College of Computer and Information Sciences (CCIS), Prince Sultan University, Riyadh, Kingdom of Saudi Arabia*

3.1 Introduction

Complex machine learning (ML) models, known as black-box learning, have internal workings and decision-making processes that humans cannot grasp. The model is a "black box" – its underlying mechanics are opaque, making it difficult for users to understand how it makes a conclusion. Complex ML algorithms like deep neural networks, ensemble approaches, and others with many interrelated components frequently lack transparency. The interactions between millions of parameters in these models are complex (Yousaf et al., 2019). The phrase "black box" contrasts

DOI: 10.1201/9781032626345-3

with plain-language models like decision trees and linear regression. Complexity may improve prediction accuracy in black-box models, but it raises questions about responsibility, trust, and hard-to-identify biases. Explainable artificial intelligence (XAI) develops tools and procedures to reveal black-box models' decision-making processes. For applications in sensitive fields like healthcare, finance, and criminal justice, where interpretability and accountability are critical, understanding how a model makes predictions is essential (Kothadiya, Bhatt, Saba, et al., 2023).

XAI is recently dominating the research field for improving the transparency of the working model with the user. The brief history of AI development relates to statistical analysis, ML, natural language processing, computer vision, and data science. Even though such developments were present, it was not able to exceed human intelligence which was later progressed by neural networks, reinforcement learning, and deep learning (DL) (Meethongjan et al., 2013). Such AI applications advancements were not only beneficial for weather forecasting analysis, self-driving cars, and the AlphaGo game capable of competing with the best humans' skills, but were also found to be of critical importance within the medical domain and its progress (Khan et al., 2020). Human–computer interaction (HCI) research is also progressing to automate many applications and provide solutions. Nevertheless, the improvements within the life expectancy have been recently improved with the use of advanced technologies and still will be beneficial to tackle the problems faced within different categories of the medical domains. Therefore, developments within the medical domain are discussed which focuses mainly on pneumonia status, bloodstream infections (BSI), acute kidney injury (AKI), and hospital mortality (HM) prediction (Kothadiya, Bhatt, Rehman, et al., 2023; Muhsin et al., 2014). XAI is necessary to be evaluated with the medical domain progression as it provides complete details of each algorithmic step thought to be trusted within the medical domain, practitioners, and experts. The three stages in XAI can be given as (i) explainable building process for facilitating acceptance, (ii) explainable decisions for enabling trust with users and administrators, and (iii) explainable decision process for the interoperability with business logic. The goal of XAI is to provide machine and DL algorithms for better performance with explainability, which further allows ease of user trust, understanding, acceptance, and management (Kothadiya, Rehman, Abbas, et al., 2023).

Nowadays, we are surrounded by black-box AI systems utilized to make decisions for us, as in autonomous vehicles, social networks, and medical systems. Most of these decisions are taken without knowing the reasons behind these decisions (Mujeeb et al., 2019). XAI refers to the concept of designing and developing AI systems in a way that their decision-making processes and outcomes are understandable, transparent, and interpretable to humans. In traditional AI models, like deep neural networks, the complex interactions and computations that drive decisions can be challenging for humans to grasp. This lack of transparency can be a significant barrier to adopting AI in critical domains such as healthcare, finance, legal systems, and more (Mughal, Muhammad, et al., 2018). In recent years, artificial intelligence (AI) has shown remarkable potential in the field of medical diagnosis, aiding healthcare professionals in accurately identifying diseases and conditions Li et al. (2023). However, as AI systems become more complex and powerful, there is a growing need to ensure transparency and understand ability in their decision-making processes (Das & Rad, 2020). This has led to the emergence of XAI in the medical domain. XAI refers to the capability of AI models to provide understandable and interpretable explanations for their decisions or predictions. In medical diagnosis (Vilone & Longo, 2020).

XAI represents a crucial evolution of AI technology, addressing the need for transparency, trustworthiness, and accountability. By providing understandable explanations for AI decisions, it enables us to harness AI's power across various industries while ensuring that the decision-making process remains accessible and comprehensible to humans (Kothadiya et al., 2022). The integration of XAI in medical diagnosis addresses the need for transparency, trust, and collaboration between AI systems and healthcare stakeholders. By offering interpretable explanations for AI decisions, we can unlock the full potential of AI technology while ensuring it aligns with the complexities and ethical considerations of the medical field. XAI has seen a significant increase in articles, conferences, and symposia (Saba, Bokhari, et al., 2018; Zhang et al., 2022). AI-based algorithms, particularly deep neural networks, are changing how humans approach real-world tasks. ML algorithms have in recent years increased in automating various aspects of science, business, and social workflow. It is partly due to a rise in research in a branch of ML known as deep learning, where thousands (even billions) of neuronal parameters are trained to generalize how to perform a specific task. As a result, a plethora of domain-dependent and context-specific methods for interpreting ML models and forming explanations for humans have emerged. The importance of comprehending trust, ethics, bias, and the effect of adversarial examples in deceiving AI classifier decisions is highlighted by the recent interest in XAI (Jiménez-Luna et al., 2020).

The recent research on medical XAI focuses completely on interpretability (Minh et al., 2022). As the medical field possesses a high level of accountability and transparency, a greater interpretability is needed to be explained by the algorithm. Even though the interpretability is treated equally across all the hospitals, it should be handled with caution; medical practices should be the prime focus for interpretability development, and data based on mathematical knowledge for technical applications are encouraged. The different interpretability categories referenced here are perceptive and mathematical structures. The perceptive interpretability is mostly a visual evidence that can be analyzed using saliency maps, i.e., LIME, class activation map (CAM) (Dieber & Kirrane, 2020), layer-wise relevance propagation (LRP), etc. In signal methods, the stimulation/collection of neurons are detected, i.e., feature maps, activation maximization, etc. The verbal interpretability is the human understandable logical statements based on the predicates, connectives, i.e., disjunctive normal form (DNF), and NLP. The mathematical structure-based interpretability is the popular mechanism used through ML and neural network

Table 3.1   Challenges in XAI

Challenge	*Remark*
Trust	In scenarios where AI influences decisions with significant consequences, like medical diagnoses or autonomous vehicles, trust is paramount. People are more likely to rely on AI recommendations if they understand the rationale behind them
Ethics and accountability	When AI is involved in sensitive areas, understanding why certain choices are made is crucial for holding the system accountable for its actions. This is especially relevant in cases where AI systems might perpetuate biases or make errors
Regulatory compliance	Many industries are subject to regulations that demand transparency in decision-making processes. XAI aids compliance by shedding light on how decisions are reached
Collaboration	In sectors like medicine, AI systems are meant to work alongside human professionals. When AI's reasoning is transparent, doctors and experts can collaborate more effectively with the technology
Insight generation	XAI can provide valuable insights into datasets, offering a better understanding of patterns, correlations, and anomalies that might not be immediately apparent to humans

algorithms, whereas the predefined models are the relation between variable to output variable that includes logistic regression, generative discriminative machine (GDM), reinforcement learning, etc. Ultimately, the feature extraction from the input source is performed by graphs presentation, clustering, frame singular value decomposition (F-SVD), etc. (Jabeen et al., 2018).

XAI aims to bridge this gap by providing insights into how AI arrives at its conclusions, making it possible for individuals, including domain experts and end users, to comprehend and trust the system's outputs. The need for explainability arises from several key reasons demonstrated in Table 3.1 (Malaviya et al., 2023; Rahevar & Ganatra, 2023).

Black-box AI systems are being utilized in many areas of our daily lives, which could be resulting in unacceptable decisions, especially those that may lead to legal effects. Thus, it poses a new challenge for the legislation. The European Union's General Data Protection Regulation (GDPR)1 is an example of why XAI is needed from a regulatory perspective. These regulations create what is called the "right to explanation," by which a user is entitled to request an explanation about the decision made by the algorithm that considerably influences them (Zhang et al., 2022). For example, if an AI system rejects one's application for a loan, the applicant is entitled to request justifications behind that decision to guarantee it is in agreement with other laws and regulations. However, the implementation of such regulations is not straightforward, challenging, and without an enabling technology that can provide explanations, the "right to explanation" is nothing more than a "dead letter" (Saba, Bokhari, et al., 2018).

Creating black-box AI models involves developing an approximation function to solve the issue. The black-box AI model becomes the base of knowledge, not the data. Accordingly, XAI can expose the scientific information gathered by black-box AI models, which might lead to innovative notions in numerous fields of research. The industry struggles to implement complicated and accurate black-box AI systems due to regulations and consumer trustworthiness. Due to legislation, the sector may favor less accurate, more interpretable models (Hussain et al., 2020). XAI can reduce the model interpretability-performance trade-off, solving these problems. However, it may raise development and deployment expenses. The model's explainability increases based on how much it supports open box architecture. The DL models, i.e., convolutional neural networks (CNN) and recurrent neural networks (RNN) are the least explainable and are the predecessor of ensemble model, i.e., random forest, XGB. The statistical models and graphical models are easy to understand and are more straightforward, i.e., SVM, Bayesian brief net, Markov models, etc. The decision trees, linear models, and rule-based models are the most explainable and completely open box architecture models. The different XAI categories explained within this reference include dimension reduction which are presented as most important input features by selecting optimal dimensions, e.g., optimal feature selection, cluster analysis, LASSO, sparse DL, and sparse balanced SVM. Figure 3.1 demonstrates different methods available for XAI, which helps to

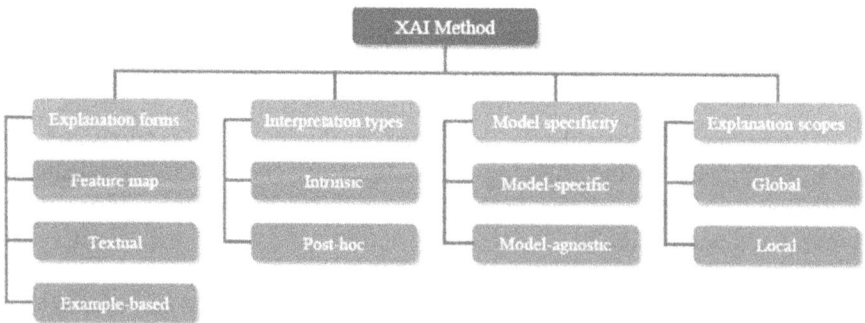

Figure 3.1 Classification of different XAI methods.

Table 3.2 Comprehensive Characteristics of XAI Models

Characteristics	Details
Importance of explainability	Explainability is crucial for building trust in AI systems, ensuring regulatory compliance, and making informed decisions based on model predictions
Types of explainability	*Model-specific explainability:* Understanding how specific types of models arrive at decisions (e.g., decision trees, linear regression) *Model-agnostic explainability:* Techniques that work with any model, providing insights into feature importance and relationships
Interpretable models	Some models are inherently interpretable, such as linear regression, decision trees, and rule-based systems. Analyze their strengths and limitations in terms of complex data and prediction accuracy
Model-agnostic techniques	Model-agnostic techniques, like LIME, SHAP, and Anchors, are crucial for making any model explainable. Analyze how these techniques work and their applicability across various models
Local versus global explanations	Differentiate between local explanations (explaining individual predictions) and global explanations (understanding overall model behavior)
Feature importance methods	Explore techniques for measuring feature importance, such as Gini impurity, permutation importance, and SHAP values. Compare their effectiveness across different scenarios
Visualizations	Visualizations play a pivotal role in making complex information understandable. Investigate the use of visual tools like partial dependence plots, ICE plots, and bar charts to communicate explanations effectively
Quantitative versus qualitative explanations	Discuss the balance between providing quantitative explanations (statistical measures) and qualitative explanations (intuitive insights) to cater to both technical and non-technical audiences
Complex models and DL	DL models, like neural networks, are often considered black boxes due to their complexity. Analyze techniques like layer-wise relevance propagation (LRP) and guided backpropagation that attempt to explain their decisions

(Continued)

Table 3.2 (Continued)

Characteristics	Details
Ethical considerations	Examine the ethical implications of XAI, including fairness, bias detection, and mitigation. Explainability can help identify discriminatory patterns and address them
Regulatory compliance	Explore how explainability is essential for complying with regulations like GDPR's "right to explanation" and various industry-specific standards
Human–AI collaboration	Discuss the concept of human–AI collaboration, where AI provides suggestions and humans make decisions based on understandable explanations
Domain-specific explanations	Different domains may require tailored explanations. Analyze the challenges and solutions for providing domain-specific insights
Trust-building	Explain how XAI fosters trust by allowing users to validate and understand model decisions, enabling better adoption and acceptance
Practices	Best practices for implementing XAI, including transparent documentation, collaboration with domain experts, and ongoing monitoring

choose appropriate model for specific application. Table 3.2 demonstrates different characteristics of explainability in DL models.

- The main objective of the proposed study is to analyze and demonstrate explainability in AI.
- The proposed study also analyzes different challenges in XAI for various DL approaches.

3.2 Literature Survey

The latest research has focused on XAI due to the growing use of complicated ML models in decision-making. As organizations and industries incorporate AI into crucial systems, transparency and interpretability are essential. The "black box" character of certain algorithms, especially DL models, is addressed by several methods for making AI models more accessible. The literature emphasizes the role of XAI in trust, ethical deployment, and regulatory compliance, laying the ground for further study (Larabi-Marie-Sainte et al., 2019; Zhang et al., 2020).

Model-specific Explainability: Research on model-specific explainability examines algorithm decision-making. Inherently interpretable decision trees and rule-based systems have been extensively studied. Researchers examine these models' strengths and weaknesses in managing various data kinds and complexity. Scholars study these models' decision routes and feature significance to understand their explainability (Dieber & Kirrane, 2020; Miller, 2019).

Model-agnostic Approaches: Literature examines model-agnostic techniques as vital to XAI. LIME and SHAP facilitate interpretability across a variety of models. These strategies are flexible enough to bridge the gap between opaque ML models and the requirement for intelligible insights, as seen subsequently. Researchers test these methods' dependability and scalability across various datasets and applications to ensure their real-world applicability (Fahad et al., 2018).

Visualizations for Interpretability: Complex knowledge is made accessible via visualizations. This literature examines the efficacy of partial dependency plots, individual conditional expectation plots, and other visuals. The topic includes how these visualizations help evaluate local forecasts and provide a comprehensive perspective of the model's global behavior. Human-centric representations help comprehend AI systems (Mughal, Sharif, et al., 2018).

Challenges in DL Models: While DL models perform well in numerous tasks, explainability is difficult. Layer-wise relevance propagation (LRP) and guided backpropagation are studied to understand neural network decision-making. Researchers critically analyze the trade-off between model complexity and transparency, noting the continuous attempts to balance accuracy and interpretability in increasingly advanced models (Kothadiya, Bhatt, Soni, et al., 2023).

Ethical Considerations and Fairness: The literature study emphasizes the necessity for XAI to address prejudice, fairness, and accountability via ethical concerns. Scholars study how explainability might discover and mitigate AI biases. The ethics of decision-making algorithms, especially in sensitive sectors, are discussed, emphasizing transparent and fair AI systems (Khan et al., 2022).

Regulatory Landscape: The literature examines AI legislation after GDPR's "right to explanation" was introduced. Researchers examine how XAI complies with these laws to ensure ethical use. This section facilitates the connection between explainability technology and its social and legal environment (Ali et al., 2023).

Real-world Applications: XAI case studies from many fields are presented in the literature. Researchers demonstrate how explainability improves AI efficiency and acceptability in healthcare diagnostics and financial decision-making. XAI's concrete advantages and implications in crucial decision systems are highlighted here (Chamola et al., 2023; Haseeb et al., 2020).

Best Practices and Future Directions: The session finishes with XAI integration recommended practices for AI projects. Transparent documentation, domain expert participation, and continual monitoring are stressed by researchers. Standardized assessment metrics, model-agnostic approaches, and toolkit and resource development are discussed as future prospects (Arrieta et al., 2020).

Rehman and Saba (2014) articulate the link between discussion in the social sciences and explainability in AI, providing an in-depth survey on research on explanations in philosophy, psychology, and cognitive science. Three major findings were highlighted. First, explanations are counterfactual, and humans tend to understand why a certain event happened instead of some other events. Second, explanations are selective and focus on one or two possible causes—instead of all possible causes—for a decision or recommendation; that is, explanations should not overwhelm the user with too much information. Third, explanations are a social conversation and interaction for the purpose of transferring knowledge, implying that the explainer must be able to leverage the mental model of the explained while engaging in the explanation process. While according to Miller (2019) these three points are key properties when building useful explanations, the different notions of explainability prevalent in XAI only recently started to take them into account (Husham et al., 2016).

Hybrid or neural-symbolic systems are those systems that combine symbolic and sub-symbolic reasoning (Samek et al., 2017). The sub-symbolic system is able to build predictive models using connectionist ML and processing large amounts of data, while the symbolic system is equipped with a rich representation of domain knowledge and can be used for higher-level, structured reasoning. These symbolic elements are used by the system to explain the decisions made by the sub-symbolic components. Also here, accuracy and fidelity are, once more, important metrics to measure the performance of an interpretable model; whereas consistency and comprehensibility are desirable properties of the produced explanations from the explainer's point of view (Islam et al., 2021).

As AI models become increasingly powerful and sophisticated, there is a growing demand for understanding the reasoning behind their predictions (Rehman, 2023). Traditional ML models, such as linear regression or decision trees, are inherently interpretable. However, the rise of complex models like deep neural networks has led to a trade-off between model performance and interpretability (Tahir et al., 2019). These complex models often operate as "black boxes," making it difficult to discern how they arrive at their decisions. This lack of transparency poses challenges in fields where trust, accountability, and regulatory compliance are critical (Javed et al., 2020). Integrated interpretability seeks to bridge this gap by combining advanced ML techniques with explainability methods. The goal is to build models that not only achieve high predictive accuracy but also provide understandable explanations for their decisions, making them suitable for use in domains where human oversight, legal compliance, and ethical considerations are paramount (Sadad et al., 2021).

3.3 Post-hoc Methods

Transparent proxy model approach finds interpretable model that globally approximates the predictions of the black-box model (Rehman et al., 2022). This approach offers both nterpretability and explainability. In XAI, a model-specific method was used to learn single decision tree from the ensemble of decision trees. The learned model was more accurate than the decision tree learned directly from the data. Rules were extracted from SVM to make more interpretable model for credit scoring. Interpretability was gained at only a small loss in performance compared to SVMs. Symbolic rules were extracted from neural network ensembles (Bhatt et al., 2023). Bayesian regression mixture with multiple elastic nets was proposed in Sevak et al. (2017) and used on DNN, SVM, and random forests to explain individual decisions and look for model vulnerabilities in image recognition and text classification. Model vulnerabilities were tested with adversarial examples. Adversarial training scheme was used on DNNs in order to increase their interpretability. Using adversarial examples, it was found that in normally trained DNNs, neurons do not detect semantic parts but only discriminative part patches. Also, representations are not robust codes of visual concepts. After adversarial training scheme, representation is more interpretable, enabling to trace the outcomes to influential neurons. This is more transparent way of making predictions.

Post-hoc interpretability methods are a subset of techniques within the field of XAI that focus on explaining the decisions and behaviors of pretrained, complex ML models. Unlike interpretable models that are inherently designed to be understandable, post-hoc methods are applied after a model is trained to shed light on its internal processes, making them more transparent and interpretable to humans (Mujahid et al., 2023). In the realm of ML, many advanced models, such as deep neural networks, operate as complex "black boxes." These models can achieve impressive accuracy but lack transparency, making it challenging to understand how they arrive at their predictions. Post-hoc interpretability methods address this limitation by providing insights into the decision-making process of these models without requiring them to be modified or retrained. Table 3.3 represents characteristics of post-hoc XAI models.

Table 3.3   Characteristics in Post-Hoc XAI Models

Feature	Remark
Model-agnostic	Post-hoc methods are designed to work with a wide range of ML models, regardless of their architecture or complexity. This agnostic nature allows these methods to be applied to various types of models, including ensemble methods, DL models, and more.
Separation of training and explanation	In a post-hoc approach, the explanation-generating process is distinct from the model training process. This separation means that explanations can be generated for existing models without the need to access or modify their training data or architecture
Interpretability techniques	Post-hoc methods encompass a variety of techniques aimed at producing explanations. These techniques include generating feature importance scores, creating surrogate models, identifying relevant input features, and highlighting critical areas of input data

3.4 XAI Challenges

XAI is an important field that aims to make AI systems more transparent and understandable to humans. While XAI offers significant benefits, there are several challenges associated with its implementation and adoption (Rehman & Saba, 2014). Some of the key challenges in explainable are discussed in Table 3.4.

Table 3.4 Model-oriented Open Challenges for Explainable Systems

Challenges	Remark
Complex model architectures	Complex models like deep neural networks often have millions of parameters and multiple layers, making it difficult to understand how they arrive at their decisions. Extracting meaningful explanations from these architectures while retaining accuracy is a challenge
Trade-off between performance and explainability	As models become more interpretable, they might sacrifice predictive performance. Finding the right balance between accuracy and explainability is crucial for practical applications
Interpretable feature representations	XAI aims to present explanations in terms of relevant features. However, translating high-dimensional, abstract features into human-interpretable representations can be challenging. Ensuring these representations are both meaningful and faithful to the underlying model is a task
Black-box models	Many advanced models, like certain DL architectures, are inherently opaque due to their complexity. Developing methods to peek into their decision-making process without compromising their efficiency is a major challenge
Contextual explanations	Effective explanations should consider not only the model's reasoning but also the specific context of the decision. Adapting explanations to different users, scenarios, or contexts adds complexity to the XAI process
User-centric explanations	Different users have different levels of technical expertise and might require explanations at varying levels of detail. Designing explanations that cater to different user needs and preferences is a significant challenge
Quantifying uncertainty	AI models often make probabilistic predictions. Translating these probabilities into understandable explanations while conveying the level of uncertainty is complex, especially to non-experts

(Continued)

Table 3.4 (Continued)

Challenges	Remark
Privacy and confidentiality	Providing explanations might inadvertently reveal sensitive information about the model or the training data, compromising privacy and confidentiality. Developing methods to provide insights without revealing sensitive details is a delicate task
Dynamic and changing models	Models are frequently updated to improve their performance. Maintaining consistent explanations across model versions while adapting to changes in the underlying architecture presents a challenge
Human bias	If the training data contains biases, explanations derived from the model's decisions can inherit these biases. Ensuring that explanations do not reinforce or perpetuate existing societal biases requires careful attention
Scalability	Generating explanations for large datasets or complex models can be computationally intensive. Efficient methods are required to make XAI feasible in real-time applications
Limited standardization	The field lacks standardized methods for generating and evaluating explanations. This lack of standardization makes it challenging to compare different XAI techniques and assess their effectiveness
Understanding global versus local explanations	Models can offer global explanations (high-level insights about their behavior) and local explanations (explanations for specific predictions). Balancing these two types of explanations effectively is a challenge
Regulatory and legal challenges	As AI systems become more integrated into various sectors, there might be regulatory requirements for providing explanations for decisions. Ensuring that XAI approaches comply with these regulations adds complexity
Educating users	Even with effective explanations, users might not fully understand the nuances of AI decision-making. Educating users about the limitations of AI systems and how to interpret explanations is essential

Addressing these challenges requires a combination of research, collaboration between disciplines, regulatory considerations, and a focus on user needs. As AI continues to advance, finding solutions to these challenges will be instrumental in building AI systems that are both accurate and transparent. Table 3.5 demonstrates detailed analysis of different challenges in explainability in black-box model (Bhatt et al., 2023; Sevak et al., 2017).

Table 3.5   Detailed Analysis of XAI Challenges

Challenges	Remark
Model complexity and interpretability	Many advanced AI models, such as deep neural networks, have complex architectures that are difficult to interpret. Balancing the need for interpretability with maintaining the model's performance is a technical challenge
Feature selection and transformation	Converting high-dimensional, abstract features used by AI models into meaningful and interpretable features that can be understood by humans is a technical challenge
Quantifying uncertainty	Translating the uncertainty inherent in AI model predictions into human-understandable explanations is technically challenging, as it involves effectively communicating probabilities and confidence levels
Black-box models	Developing techniques to extract insights from opaque, "black-box" models like deep neural networks, where internal workings are not readily understandable, is a significant technical hurdle
Model-agnostic methods	Creating methods that can provide explanations for a wide range of AI models rather than just one specific model is a technical challenge, as different models may require different approaches for explainability
Local versus global explanations	Balancing the need for local explanations (explaining individual predictions) and global explanations (describing the overall behavior of a model) presents a technical challenge, as different techniques might be needed for each
Contextual explanations	Developing methods to incorporate contextual information into explanations, considering the specific scenario or context in which the AI system is making decisions, requires sophisticated technical approaches

(Continued)

Table 3.5 (Continued)

Challenges	Remark
Feature importance and contribution	Determining the relative importance of different features or inputs in influencing the AI model's decisions, and conveying this information in a clear and understandable manner, poses a technical challenge
Adversarial attacks and robustness	Ensuring that explanations are robust to adversarial attacks, where intentionally crafted inputs could mislead the AI model or its explanations, requires advanced technical solutions
Efficiency and scalability	Generating explanations in a computationally efficient manner for large datasets and complex models is a technical challenge, particularly for real-time applications
Dynamic models and updates	Maintaining consistent and meaningful explanations as AI models are updated or retrained requires technical solutions that can adapt to changing model architectures
Combining multiple explanations	Integrating and presenting explanations from multiple sources or techniques in a coherent and informative manner can be technically challenging
Interpretable interfaces	Designing user interfaces that effectively convey complex explanations in an understandable way is a technical challenge, requiring expertise in human–computer interaction
Automating explanation generation	Developing automated methods to generate explanations that are accurate, informative, and tailored to specific user needs requires technical innovation
Standardization and benchmarking	Establishing standardized methods and benchmarks for evaluating the effectiveness of different XAI techniques is technically challenging due to the diversity of AI models and applications

3.5 Model-specific XAI

XAI is a significant area in AI that bridges complicated ML models with human comprehension. Interpreting and explaining AI judgments is crucial as they become part of decision-making in numerous fields. Model-specific XAI models are unique methods that give insightful and interpretable explanations for particular ML models. Users can understand what AI models predict and why, creating trust, transparency, and responsibility (Surati et al., 2023).

The incomprehensible nature of big ML models has become a major issue as AI permeates our lives. Model-specific XAI investigates algorithm decision-making to overcome this issue. In AI, where models are frequently "black boxes," understanding decision-making is essential for transparency, trust, and accountability. Model-specific XAI analyzes certain algorithms' decision pathways and predictors to explain them. This approach emphasizes interpretable models like decision trees and rule-based systems. These models' judgments are based on clear criteria, ensuring transparency. While XAI methods span a broad spectrum, model-specific approaches stand out for their ability to uncover nuances hidden within each model's architecture. These approaches recognize that different types of models operate on distinct principles and data representations. By leveraging this knowledge, model-specific XAI models enhance our ability to extract meaningful insights from various AI models. Table 3.6 represent model-wise explainability.

Table 3.6   Model Wise Features Analysis for XAI Systems

Model	Explainability	Remark
Decision trees and random forests	Feature importance	For decision trees and random forests, you can calculate feature importance scores based on how much a feature contributes to the overall decision-making process. This information can be visualized to show which features have the most influence on predictions
Linear regression	Coefficients and relationships	In linear regression, you can interpret the coefficients of each feature to understand the direction and magnitude of their impact on the predicted outcome. Positive coefficients indicate a positive relationship, while negative coefficients indicate a negative relationship
Support vector machines (SVM)	Support vectors and margins	For SVMs, we can identify the support vectors and examine the margins between different classes. These explain how the model separates classes and why certain data points were considered important for the classification decision

(Continued)

Table 3.6   (Continued)

Model	Explainability	Remark
Naive Bayes	Conditional probabilities	Naive Bayes models are based on conditional probabilities. You can provide explanations by showing how the probabilities of different features contribute to the overall probability of a particular class
Neural networks	Gradient-based methods	For neural networks, you can use gradient-based methods to compute the importance of input features for a specific prediction. These methods, such as gradient-weighted class activation mapping (Grad-CAM) for image data, highlight which parts of the input had the greatest influence on the model's decision
Recurrent neural networks (RNNs) and LSTMs	Attention mechanisms	RNNs and LSTMs often use attention mechanisms to focus on specific parts of the input sequence. These mechanisms can be used to show which parts of the sequence were more influential in generating the output
Transformer models	Attention heads	Attention heads used encoder–decoder architecture to learn internal dependency of set of words
Time series models	Lagged features and trends	For time series models, explanations might involve showing the significance of lagged features and identifying underlying trends that influenced the model's predictions
Ensemble models	Combining explanations	Ensemble models like AdaBoost or XGBoost combine multiple weak learners. Explanations could involve combining the individual explanations from each weak learner to provide an ensemble-level explanation

(Continued)

Table 3.6 (Continued)

Model	Explainability	Remark
Rule-based systems	Rule interpretation	Rule-based systems generate decisions based on a set of predefined rules. Explanations can involve displaying which rules were triggered for a specific input and how they collectively led to the decision

3.6 Model-agnostic XAI

In the era of complex ML models, understanding the decisions made by these models has become a paramount concern. Model-agnostic XAI methods have emerged as a versatile solution to address this challenge. Unlike model-specific approaches that tailor explanations to a particular type of model, model-agnostic XAI methods are designed to provide insights into a wide range of ML models, irrespective of their complexity or architecture. This flexibility makes them a valuable toolkit for ensuring transparency, accountability, and trust in AI systems.

3.6.1 SHAP

SHAP (SHapley Additive exPlanations) is a powerful method in XAI that helps explain the output of ML models by attributing contributions to individual features. It is based on cooperative game theory and provides a unified framework for understanding the importance of each feature in a prediction. Explaining SHAP in complete detail would be quite extensive (Iftikhar et al., 2017).

The basic idea behind SHAP is to assign each feature an importance value that represents its contribution to the difference between the actual model output and a baseline output. Here is a simplified explanation along with Equation (3.1), The foundation of SHAP is Shapley values from cooperative game theory. These values fairly distribute the total contribution of a player (feature) across different coalitions (combinations of features). In the context of SHAP, Shapley values represent the average contribution of a feature across all possible orders in which the features could be added to the prediction. Shapley value for features i can be calculated as Equation (3.1).

$$\varnothing_i(x) = \sum_{s \subseteq N} \frac{|S|!(|N|-|S|-1)!}{|N|!} \left[f(x_{S \cup \{i\}}) - f(x_S) \right] \tag{3.1}$$

Here, N stands for all feature sets, S stands for subset feature without i; $f(x_{S \cup \{i\}})$ is the models prediction when adding feature i to subset S, SHAP values combine Shapley values with the concept of a baseline. A baseline is a reference point that serves as the starting point for explaining the model's prediction. For a given instance (x), the SHAP value for feature (i) is calculated as the average difference in model outputs when adding feature (i) to different subsets of features, compared to the baseline output as Equation (3.2).

$$\emptyset_i(x) = \frac{1}{M} \sum_{m=1}^{M} \left[f(x_m) - f(z) \right] \qquad (3.2)$$

x_m is permuted instance where feature I is replaced with a value from a reference dataset; M is the number of permutations, and z is the baseline instance. Equation (3.2) represents the core ideas behind SHAP's architecture. The method computes feature importance values that are consistent, individually fair, and have solid theoretical grounding in cooperative game theory. While the actual implementation of SHAP involves additional optimizations and adjustments, these equations capture the essence of how SHAP explains the contributions of individual features to a ML model's predictions (Arrieta et al., 2020).

3.6.2 LIME

LIME (local interpretable model-agnostic explanations) is another popular method in the field of XAI that focuses on creating locally faithful explanations for individual predictions made by complex ML models. LIME approximates the model's behavior around a specific instance by training a simpler, interpretable model, which can then be used to explain the model's prediction formulated as Equation (3.3) (Nguyen et al., 2020).

$$\emptyset(x) = \arg\min \sum_{x'} L\big(f(x), \emptyset(x') \big) + \Omega(\emptyset) \qquad (3.3)$$

Here $\emptyset(x)$ is the explainable instance; $f(x)$ is the prediction by DL model; L is the loss function to measure the discrepancy between prediction and actual result; and Ω is the regulation term that encourages the interpretability of the local model.

3.7 Feature Scope of XAI

XAI's wide range of methods may help explain AI models' decision-making. Key among these characteristics is feature importance, which helps stakeholders understand how attributes affect model predictions. Local explanations explain individual predictions, whereas global explanations examine the model's overall behavior. Visualizations like partial dependency plots and attention processes simplify complicated information. Rule-based explanations clarify judgments using clear rules.

Counterfactual explanations show how changing input attributes changes model outputs. Model-agnostic LIME and SHAP provide many model designs, enabling adaptability. Fairness and prejudice are addressed ethically to ensure responsible AI implementation. Interactive explanations make material accessible to non-experts and enable dynamic inquiry. Domain-specific explanations address application domain specifics, increasing relevance.

3.8 Conclusion and Future Work

The exploration of visualizations, both at the local and global levels, has demonstrated their pivotal role in bridging the gap between complex algorithms and human understanding. As we navigate the intricate terrain of DL models, the quest for balancing complexity with transparency remains an ongoing challenge, yet one that is met with innovative solutions aimed at demystifying the "black box." Real-world case studies across diverse domains have demonstrated the tangible impact of XAI, from facilitating medical diagnoses to enhancing financial decision-making. As we navigate the intersection of technology and humanity, the trust engendered by explainability becomes foundational for the widespread acceptance and ethical use of AI. This survey serves as a comprehensive guide for researchers, practitioners, and policymakers navigating the intricate landscape of XAI. As AI continues its march into various facets of our lives, the torch of transparency and accountability, carried by explainability, becomes increasingly indispensable for building a future where AI augments human potential ethically and responsibly. XAI has great potential as it evolves to address the rising need for transparency, interpretability, and accountability in AI systems.

References

Ali, S., Abuhmed, T., El-Sappagh, S., Muhammad, K., Alonso-Moral, J. M., Confalonieri, R., Guidotti, R., Del Ser, J., Díaz-Rodríguez, N., & Herrera, F. (2023). Explainable Artificial Intelligence (XAI): What we know and what is left to attain Trustworthy Artificial Intelligence. *Information Fusion, 99,* 101805.

Arrieta, A. B., Díaz-Rodríguez, N., Del Ser, J., Bennetot, A., Tabik, S., Barbado, A., García, S., Gil-López, S., Molina, D., & Benjamins, R. (2020). Explainable Artificial Intelligence (XAI): Concepts, taxonomies, opportunities and challenges toward responsible AI. *Information Fusion, 58,* 82–115.

Bhatt, C. M., Patel, P., Ghetia, T., & Mazzeo, P. L. (2023). Effective heart disease prediction using machine learning techniques. *Algorithms, 16*(2), 88.

Chamola, V., Hassija, V., Sulthana, A. R., Ghosh, D., Dhingra, D., & Sikdar, B. (2023). A review of trustworthy and explainable artificial intelligence (XAI). *IEEE Access, 11,* 78994–79015. https://ieeexplore.ieee.org/abstract/document/10188681/

Das, A., & Rad, P. (2020). *Opportunities and challenges in explainable artificial intelligence (XAI): A survey.* http://arxiv.org/abs/2006.11371

Dieber, J., & Kirrane, S. (2020). *Why model why? Assessing the strengths and limitations of LIME.* http://arxiv.org/abs/2012.00093

Fahad, H. M., Ghani Khan, M. U., Saba, T., Rehman, A., & Iqbal, S. (2018). Microscopic abnormality classification of cardiac murmurs using ANFIS and HMM. *Microscopy Research and Technique, 81*(5), 449–457. https://doi.org/10.1002/jemt.22998

Haseeb, K., Islam, N., Saba, T., Rehman, A., & Mehmood, Z. (2020). LSDAR: A lightweight structure based data aggregation routing protocol with secure Internet of Things integrated next-generation sensor networks. *Sustainable Cities and Society, 54,* 101995.

Husham, A., Hazim Alkawaz, M., Saba, T., Rehman, A., & Saleh Alghamdi, J. (2016). Automated nuclei segmentation of malignant using level sets. *Microscopy Research and Technique, 79*(10), 993–997. https://doi.org/10.1002/jemt.22733

Hussain, N., Khan, M. A., Sharif, M., Khan, S. A., Albesher, A. A., Saba, T., & Armaghan, A. (2020). A deep neural network and classical features based scheme for objects recognition: An application for machine inspection. *Multimedia Tools and Applications, 83,* 14935–14957.

Iftikhar, S., Fatima, K., Rehman, A., Almazyad, A. S., & Saba, T. (2017). An evolution based hybrid approach for heart diseases classification and associated risk factors identification. *Biomedical Research, 28*(8), 3451–3455.

Islam, S. R., Eberle, W., Ghafoor, S. K., & Ahmed, M. (2021). *Explainable artificial intelligence approaches: A survey.* http://arxiv.org/abs/2101.09429

Jabeen, S., Mehmood, Z., Mahmood, T., Saba, T., Rehman, A., & Mahmood, M. T. (2018). An effective content-based image retrieval technique for image visuals representation based on the bag-of-visual-words model. *PLoS One, 13*(4), e0194526.

Javed, R., Rahim, M. S. M., Saba, T., & Rehman, A. (2020). A comparative study of features selection for skin lesion detection from dermoscopic images. *Network Modeling Analysis in Health Informatics and Bioinformatics, 9,* 1–13.

Jiménez-Luna, J., Grisoni, F., & Schneider, G. (2020). Drug discovery with explainable artificial intelligence. *Nature Machine Intelligence, 2*(10), 573–584.

Khan, M. A., Akram, T., Sharif, M., Javed, K., Raza, M., & Saba, T. (2020). An automated system for cucumber leaf diseased spot detection and classification using improved saliency method and deep features selection. *Multimedia Tools and Applications, 79*(25–26), 18627–18656. https://doi.org/10.1007/s11042-020-08726-8

Khan, M. A., Sharif, M. I., Raza, M., Anjum, A., Saba, T., & Shad, S. A. (2022). Skin lesion segmentation and classification: A unified framework of deep neural network features fusion and selection. *Expert Systems, 39*(7), e12497. https://doi.org/10.1111/exsy.12497

Kothadiya, D. R., Bhatt, C. M., Rehman, A., Alamri, F. S., & Saba, T. (2023). SignExplainer: An explainable AI-enabled framework for sign language recognition with ensemble learning. *IEEE Access, 11,* 47410–47419. https://ieeexplore.ieee.org/abstract/document/10122570/

Kothadiya, D. R., Bhatt, C. M., Saba, T., Rehman, A., & Bahaj, S. A. (2023). SignFORMER: DeepVision transformer for sign language recognition. *IEEE Access, 11,* 4730–4739.

Kothadiya, D., Bhatt, C., Sapariya, K., Patel, K., Gil-González, A.-B., & Corchado, J. M. (2022). Deepsign: Sign language detection and recognition using deep learning. *Electronics, 11*(11), 1780.

Kothadiya, D., Bhatt, C., Soni, D., Gadhe, K., Patel, S., Bruno, A., & Mazzeo, P. L. (2023). Enhancing fingerprint liveness detection accuracy using deep learning: A comprehensive study and novel approach. *Journal of Imaging, 9*(8), 158.

Kothadiya, D., Rehman, A., Abbas, S., Alamri, F. S., & Saba, T. (2023). Attention-based deep learning framework to recognize diabetes disease from cellular retinal images. *Biochemistry and Cell Biology, 101*(6), 550–561. https://doi.org/10.1139/bcb-2023-0151

Larabi-Marie-Sainte, S., Aburahmah, L., Almohaini, R., & Saba, T. (2019). Current techniques for diabetes prediction: Review and case study. *Applied Sciences, 9*(21), 4604.

Li, M., Jiang, Y., Zhang, Y., & Zhu, H. (2023). Medical image analysis using deep learning algorithms. *Frontiers in Public Health, 11*, 1273253.

Malaviya, N., Rahevar, M., Virani, A., Ganatra, A., & Bhuva, K. (2023). LViT: Vision transformer for lung cancer detection. *2023 International Conference on Artificial Intelligence and Smart Communication (AISC)*, 93–98. https://ieeexplore.ieee.org/abstract/document/10085230/

Meethongjan, K., Dzulkifli, M., Rehman, A., Altameem, A., & Saba, T. (2013). An intelligent fused approach for face recognition. *Journal of Intelligent Systems, 22*(2), 197–212. https://doi.org/10.1515/jisys-2013-0010

Miller, T. (2019). Explanation in artificial intelligence: Insights from the social sciences. *Artificial Intelligence, 267*, 1–38.

Minh, D., Wang, H. X., Li, Y. F., & Nguyen, T. N. (2022). Explainable artificial intelligence: A comprehensive review. *Artificial Intelligence Review, 55*(5), 3503–3568. https://doi.org/10.1007/s10462-021-10088-y

Mughal, B., Muhammad, N., Sharif, M., Rehman, A., & Saba, T. (2018). Removal of pectoral muscle based on topographic map and shape-shifting silhouette. *BMC Cancer, 18*(1), 778. https://doi.org/10.1186/s12885-018-4638-5

Mughal, B., Sharif, M., Muhammad, N., & Saba, T. (2018). A novel classification scheme to decline the mortality rate among women due to breast tumor. *Microscopy Research and Technique, 81*(2), 171–180. https://doi.org/10.1002/jemt.22961

Muhsin, Z. F., Rehman, A., Altameem, A., Saba, T., & Uddin, M. (2014). Improved quadtree image segmentation approach to region information. *The Imaging Science Journal, 62*(1), 56–62. https://doi.org/10.1179/1743131X13Y.0000000063

Mujahid, M., Rehman, A., Alam, T., Alamri, F. S., Fati, S. M., & Saba, T. (2023). An efficient ensemble approach for Alzheimer's disease detection using an adaptive synthetic technique and deep learning. *Diagnostics, 13*(15), 2489.

Mujeeb, S., Alghamdi, T. A., Ullah, S., Fatima, A., Javaid, N., & Saba, T. (2019). Exploiting deep learning for wind power forecasting based on big data analytics. *Applied Sciences, 9*(20), 4417.

Nguyen, T. G., Phan, T. V., Hoang, D. T., Nguyen, T. N., & So-In, C. (2020). Efficient SDN-based traffic monitoring in IoT networks with double deep Q-network. In S. Chellappan, K.-K. R. Choo, & N. Phan (Eds.), *Computational Data and Social Networks* (Vol. 12575, pp. 26–38). Springer International Publishing. https://doi.org/10.1007/978-3-030-66046-8_3

Rahevar, M., & Ganatra, A. (2023). Spatial–temporal gated graph attention network for skeleton-based action recognition. *Pattern Analysis and Applications, 26*(3), 929–939. https://doi.org/10.1007/s10044-023-01179-3

Rehman, A. (2023). Brain stroke prediction through deep learning techniques with ADASYN strategy. *2023 16th International Conference on Developments in eSystems Engineering (DeSE)*, Istanbul, Turkiye, 679–684.

Rehman, A., & Saba, T. (2014). Features extraction for soccer video semantic analysis: Current achievements and remaining issues. *Artificial Intelligence Review, 41*(3), 451–461. https://doi.org/10.1007/s10462-012-9319-1

Rehman, A., Saba, T., Kashif, M., Fati, S. M., Bahaj, S. A., & Chaudhry, H. (2022). A revisit of Internet of Things technologies for monitoring and control strategies in smart agriculture. *Agronomy, 12*(1), 127.

Saba, T., Bokhari, S. T. F., Sharif, M., Yasmin, M., & Raza, M. (2018). Fundus image classification methods for the detection of glaucoma: A review. *Microscopy Research and Technique, 81*(10), 1105–1121.

Sadad, T., Rehman, A., Munir, A., Saba, T., Tariq, U., Ayesha, N., & Abbasi, R. (2021). Brain tumor detection and multi-classification using advanced deep learning techniques. *Microscopy Research and Technique, 84*(6), 1296–1308. https://doi.org/10.1002/jemt.23688

Samek, W., Wiegand, T., & Müller, K.-R. (2017). Explainable artificial intelligence: Understanding, visualizing and interpreting deep learning models. http://arxiv.org/abs/1708.08296

Sevak, J. S., Kapadia, A. D., Chavda, J. B., Shah, A., & Rahevar, M. (2017). Survey on semantic image segmentation techniques. *2017 International Conference on Intelligent Sustainable Systems (ICISS)*, 306–313. https://doi.org/10.1109/ISS1.2017.8389420

Surati, S., Trivedi, H., Shrimali, B., Bhatt, C., & Travieso-González, C. M. (2023). An enhanced diagnosis of monkeypox disease using deep learning and a novel attention model SENet on diversified dataset. *Multimodal Technologies and Interaction, 7*(8), 75.

Tahir, B., Iqbal, S., Usman Ghani Khan, M., Saba, T., Mehmood, Z., Anjum, A., & Mahmood, T. (2019). Feature enhancement framework for brain tumor segmentation and classification. *Microscopy Research and Technique, 82*(6), 803–811. https://doi.org/10.1002/jemt.23224

Vilone, G., & Longo, L. (2020). *Explainable artificial intelligence: A systematic review.* http://arxiv.org/abs/2006.00093

Yousaf, K., Mehmood, Z., Saba, T., Rehman, A., Munshi, A. M., Alharbey, R., & Rashid, M. (2019). Mobile-health applications for the efficient delivery of health care facility to people with dementia (PwD) and support to their carers: A survey. *BioMed Research International, 2019*, 7151475. https://www.hindawi.com/journals/bmri/2019/7151475/abs/

Zhang, K., Xu, P., & Zhang, J. (2020). Explainable AI in deep reinforcement learning models: A SHAP method applied in power system emergency control. *2020 IEEE 4th Conference on Energy Internet and Energy System Integration (EI2)*, 711–716. https://ieeexplore.ieee.org/abstract/document/9347147/

Zhang, Y., Weng, Y., & Lund, J. (2022). Applications of explainable artificial intelligence in diagnosis and surgery. *Diagnostics, 12*(2), 237.

Chapter 4

Explainable Artificial Intelligence Techniques in Healthcare Applications

Hareem Ayesha[1], Sajid Iqbal[2], Mehreen Tariq[3],
Abdullah Alaulamie[2], and Aiesha Ahmad[1]

[1]*Institute of Computer Science and Information Technology,
The Women University, Multan, Pakistan*

[2]*Department of Information Systems, College of Computer
Science and Information Technology, King Faisal University,
Kingdom of Saudi Arabia*

[3]*Department of Computer Science, Bahauddin Zakariya University,
Multan, Pakistan*

4.1 Introduction

Deep learning has played a prominent role in performance enhancement of various artificial intelligence (AI)-based tasks like classification, regression, object detection, and image segmentation and may often surpass the domain-specific human experts (Iqbal et al., 2021). This remarkable performance of deep models has significantly elevated during the past few years; however, this improvement is usually attained by increasing the complexity of model, which induces opaqueness in the model's functionality that ultimately makes it challenging to completely trust the decisions made by the model. Moreover, opacity of deep models makes it challenging to execute amendments in the model for its optimization or performance enhancement (Zhang et al., 2021). The lack of reliable explanations that precisely

DOI: 10.1201/9781032626345-4

depict the underlying processes of current AI-based systems contributes to human uncertainty about their trustworthiness. When implementing AI applications in critical real-world environments (i.e., in medical domain), various dynamics and uncertainties make its users perceive AI as untrustworthy (Tomsett et al., 2020; Yousaf et al., 2019). This highlights the necessity that AI systems should be explainable, aiding in confirming critical decisions for human users.

Apart from this, the self-learning capability of AI-based systems made them highly compatible for performing various critical tasks in medical AI-based systems, e.g., automated diagnosis of fatal disease, automated detection and segmentation of malignancies in medical images, in automated treatment recommendation and computer-aided surgeries. However, the integration of AI in medical domain possesses a prominent yet untapped potential, as the medical AI community is already grappling with diverse challenges for making their systems secure and efficient. The key root of these challenges is the opacity of AI algorithms and the inability of these predictive models to provide their forecasting in a human comprehensible (Meethongjan et al., 2013).

4.2 Need of XAI

The essence or cruciality of explainable artificial intelligence (XAI) could be determined by analyzing its commercial benefits, i.e., coping with ethical concerns, building up user's trust, and providing efficient comprehension of AI-based predictions. By performing a comprehensive analysis of existing literature studies, we have explored and summated the four primary motivations of introducing explainability in AI, which have been briefly discussed below.

4.2.1 Explainability

Due to the opaqueness of AI-based algorithms, significant objections and disagreements have been seen regarding the biasness of predictive models, during past few years (Howard et al., 2017). Hence, to authenticate the predictions of AI-based models, it is crucial to provide its comprehensive explanation. The term explanation refers to the comprehension or validation of a particular model's prediction, while the elucidation about the logical reasoning or internal model's processing is out of the scope of explainability. XAI-based systems provide assistance in justifying the model's forecasting, especially when the unanticipated predictions are made by the predictive model. Additionally, for acquiring the trust of end users, explainability of AI pledges that the decisions made by the predictive algorithm are entirely ethical and impartial, i.e., in a verifiable and auditable way. Moreover, in order to fulfill legal concerns regarding data privacy and safety defined by General Data Protection Regulation (GDPR) (Regulation, 2023), it is essential to provide proper explanation or reasoning about the predictions of AI.

4.2.2 Error Control

The concept of explainability in AI also plays an eminent role in the detection and prevention of erroneous activities. Gaining ample knowledge and understanding about the behavior of AI-based systems provides significant discernibility to the indefinite errors and vulnerabilities of the system, which also assist in the detection and rectification of errors at an early (less critical) stage. Thus, explainability of AI provides better error control (Hussain et al., 2020; Khan et al., 2022).

4.2.3 Performance Improvement

Improving the performance of AI-based predictive models is a major concern of researchers nowadays. To do so, highlighting and understanding the weaknesses of existing models is the first step. However, such analysis could not be done on black-box models of AI. Whereas a well-explained predictive model embraces better capability of performance improvement. Hence, introducing explainability in AI models provides researchers with an eminent opportunity to achieve their intended goal.

By knowing the justification behind the forecasting of predictive models, it became easier for the user to improve the outcomes. Therefore, XAI could play a primary role in the ongoing iterative enhancement of machine algorithms (Iftikhar et al., 2017; Khan et al., 2022).

4.2.4 Discovery of New Facts

One of the promising ways for discovering new facts and gaining advance knowledge regarding AI models is to acquire explanation of predictive models. For instance, given that the DeepMind Software, namely, AlphaGo Zero (Jabeen et al., 2018; Silver et al., 2017), has better performance as compared to human players, in games like "Go," in such cases it would be required to know the knowledge that has been learned by the machine for getting this ability. Hence for unearthing of new facts, XAI systems play an eminent role (Jamal et al., 2017; Javed et al., 2020).

4.3 Characteristics of XAI

4.3.1 Explainable AI

According to DARPA XAI-based program, XAI refers to the systems that incorporate the ability to describe or explain its foundation to the end users, illustrates its weaknesses and strengths, and also provides information about its future behavior (Figure 4.1). The aim of DARPA behind referring this program as XAI is to provide human-understandable AI-based systems with the assistance of effective explanation (Gunning & Aha, 2019; Larabi-Marie-Sainte et al., 2019).

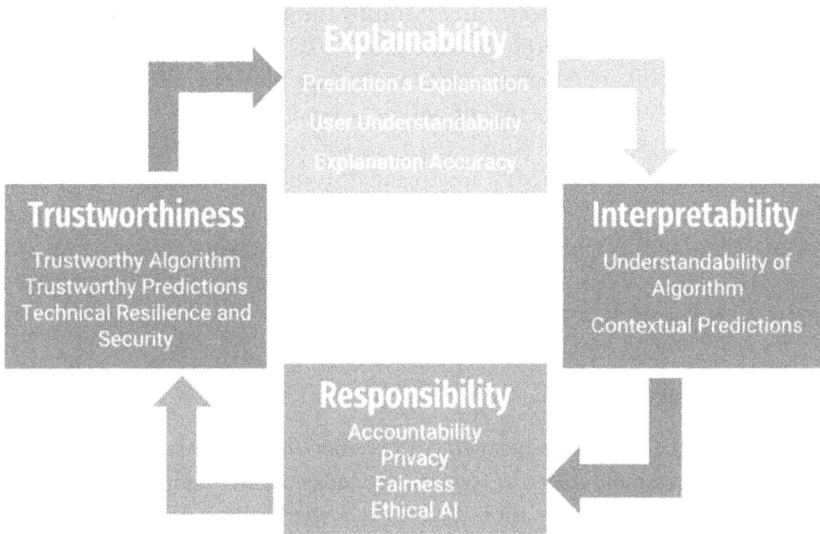

Figure 4.1 Characteristics of XAI.

The term explanation here refers to a comprehensive description about the internal working or mechanism of the algorithm that leads to the outcome. This description or explanation can provide significant assistance in the performance improvement of intended algorithm (Broniatowski, 2021).

According to Phillips et al. (2020), the four primary principles of XAI are as follows:

- *Prediction's Explanation:* The forecasting or predictions made by the AI algorithm needs to be properly justified with the aid of supplementary information and evidence (Mughal 2018a).
- *User Understandability:* The provided system's explanation needs to be comprehensive and highly understandable by the intended human user (Muhsin et al., 2014).
- *Explanation Accuracy:* The provided explanation should precisely justify or explain the system's processes.
- *Controlled Operations:* The AI system must operate only in those specific circumstances for which it is designed for, particularly when it approaches adequate confidence.

4.3.2 Interpretable AI

The term "Interpretability" regarding XAI has been referred differently by different researchers, such that according to Doran et al. (2017), an AI-based system is said to be interpretable if it not only provides outputs but also facilitates the user with the capability to understand how mathematically the model input gets mapped with its output (Mughal et al., 2018b, Ayesha, et al., 2021). According to Broniatowski (2021), interpretability of AI models refers to the capability to contextualize the predictions of algorithm, i.e., whether or not it corresponds to the functional requirements of designed system and fulfills the goals and preferences of end users. In the context of machine learning (ML), interpretability refers to understanding the data processing logic of ML algorithms. In some studies, it has also been seen that both "explainability" and "interpretability" are being employed synonymously, even when some researchers have acknowledged about the essence of an evident taxonomy for the two terms (Bojarski et al., 2017; Lipton, 2018; Naz et al., 2019).

4.3.3 Responsible AI

Responsible AI focuses on the behavior and predictions of AI systems that may lead to ethical repercussions. As such, system may cause negative impact over the societal welfare and human prosperity, even if the system is declared to be secure and comply with legislations. Regardless of their level of independence and learning capability, these systems should be considered as a human-created tool that could not absolutely replace human responsibility.

The major concerns of responsible AI include:

- Establishment of principles regarding AI-based ethical and cultural issues.
- Ensuring accountability, privacy, fairness, bias reduction, privacy, and explainability of AI (Tomsett et al., 2020).

4.3.4 Trustworthy AI

Trust is a fundamental concern of XAI. The major aim behind introducing explainability and transparency in AI is to gain trust of its stakeholders. According to Molnar et al. (2020), trust in AI could be characterized in two ways: (1) trust in model's predictions and (2) trust in the predictive model. In medical field, the trust of patient is usually relying upon predictions of model, while the trust of data scientist relies upon the predictive model.

The AI-based Expert Group of European Union (Brunese et al., 2020) has defined the seven primary guidelines that must be followed during the life cycle of AI system for ensuring trustworthiness:

- Supervision and control of human
- Technical resilience and security
- Efficient data management and privacy
- Process transparency
- Social and environmental prosperity
- Fair and assorted model
- Accountability

4.4 Challenges in XAI

As a matter of fact, XAI grasps a promising commitment for improving accountability, trust, and adoption of AI-based systems, but it also comes up with several challenges, i.e., designing of decisive predictive models that engender precise outcomes and oblige apprehensive explanation. In addition to this, fulfilling the key concerns of AI-based systems, including robustness, quality of explanation, completeness, fairness, and transparency, is also considered to be challenging. Some of the pivotal challenges regarding XAI are analyzed further in the subsequent section.

4.4.1 Quality of Explanation

For getting the insights and apprehension regarding an AI-based system, the major focus of experts is to gauge their reliability, validation, and debugging power. The provided explanation regarding these perturbations is often not adequate, e.g.: What is the reason behind the veracity of a model's prediction? Several researchers have dispensed their ideas for assuring the quality of explanation, such as Gilpin et al. (2018) have recommended to provide a holistic, human interpretable outside explanation that also answers the why questions regarding XAI-based system. The purpose of this explanation is to develop trust within the specialized technical and non-technical end users of the system (Saba & Rehman, 2013).

Nevertheless, meticulous explanations are often unaccountable for end users, while the most explicable descriptions often do not stipulate predictive power. Hence, XAI is facing a momentous challenge of providing adequate explanation of the system that is both decipherable and absolute.

4.4.2 Trade-off between Interpretability and Performance

A significant challenge in XAI is to balance the traditional trade-off between the performance (i.e., accuracy) and the accountability of predictive ML-based models (Molnar et al., 2020). An intrinsic and integral fact about predictive models is that the more explicable ML models (i.e., KNN and decision tree) often stipulate less accuracy as compared to opaque or black-box-based models like deep neural networks and convolutional neural networks (CNN). In several recent publications, researchers have dispensed novel anticipation models that are both accurate and comprehensible like novel rule-based models (Letham et al., 2015), GA2M (Muhsin et al., 2014), and distillation model (Che et al., 2016; Saba et al., 2012).

4.4.3 Maintaining Trust in AI

For the ubiquitous acceptance of AI-based technologies across assorted domains, it is crucial to ensure trustworthiness of AI. Trust in traditional software development gets built by the employment of approaches like software testing, documentation, and auditability, while a set of explicit rules are defined for decreeing the behavior of a system. However, the behavior of AI-based systems could not be explicitly defined, as it is based upon continuously evolving knowledge, hence building trust in such system is challenging. IBM has acquainted their approach for the institution of trust in AI-based systems (Arnold et al., 2019); while for ensuring trust in XAI-based systems, European Union has presented a set of regulations that need to be considered during designing of such systems (Ethics Guidelines for Trustworthy AI, 2019). The primary guidelines defined by IBM and EU focused upon security, reliability, trustworthiness, robustness, diversity, explainability, fairness, transparency, accountability, and lineage of designed system (Saba et al., 2018).

4.4.4 User-centered Explanation

A major challenge in XAI is to provide a human interpretable or intelligible explanation about the forecasting of predictive models. According to Ko et al. (2011), a programmer never codes a software application by keeping in view user's understanding, hence it is often poorly designed. Additionally, another significant limitation in literature is that majority of the existing studies are convergent toward the researcher's perspective of model's explanation rather than focusing upon the users without significant background knowledge.

Miller et al. (2017) have acquainted that the prosperity of XAI could be eminently enhanced if the researchers get interpret, adopt, deploy and improve the predictive models by taking in account vast research in the fields of cognitive science and psychology. According to them, explanation of a system is basically a part of social interaction between the system's explainer and the end user. Therefore, by focusing upon the social context, the content and the nature of explanation could be improved.

4.4.5 Black-box Problem

Terms like black-box, white-box, and gray-box referred to the degree of opaqueness of the internal essence of a component (Le Merrer et al., 2020). The black-box models are usually the opaquest and do not divulge the internal design and processing of the model. On the contrary, the white-box or glass-box models are completely transparent or disclosed to its end users. In between the black-box and white-box, the model with limited opaqueness exists, which is termed as gray-box model.

The primary limitation of AI-based systems is that they are highly opaque due to which it is hard to provide explanation regarding the input–output mapping procedure of the model. This issue is usually termed as black-box problem of AI. The major motive of XAI is to evolve from black-box to a white-box model (Gilpin et al., 2018).

Models like linear regression and decision tree are known as glass-box models, as their internal processing of mapping input to output is entirely transparent. On the other hand, deep learning–based models like CNN and RNN show transparency up to a certain degree, due to which they are termed as black-box or translucent glass box models (Yang et al., 2022). As transparent or less-opaque models provide better explainability, they also assist in gaining trust of end users.

4.4.6 Challenges in Medical Field

The opaqueness of AI-based algorithms raise significant concerns and challenges, while embedding them in medical field. Some of the major challenges have been mentioned below:

1. ***Trade-off between Security and Transparency:*** Nevertheless, XAI has significantly assisted in tackling with the security concerns of AI-based systems by discernment of malicious activities and system errors (Sharif et al., 2019). However, its ability of providing fully transparent explanation about the decisions made by predictive models has also given rise to critical security and privacy threats, i.e., attackers may access the sensitive medical information or may cause malicious activities by employing techniques like reverse engineering (Sadad et al., 2021; Tramèr et al., 2016). Hence, providing absolute transparency in medical XAI-based systems may render an endless system access to the nonlegitimate users. Therefore, for cushioning sensitive clinical and personal data of patients, it is crucial to apply befitting measures for the mitigation of risk regarding security and privacy of XAI-based medical applications. In this regard, methods like federated learning (Kaissis et al., 2020) could significantly assist, i.e., by providing enough explanation of predictive algorithms in combination with techniques for privacy-preserving. According to a study (Khan et al., 2020), the two significant research areas, including privacy preserving machine learning (PPML) and XAI, have not yet acquired evidential research attention.

2. ***Trust Issues in Healthcare:*** Building trust in the end users is the primary concern of the explanation provided by the XAI-based systems. Occasionally, the end user of the XAI-based application may not trust the system, even if an apprehensive explanation has been provided. In such cases, the quality of explanation could be enhanced, i.e., by providing graphical depictions related to the performance of predictive models and their corresponding narrative explanation (Le Merrer et al., 2020; Tahir et al., 2019).

   In healthcare, the outputs of AI-based predictive models play a noteworthy role in taking important and critical medical decisions, due to which trust is a fundamental concern in this field. Lack of trust may cause overlooking of absolute predictions. On the contrary, over-trust may lead to reliance upon inaccurate predictions. For coping up with these issues, it is crucial to provide a honest and open-ended information about the capabilities and weaknesses of employed AI algorithm to the end user (Hulsen, 2023; Fahad et al., 2018).

3. ***Legal Challenges:*** Integration of XAI in healthcare may arise significant legal considerations and challenges:
   - ■ *Follow Data Privacy Standards:* The patient's health records are highly sensitive and need to be protected by following strict privacy concerns such as defined by Health Insurance Portability and Accountability Act (HIPAA) in the United States and the GDPR in the European Union.
   - ■ *Patient's Conscious Consent:* It refers to the concept that before the utilization of patient's data, the corresponding predictive algorithm should be completely explained to the patient in advance.
   - ■ *Certificate or Endorsement as a Medical Device:* The underlying medical device should be certified with the European Commission (MDR) and U.S. Food and Drug Administration (FDA) (Sampson et al., 2019) by introducing the requirements to legalize the necessity for AI-based medical devices.

4.5 Explainability Approaches

For making the AI-based systems more transparent and interpretable for the end users, various explainability techniques have been dispensed so far. These approaches have been categorized differently by different researchers in literature. However, in general, there is no fixed or absolute categorization that exists. Prior to delving into these taxonomies or explainability techniques, we have established a common terminology for distinguishing various types of approaches used for explaining AI models (Figure 4.2). Below, you will find a concise description of these approaches.

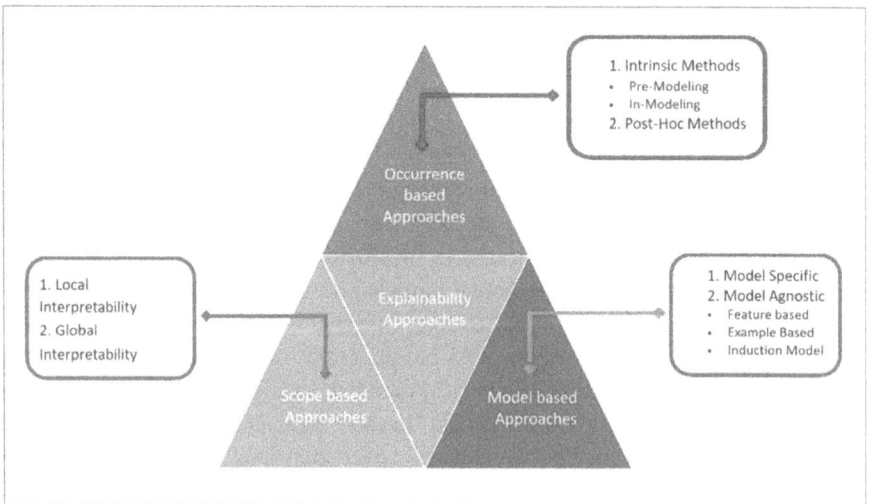

Figure 4.2   Explainability approaches.

4.5.1 Occurrence-based Methods

The discrimination of XAI methods could be done based upon the manifestation of model's interpretability criteria, i.e., whether the explainability mechanism have been deployed within the model's internal architecture (within development phase) or outside the architecture (after model's development and training phase). Based upon this criterion, the explainability methods could be categorized into two types (Adadi & Berrada, 2020):

1. Intrinsic methods
2. Post-hoc methods

1. ***Intrinsic Methods***
   Intrinsic methods are characterized by their ability to comprehend a decision-making process or the underlying principles of a predictive algorithm, without requiring additional information. These methods are also referred to as "transparent models" or "interpretable models." The interpretable models incorporate inherent self-explanatory features, due to the low design complexity of their structure. These models offer more precise explanations, albeit with a slight compromise on prediction performance. Some of the commonly employed intrinsic models encompass linear regression (LR), k-nearest neighbor, logistic regression, rule-based learners, Bayesian models, general additive models, decision tree set, etc. The transparent or intrinsic explainability methods could further be characterized into two categories (Elshawi et al., 2019):
   - ***Pre-modeling Intrinsic Methods:*** The primary motive of these explainability approaches is to apprehend and delineate the input data provided to the predictive model. These methods are autonomous and can be utilized without reliance on a specific model architecture. t-Distributed *stochastic neighbor embedding*(t-SNE) (Van der Maaten & Hinton, 2008) and principal component analyzer (PCA) (Wold et al., 1987) are common pre-modeling explainability methods.
   - ***In-modeling Intrinsic Methods:*** In-modeling or during-modeling explainability approaches are dedicated for designing more explainable structure of predictive models inherently.

2. ***Post-hoc Methods***
   In contrary to the transparent ML models, there exist another class of uninterpretable and highly intricate black-box models that are particularly known for their precision. For explaining these models, a distinctive class of explainability methods are utilized after the building of complex AI models, which are known as post-hoc methods (Lipton, 2018). Post-hoc methods provide the decisive explanation of black-box models, without getting insights of model's internal mechanism and without performing any significant alteration in model's architecture. According to Adadi et al. (2018), majority of recent

developments in the field of XAI regarding explainability approaches fall into the post-hoc category, i.e., example-based, visualization-based, and language-based explanations (Krening et al., 2016).

4.5.2 Model-based Methods

The model interpretability or explainability methods could be categorized into two groups based upon the type of model to which they are envisioned (Haseeb et al., 2020):

1. Model-agnostic interpretability methods
2. Model-specific interpretability methods

Further details of these techniques are mentioned below:

1. *Model-agnostic Techniques*
   Model-agnostic techniques are independent and do not depend on specific types of ML models. In essence, this category of interpretability approaches decouples the prediction process from the model's explanation process. These interpretation approaches typically come under the category of post-hoc explainability methods, and pertain the ability of both local and global interpretable models. To enhance the interpretability of AI models, a significant number of model-agnostic methods have been recently developed. These methods draw on a wide range of techniques: statistics, ML, and data science. Model-agnostic explainability approaches could be broadly classified into three distinct groups:
   - *Features-based Explanation:* These approaches are dedicated for evaluating relevance or contribution of the input features, for which it assigns a score to input features that signify their relative implication in relation to the model's prediction function. By doing so, the input features provide explanatory insights into the prediction process (Mughal et al., 2018a). Partial dependent plots (PDP), perturbation-based features significance, and Shapely additive method (SHAP) (Saba et al., 2012) are some of the well-known features-based XAI approaches.
   - *Example-based Explanation:* Example-based explainability approaches (Mughal et al., 2018b) choose specific data instances from the input dataset to deliver explanations regarding the model's predictions.
   - *Induction Models–based Explanation:* Model induction approaches refer to the techniques which construct simplified and interpretable models, with the purpose of elucidating the functioning of intricate or opaque ML models. The primary purpose of model induction methods is to enhance the transparency of opaque models with the aid of new models that encapsulate the fundamental characteristics and decision-making mechanisms of black-box models (Ribeiro et al., 2016).

2. *Model-specific*

Contrary to model-agnostic methods, the model-specific methods are inherently constrained and refer to a class of explainability approaches that are tailored for specific predictive algorithms. Intrinsic methods also came under this category of explainability approaches. The downside of this approach is that it provided limited choices when we need a specific type of interpretation. This limitation may force us to select models that offer the desired interpretability, possibly at the cost of sacrificing the use of more efficient predictive and comprehensive models. Consequently, there has been a growing interest in model-agnostic interpretability methods, as they do not depend on a particular model and offer a more flexible approach.

4.5.3 Scope-based Methods

The explainability methods for the comprehension of XAI-based models could be broadly categorized into two groups based upon their scope of explanation: (1) *Global explanation:* This involves understanding of entire predictive model; (2) *Local explanation:* This encompasses the comprehension of a single model's prediction.

We have distinguished between the two subclasses in the subsequent sections.

1. *Local Interpretability-based Methods*

Local interpretability-based methods are responsible for elucidating a particular prediction of the model, i.e., by explaining why the model has made a certain forecasting over a particular data instance. For example, a local explanation–based method may involve a brain magnetic resonance imaging (MRI) scan highlighting the brain tumor with the aid saliency map. This map explains which specific portion of the MRI image predominantly influenced the classifier's output. As it clarifies which part of the image leads the classifier to classify it as "tumor" for an individual data instance, this example falls under the category of a local explanation (Van der Velden et al., 2022).

2. *Global Interpretability-based Methods*

The focus of global interpretability–based methods is upon getting comprehensive knowledge about the logic of the predictive algorithms, including the information about the utilized dataset and the whole training process. These models attempt to distinguish the general behavior and reasoning process of a model to predict its possible outcomes. Feature importance is considered to be a prominent example of global interpretability methods, i.e., discriminating that particular feature responsible for achieving improved performance from the whole dataset (Singh et al., 2020). Getting the insights from a neural network about the degree to which high blood pressure elevates the likelihood of a cardiac event is another global interpretation method (Jabeen et al., 2018).

4.6 XAI Pipeline in Medical Domain

An abstract outline and description of the general XAI pipeline in medical domain has been provided below (see Figure 4.3):

1. *Input Dataset*

   In the first phase of this pipeline, the medical dataset has been gathered and prepared, i.e., either by affiliation from any hospital or through public data repositories. This dataset could be either medical image–based electronic health records or textual medical reports. However, the quantity of data should be enough for the training of an AI predictive model.

2. *Data Preparation*

   Data preparation is the second major stage of XAI pipeline that involves pre-processing of input data to ensure its compatibility with the XAI-based predictive model. In this phase, a variety of explanation approaches known as *pre-model XAI methods* are utilized to enhance the comprehension of input data. The need for data explainability arises from the profound impact the training dataset exerts on an AI model's behavior. The quality of the data is paramount, as it is impossible to construct a high-performing model with poor input. Hence, thorough scrutiny of the collected data is imperative for which various pre-model explainability methods have been introduced so far:

   i. *t*-SNE (Van der Maaten & Hinton, 2008)
   ii. Parallel coordinate plots (PCP) (Tilouche et al., 2021)
   iii. Principal component analysis (PCA)

3. *Model Training*

   The subsequent phase entails the selection of a suitable ML model and training it with the prepared dataset. The interpretability of selected ML model is crucial for achieving better results in the training phase, such as the developers may leverage their domain knowledge efficiently in performance enhancement, if the model is understandable. Hence, in addition to data explainability, the significance of model explainability could not be overstated. The phrase

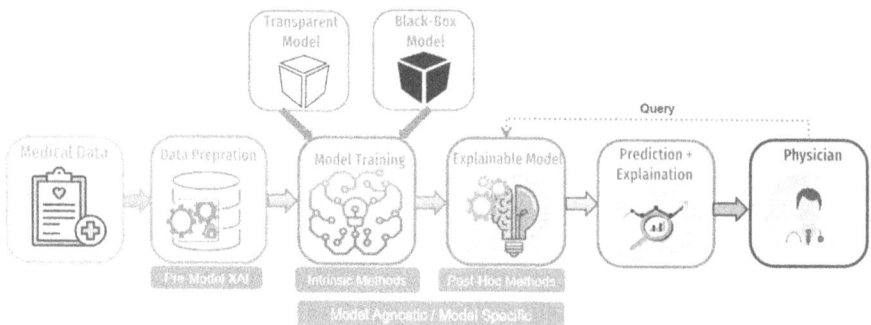

Figure 4.3   XAI pipeline.

model explainability refers to the ML models that are intrinsically (i.e., by design) more understandable. These models are also referred to as *transparent models* or *intrinsic methods* (as mentioned in Figure 4.3). Some of the renowned intrinsic ML models are as follows:

    i. Linear regression (Ustun & Rudin, 2016)
    ii. Decision sets (Lakkaraju et al., 2016)
    iii. Decision tree
    iv. Case-based reasoning
    v. Rule sets (Jung et al., 2017)

4. *Explainable Model*
   In case if the explainability criteria are not intrinsically indulged in the predictive model, a post-hoc explainability model is employed after the training of actual predictive model. This post-hoc approach could be either model-agnostic or model-specific; however, the primary goal of this approach is to formulate interpretability or understandability of the predictions made by the trained model.

5. *Predictions with Explanation Generation*
   In this phase, the predictions made by the trained model together with the explanation generated by the explainability method have been given as output to the end user. In the case of healthcare application, it could be either a patient or an expert medical practitioner.

6. *Physician/End User*
   In the final phase of XAI pipeline, the quality of explanation has been gauged by the end user or physician utilizing the XAI-based system. The end user can either make a query from the system or provide a feedback based upon the provided prediction's explanation.

4.7 XAI in Medical Image Analysis for Disease Diagnosis

4.7.1 X-rays-based Pulmonary Disease Diagnosis

Chest X-ray (CXR) is a cost-effective and easily accessible imaging method (Singh et al., 2021). It has been widely employed for the automated diagnosis of lungs disease like pneumonia and COVID-19, such as by Iqbal et al. (2022), who have presented a deep CNN algorithm for the discrimination of COVID-19, pneumonia, and normal cases with the aid of CXR images. Nine distinct datasets that incorporate over 3,200 COVID-19 CXR images have been utilized for gauging the efficacy of the proposed method. To comprehend the learning process of the model in identifying pneumonia pathology, including signs of COVID-19, an explainability algorithm based on gradient-weighted class activation mapping (Grad-CAM) (Selvaraju et al., 2017) has been utilized, which primarily aid in the generation of visual representation regarding the detected lung-infected areas by the proposed

CNN model. The achieved results demonstrate high performance, with an area under curve (AUC) of 0.97 for multiclass classification and 0.98 for the binary classification. The presented explainability model illustrates the model's proficiency in identifying COVID-19 indicators.

A deep CNN-based ensemble learning approach has been presented by Singh et al. (2021) for the automated diagnosis of COVID-19 and pneumonia disease using CXRs. The authors have employed four CNN models and SVM as a meta-classifier for the discrimination of input CXRs into three classes (i.e., COVID, pneumonia, and normal). For reducing the model's complexity and for enhancing its performance, effective model-pruning criteria have also been devised. Explainability and trust in model have been introduced with the aid of Grad-CAM visualization method.

4.7.2 MRI-based Diagnosis

For highlighting the predictive markers of Parkinson's disease (PD), Shinde et al. (2019) have presented a deep CNN-based classification approach. The training and performance evaluation of proposed CNN architecture has been done using neuromelanin-sensitive magnetic resonance imaging (NMS-MRI), gathered from 55 patients. The testing accuracy attained by the presented CNN has outperformed the prevailing radiomics-based and Contrast ratio techniques, by achieving an accuracy of 85.7%. Interpretability in the presented approach has been introduced with the aid of CAM, which highlights or discriminates the most prominent features contributed in the decision-making process.

Levakov et al. (2020) have presented a 3D CNN-based ensemble approach for the automated brain aging prediction using T1-weighted brain MRI images. To perform this task, a total of 10,176 brain MRI scans have been gathered from 15 distinct data repositories. After employing data preprocessing and data augmentation techniques, the input images are fed to an ensemble of 10 2D CNN architectures, with the aim of predicting the age of input subject. The ten resultant predictions made by the ensemble are then fed to the linear regression model to predict the final outcome. At the second phase of this study, author has employed an explainability approach for highlighting the specific anatomical regions of the brain that significantly contributes in brain age prediction. To do so, a gradient-based interpretability method known as SmoothGRAD (Smilkov et al., 2017) has been exploited with the assistance of investigate (Alber et al., 2019). By the analysis of aggregated explanation map, it has been concluded that age predictions were primarily influenced by cisterns and ventricle.

4.7.3 Other Modalities

In addition to the state-of-the-art medical imaging modalities (i.e., CXR, CT scan, MRI, and ultrasound), various XAI approaches have also been introduced for disease diagnosis using less familiar imaging modalities, i.e., optical imaging and nuclear imaging (Tariq et al., 2021). Various applications of nuclear imaging have been found in the diagnosis of disease regarding dermatology, cancer, and diabetic retinopathy, while a limited number of studies have also utilized nuclear imaging modality for the diagnosis of Parkinson's disease (Javed et al., 2020).

4.8 Conclusion and Future Directions

In this chapter, we have presented a review of the emerging field of XAI approaches and their respective applications for enhancing the interpretability of image classification and segmentation tasks in the field of medical image analysis. The amalgamation of XAI methods with deep neural network models holds the potential to assist in both disease detection and diagnosis, while also offering additional insights to the medical practitioners. However, there is a significant need of making effort to devise new algorithms that incorporate reasoning and explainability, taking into account clinical parameters and the factors leading to specific findings.

We conducted an extensive investigation into the innovative application of XAI in disease diagnosis using diverse medical imaging modalities, including CXRs, ultrasound, MRI, etc. Through this analysis, we discovered that numerous explainability approaches have been applied in the diagnosis of various diseases such as COVID-19, Parkinson's, breast cancer, liver disease, kidney disease, dermatology, and more. However, the predominant approach in many of these image-based diagnostic methods has been the use of visual explanation-based methods, as opposed to other explainability techniques. Furthermore, a significant portion of the studies has relied on established visual explainability approaches instead of introducing novel XAI methodologies. Among the employed visual explainability methods, CAM and Grad-CAM are the most commonly utilized.

References

Adadi, A., & Berrada, M. (2018). Peeking inside the black-box: A survey on explainable artificial intelligence (XAI). IEEE Access, 6, 52138–52160.

Adadi, A., & Berrada, M. (2020). Explainable AI for healthcare: From black box to interpretable models. In Embedded Systems and Artificial Intelligence: Proceedings of ESAI 2019, Fez, Morocco (pp. 327–337). Springer, Singapore. https://doi.org/10.1007/978-981-15-0947-6_31

Alber, M., Lapuschkin, S., Seegerer, P., Hägele, M., Schütt, K. T., Montavon, G., ..., & Kindermans, P. J. (2019). iNNvestigate neural networks! Journal of Machine Learning Research, 20(93), 1–8.

Arnold, M., Bellamy, R. K., Hind, M., Houde, S., Mehta, S., Mojsilović, A., ..., & Varshney, K. R. (2019). FactSheets: Increasing trust in AI services through supplier's declarations of conformity. IBM Journal of Research and Development, 63(4/5), 6:1–6:13. https://doi.org/10.1147/JRD.2019.2942288

Arrieta, A. B., Díaz-Rodríguez, N., Del Ser, J., Bennetot, A., Tabik, S., Barbado, A., ..., & Herrera, F. (2020). Explainable artificial intelligence (XAI): Concepts, taxonomies, opportunities and challenges toward responsible AI. Information Fusion, 58, 82–115. https://doi.org/10.1016/j.inffus.2019.12.012

Ayesha, H., Iqbal, S., Tariq, M., Abrar, M., Sanaullah, M., Abbas, I., …, & Hussain, S. (2021). Automatic medical image interpretation: State of the art and future directions. Pattern Recognition, 114, 107856.

Bojarski, M., Yeres, P., Choromanska, A., Choromanski, K., Firner, B., Jackel, L., & Muller, U. (2017). Explaining how a deep neural network trained with end-to-end learning steers a car. arXiv:1704.07911.

Broniatowski, D. A. (2021). Psychological foundations of explainability and interpretability in artificial intelligence. NIST, Technical Report. doi: 10.6028/NIST.IR.8367

Brunese, L., Mercaldo, F., Reginelli, A., & Santone, A. (2020). Explainable deep learning for pulmonary disease and coronavirus COVID-19 detection from X-rays. Computer Methods and Programs in Biomedicine, 196, 105608. https://doi.org/10.1016/j.cmpb.2020.105608

Che, Z., Purushotham, S., Khemani, R., & Liu, Y. (2016). Interpretable deep models for ICU outcome prediction. In AMIA Annual Symposium Proceedings (Vol. 2016, p. 371). American Medical Informatics Association.

Chen, X., Lin, L., Liang, D., Hu, H., Zhang, Q., Iwamoto, Y., …, & Wu, J. (2019, September). A dual-attention dilated residual network for liver lesion classification and localization on CT images. In 2019 IEEE International Conference on Image Processing (ICIP) (pp. 235–239). IEEE.

Doran, D., Schulz, S., & Besold, T. R. (2017). What does explainable AI really mean? A new conceptualization of perspectives. arXiv:1710.00794.

Elshawi, R., Al-Mallah, M. H., & Sakr, S. (2019). On the interpretability of machine learning-based model for predicting hypertension. BMC Medical Informatics and Decision Making, 19(1), 1–32. https://doi.org/10.1186/S12911-019-0874-0

Ethics guidelines for trustworthy AI. (2019, April 8). Shaping Europe's Digital Future. https://digital-strategy.ec.europa.eu/en/library/ethics-guidelines-trustworthy-ai (accessed September 30, 2023).

Fahad, H. M., Ghani Khan, M. U., Saba, T., Rehman, A., & Iqbal, S. (2018). Microscopic abnormality classification of cardiac murmurs using ANFIS and HMM. Microscopy Research and Technique, 81(5), 449–457.

Gilpin, L. H., Bau, D., Yuan, B. Z., Bajwa, A., Specter, M., & Kagal, L. (2018, October). Explaining explanations: An overview of interpretability of machine learning. In 2018 IEEE 5th International Conference on Data Science and Advanced Analytics (DSAA) (pp. 80–89). IEEE. https://doi.org/10.1109/DSAA.2018.00018

Gunning, D., & Aha, D. (2019). DARPA's explainable artificial intelligence (XAI) program. AI Magazine, 40(2), 44–58. https://doi.org/10.1609/AIMAG.V40I2.2850

Haseeb, K., Islam, N., Saba, T., Rehman, A., & Mehmood, Z. (2020). LSDAR: A lightweight structure based data aggregation routing protocol with secure Internet of Things integrated next-generation sensor networks. Sustainable Cities and Society, 54, 101995.

Hassan, M. R., Islam, M. F., Uddin, M. Z., Ghoshal, G., Hassan, M. M., Huda, S., & Fortino, G. (2022). Prostate cancer classification from ultrasound and MRI images using deep learning based explainable artificial intelligence. Future Generation Computer Systems, 127, 462–472.

Howard, A., Zhang, C., & Horvitz, E. (2017, March). Addressing bias in machine learning algorithms: A pilot study on emotion recognition for intelligent systems. In 2017 IEEE Workshop on Advanced Robotics and Its Social Impacts (ARSO) (pp. 1–7). IEEE. https://doi.org/10.1109/ARSO.2017.8025197.

Hulsen, T. (2023). Explainable Artificial Intelligence (XAI): Concepts and challenges in healthcare. AI, 4, 652–666. https://doi.org/10.3390/AI4030034

Husham, A., Hazim Alkawaz, M., Saba, T., Rehman, A., & Saleh Alghamdi, J. (2016). Automated nuclei segmentation of malignant using level sets. Microscopy Research and Technique, 79(10), 993–997.

Hussain, N., Khan, M. A., Sharif, M., Khan, S. A., Albesher, A. A., Saba, T., & Armaghan, A. (2020). A deep neural network and classical features based scheme for objects recognition: An application for machine inspection. Multimedia Tools and Applications, 83, 14935–14957.

Iftikhar, S., Fatima, K., Rehman, A., Almazyad, A. S., & Saba, T. (2017). An evolution based hybrid approach for heart diseases classification and associated risk factors identification. Biomedical Research, 28(8), 3451–3455.

Iqbal, S., Ayesha, H., Farooq Khan Niazi, M., Ayesha, N., & Tehseen Ahmad, K. (2022). COVID-19 prediction, diagnosis and prevention through computer vision. In T. Saba, A. Rehman, S. Roy (eds), Prognostic Models in Healthcare: AI and Statistical Approaches (pp. 79–113). Springer, Singapore.

Iqbal, S., Tariq, M., Ayesha, H., & Ayesha, N. (2021). AI technologies in health-care applications. In L. M. Goyal, T. Saba, A. Rehman, S. Larabi-Marie-Sainte (eds), Artificial Intelligence and Internet of Things (pp. 3–44). CRC Press.

Jabeen, S., Mehmood, Z., Mahmood, T., Saba, T., Rehman, A., & Mahmood, M. T. (2018). An effective content-based image retrieval technique for image visuals representation based on the bag-of-visual-words model. PLoS One, 13(4), e0194526.

Jamal, A., Hazim Alkawaz, M., Rehman, A., & Saba, T. (2017). Retinal imaging analysis based on vessel detection. Microscopy Research and Technique, 80(7), 799–811.

Javed, R., Rahim, M. S. M., Saba, T., & Rehman, A. (2020). A comparative study of features selection for skin lesion detection from dermoscopic images. Network Modeling Analysis in Health Informatics and Bioinformatics, 9, 1–13.

Jung, J., Concannon, C., Shroff, R., Goel, S., & Goldstein, D. G. (2017). Simple rules for complex decisions. arXiv:1702.04690. https://doi.org/10.2139/ssrn.2919024

Kaissis, G. A., Makowski, M. R., Rückert, D., & Braren, R. F. (2020). Secure, privacy-preserving and federated machine learning in medical imaging. Nature Machine Intelligence, 2(6), 305–311. https://doi.org/10.1038/s42256-020-0186-1

Khan, M. A., Akram, T., Sharif, M., Javed, K., Raza, M., & Saba, T. (2020). An automated system for cucumber leaf diseased spot detection and classification using improved saliency method and deep features selection. Multimedia Tools and Applications, 79, 18627–18656.

Khan, M. A., Sharif, M. I., Raza, M., Anjum, A., Saba, T., & Shad, S. A. (2022). Skin lesion segmentation and classification: A unified framework of deep neural network features fusion and selection. Expert Systems, 39(7), e12497.

Ko, A. J., Abraham, R., Beckwith, L., Blackwell, A., Burnett, M., Erwig, M., …, & Wiedenbeck, S. (2011). The state of the art in end-user software engineering. ACM Computing Surveys (CSUR), 43(3), 1–44.

Komatsu, M., Sakai, A., Dozen, A., Shozu, K., Yasutomi, S., Machino, H., …, & Hamamoto, R. (2021). Towards clinical application of artificial intelligence in ultrasound imaging. Biomedicines, 9(7), 720. https://doi.org/10.3390/biomedicines9070720

Krening, S., Harrison, B., Feigh, K. M., Isbell, C. L., Riedl, M., & Thomaz, A. (2016). Learning from explanations using sentiment and advice in RL. IEEE Transactions on Cognitive and Developmental Systems, 9(1), 44–55. https://doi.org/10.1109/TCDS.2016.2628365

Kumar, A., Manikandan, R., Kose, U., Gupta, D., & Satapathy, S. C. (2021). Doctor's dilemma: Evaluating an explainable subtractive spatial lightweight convolutional neural network for brain tumor diagnosis. ACM Transactions on Multimedia Computing, Communications, and Applications (TOMM), 17(3s), 1–26. https://doi.org/10.1145/3457187

Lakkaraju, H., Bach, S. H., & Leskovec, J. (2016, August). Interpretable decision sets: A joint framework for description and prediction. In Proceedings of the 22nd ACM SIGKDD International Conference on Knowledge Discovery and Data Mining (pp. 1675–1684). https://doi.org/10.1145/2939672.2939874

Larabi-Marie-Sainte, S., Aburahmah, L., Almohaini, R., & Saba, T. (2019). Current techniques for diabetes prediction: Review and case study. Applied Sciences, 9(21), 4604.

Le Merrer, E., & Trédan, G. (2020). Remote explainability faces the bouncer problem. Nature Machine Intelligence, 2(9), 529–539. https://doi.org/10.1038/s42256-020-0216-z

Letham, B., Rudin, C., McCormick, T. H., & Madigan, D. (2015). Interpretable classifiers using rules and Bayesian analysis: Building a better stroke prediction model. Annals of Applied Statistics, 9(3), 1350–1371. https://doi.org/10.1214/15-AOAS848

Levakov, G., Rosenthal, G., Shelef, I., Raviv, T. R., & Avidan, G. (2020). From a deep learning model back to the brain: Identifying regional predictors and their relation to aging. Human Brain Mapping, 41(12), 3235–3252. https://doi.org/10.1002/hbm.25011

Lipton, Z. C. (2018). The mythos of model interpretability: In machine learning, the concept of interpretability is both important and slippery. Queue, 16(3), 31–57. https://doi.org/10.1145/3233231

Meethongjan, K., Dzulkifli, M., Rehman, A., Altameem, A., & Saba, T. (2013). An intelligent fused approach for face recognition. Journal of Intelligent Systems, 22(2), 197–212.

Miller, T., Howe, P., & Sonenberg, L. (2017). Explainable AI: Beware of inmates running the asylum or: How I learnt to stop worrying and love the social and behavioural sciences. arXiv:1712.00547v2

Molnar, C., Casalicchio, G., & Bischl, B. (2020, September). Interpretable machine learning: A brief history, state-of-the-art and challenges. In Joint European Conference on Machine Learning and Knowledge Discovery in Databases (pp. 417–431). Springer International Publishing, Cham. https://doi.org/10.1007/978-3-030-65965-3_28

Mughal, B., Muhammad, N., Sharif, M., Rehman, A., & Saba, T. (2018a). Removal of pectoral muscle based on topographic map and shape-shifting silhouette. BMC Cancer, 18(1), 1–1.

Mughal, B., Sharif, M., Muhammad, N., & Saba, T. (2018b). A novel classification scheme to decline the mortality rate among women due to breast tumor. Microscopy Research and Technique, 81(2), 171–180.

Muhsin, Z. F., Rehman, A., Altameem, A., Saba, T., & Uddin, M. (2014). Improved quadtree image segmentation approach to region information. The Imaging Science Journal, 62(1), 56–62.

Naz, A., Javed, M. U., Javaid, N., Saba, T., Alhussein, M., & Aurangzeb, K. (2019). Short-term electric load and price forecasting using enhanced extreme learning machine optimization in smart grids. Energies, 12(5), 866.

Phillips, P. J., Hahn, C. A., Fontana, P. C., Broniatowski, D. A., & Przybocki, M. A. (2020). Four principles of explainable artificial intelligence. NIST, Gaithersburg, Maryland, p. 18.

Regulation, G. D. P. (2023). General Data Protection Regulation (GDPR): Official legal text.

Rehman, A. (2023). Brain stroke prediction through deep learning techniques with ADASYN strategy. 2023 16th International Conference on Developments in eSystems Engineering (DeSE), Istanbul, Turkiye, pp. 679–684.

Ribeiro, M. T., Singh, S., & Guestrin, C. (2016, August). "Why should I trust you?" Explaining the predictions of any classifier. In Proceedings of the 22nd ACM SIGKDD International Conference on Knowledge Discovery and Data Mining (pp. 1135–1144). https://doi.org/10.1145/2939672.2939778

Saba, T., Al-Zahrani, S., & Rehman, A. (2012). Expert system for offline clinical guidelines and treatment. Life Science Journal, 9(4), 2639–2658.

Saba, T., Bokhari, S. T. F., Sharif, M., Yasmin, M., & Raza, M. (2018). Fundus image classification methods for the detection of glaucoma: A review. Microscopy Research and Technique, 81(10), 1105–1121.

Saba, T., & Rehman, A. (2013). Effects of artificially intelligent tools on pattern recognition. International Journal of Machine Learning and Cybernetics, 4, 155–162.

Saba, T., Rehman, A., Mehmood, Z., Kolivand, H., & Sharif, M. (2018). Image enhancement and segmentation techniques for detection of knee joint diseases: A survey. Current Medical Imaging, 14(5), 704–715.

Sadad, T., Rehman, A., Munir, A., Saba, T., Tariq, U., Ayesha, N., & Abbasi, R. (2021). Brain tumor detection and multi-classification using advanced deep learning techniques. Microscopy Research and Technique, 84(6), 1296–1308.

Sampson, D. K., Dwyer, L. M., Tseng, E. H., Lorell, B. H., & Kavi, K. J. (2019). FDA proposes regulatory framework for artificial intelligence/machine learning software as a medical device. J tl, 31(7), 12–6. (accessed September 30, 2023).

Selvaraju, R. R., Cogswell, M., Das, A., Vedantam, R., Parikh, D., & Batra, D. (2017). Grad-CAM: Visual explanations from deep networks via gradient-based localization. In Proceedings of the IEEE International Conference on Computer Vision (pp. 618–626). doi: 10.1007/s11263-019-01228-7

Sharif, U., Mehmood, Z., Mahmood, T., Javid, M. A., Rehman, A., & Saba, T. (2019). Scene analysis and search using local features and support vector machine for effective content-based image retrieval. Artificial Intelligence Review, 52, 901–925.

Shinde, S., Prasad, S., Saboo, Y., Kaushick, R., Saini, J., Pal, P. K., & Ingalhalikar, M. (2019). Predictive markers for Parkinson's disease using deep neural nets on neuromelanin sensitive MRI. NeuroImage: Clinical, 22, 101748. https://doi.org/10.1016/j.nicl.2019.101748

Silver, D., Schrittwieser, J., Simonyan, K., Antonoglou, I., Huang, A., Guez, A., …, & Hassabis, D. (2017). Mastering the game of go without human knowledge. Nature, 550(7676), 354–359. https://doi.org/10.1038/nature24270

Singh, R. K., Pandey, R., & Babu, R. N. (2021). COVIDScreen: Explainable deep learning framework for differential diagnosis of COVID-19 using chest X-rays. Neural Computing and Applications, 33, 8871–8892. https://doi.org/10.1007/S00521-020-05636-6/FIGURES/9

Singh, A., Sengupta, S., & Lakshminarayanan, V. (2020). Explainable deep learning models in medical image analysis. Journal of Imaging, 6(6), 52. https://doi.org/10.3390/JIMAGING6060052

Smilkov, D., Thorat, N., Kim, B., Viégas, F., & Wattenberg, M. (2017). SmoothGrad: Removing noise by adding noise. arXiv:1706.03825

Tahir, B., Iqbal, S., Usman Ghani Khan, M., Saba, T., Mehmood, Z., Anjum, A., & Mahmood, T. (2019). Feature enhancement framework for brain tumor segmentation and classification. Microscopy Research and Technique, 82(6), 803–811.

Tariq, M., Iqbal, S., Ayesha, H., Abbas, I., Ahmad, K. T., & Niazi, M. F. K. (2021). Medical image based breast cancer diagnosis: State of the art and future directions. Expert Systems with Applications, 167, 114095.

Tilouche, S., Partovi Nia, V., & Bassetto, S. (2021). Parallel coordinate order for high-dimensional data. Statistical Analysis and Data Mining: The ASA Data Science Journal, 14(5), 501–515. https://doi.org/10.1002/SAM.11543

Tomsett, R., Preece, A., Braines, D., Cerutti, F., Chakraborty, S., Srivastava, M., …, & Kaplan, L. (2020). Rapid trust calibration through interpretable and uncertainty-aware AI. Patterns, 1(4), 100049. https://doi.org/10.1016/j.patter.2020.100049

Tramèr, F., Zhang, F., Juels, A., Reiter, M. K., & Ristenpart, T. (2016). Stealing machine learning models via prediction APIs. In 25th USENIX Security Symposium (USENIX Security 16) (pp. 601–618). https://arxiv.org/abs/1609.02943v2

Ustun, B., & Rudin, C. (2016). Supersparse linear integer models for optimized medical scoring systems. Machine Learning, 102, 349–391. https://doi.org/10.1007/s10994-015-5528-6

van der Maaten, L., & Hinton, G. (2008). Visualizing data using t-SNE. Journal of Machine Learning Research, 9(86), 2579–2605 (accessed October 19, 2023). http://jmlr.org/papers/v9/vandermaaten08a.html

van der Velden, B. H., Kuijf, H. J., Gilhuijs, K. G., & Viergever, M. A. (2022). Explainable artificial intelligence (XAI) in deep learning-based medical image analysis. Medical Image Analysis, 79, 102470. https://doi.org/10.1016/J.MEDIA.2022.102470

Wold, S., Esbensen, K., & Geladi, P. (1987). Principal component analysis. Chemometrics and Intelligent Laboratory Systems, 2(1–3), 37–52. https://doi.org/10.1016/0169-7439(87)80084-9

Yang, G., Ye, Q., & Xia, J. (2022). Unbox the black-box for the medical explainable AI via multi-modal and multi-centre data fusion: A mini-review, two showcases and beyond. Information Fusion, 77, 29–52.

Yousaf, K., Mehmood, Z., Saba, T., Rehman, A., Munshi, A. M., Alharbey, R., & Rashid, M. (2019). Mobile-health applications for the efficient delivery of health care facility to people with dementia (PwD) and support to their carers: A survey. BioMed Research International, 2019, 7151475.

Zhang, Y., Tiňo, P., Leonardis, A., & Tang, K. (2021). A survey on neural network interpretability. IEEE Transactions on Emerging Topics in Computational Intelligence, 5(5), 726–742. https://doi.org/10.1109/TETCI.2021.3100641

Chapter 5

Automatic Detection of Leukemia through Explainable AI-Based Machine Learning Approaches: Directional Review

Rida Arif[1], Shahzad Akbar[1], Sahar Gull[1], Qurat Ul Ain[1], and Noor Ayesha[2]

[1]Riphah College of Computing, Riphah International University, Faisalabad Campus, Faisalabad, Pakistan

[2]Center of Excellence in Cyber Security (CYBEX), Prince Sultan University Riyadh, Kingdom of Saudi Arabia

5.1 Introduction

Blood is an essential component of human body that performs various important functions in the body like the circulation of oxygen, minerals, and carbon dioxide to sustain metabolism. Blood has three vital components: white blood cells (WBCs), red blood cells (RBCs), and platelets (Supardi, Mashor, Harun, Bakri, & Hassan, 2012). The primary function of WBCs or leukocytes is to fight against disease and infection, RBCs or erythrocytes transport oxygen from the lungs to the

DOI: 10.1201/9781032626345-5

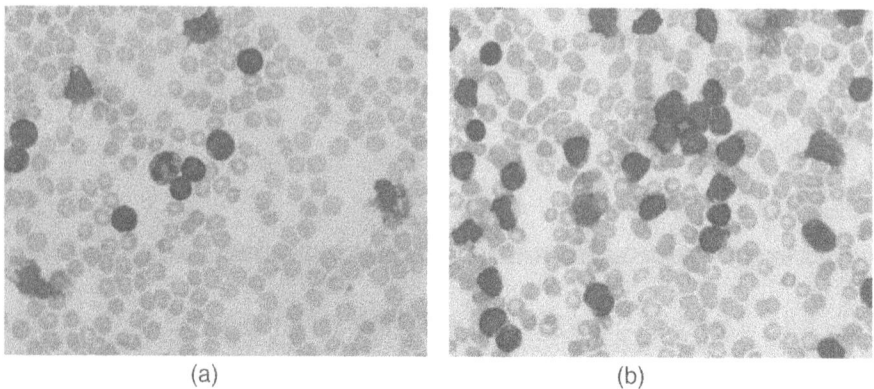

(a)   (b)

Figure 5.1   Leukemia-affected blood cells.

rest of the body, and platelets or thrombocytes help in the formation of blood clots and stop bleeding (Felman, 2024). A microliter of blood includes the WBC count normally between 3,700 and 10,500, the RBCs range between 4.0 and 5.2 million in women and 4.5 and 6.2 million in men, and the platelets range between 150,000 and 400,000 (Howard, 2013).

The human body creates billions of new blood cells every day, the bulk being red blood cells. Blood cancer is also called hematologic cancer. Blood cancer is shown to be very threatening if not treated appropriately. The bone marrow produces the vast bulk of blood cells, thus blood cancer begins there (Howard, 2013). Leukemia is a cancer of WBCs, which occurs when the malignant WBCs start growing uncontrollably, as shown in Figure 5.1. The malignant WBCs are also called blast cells, whose irregular production in the bone marrow causes leukemia. Blood cancer diminishes the body's immune system (Sadler, 2015). In the UK, about 9,900 new cases are reported every year (Chen et al., 2021). Leukemia is divided into two classes: (1) acute leukemia and (2) chronic leukemia. Acute and chronic leukemia are further classified into four different classes based on the cell type, namely, acute lymphocytic leukemia (ALL), acute myeloid leukemia (AML), chronic myeloid leukemia (CML), and chronic lymphocytic leukemia (CLL).

5.1.1 Acute Lymphocytic Leukemia

The keyword "acute" in the context of ALL refers to how quickly the disease progresses and produces immature cells. In ALL, immature blast cells (irregular WBCs) develop repeatedly and worsen the condition of the patient if not treated early (Kessenbrock, Plaks, & Werb, 2010). Therefore, these blasts function improperly; this type of blood cancer is most common in kids between the ages of 2 and 10. People with ALL commonly reveal symptoms of temperature, exhaustion, bleeding, leg discomfort, headaches, nausea, etc. ALL is that type of leukemia in which an enormous number of lymphocytes are produced in the bone marrow. This rapid production of lymphocytes badly affects the working of the bone marrow which causes cancer (Abdeldaim, Sahlol, Elhoseny, & Hassanien, 2018).

5.1.2 Acute Myeloid Leukemia

It is acute leukemia kind that is produced by an excess of WBCs in the bone marrow. This type of cancer can also produce immature RBCs and platelets. However, AML is mostly found in adults, it occurs due to abnormal myeloblasts and some bad effects on bone marrow. A patient having this type of cancer may encounter some symptoms like breathing difficulties and bleeding (Oostindjer et al., 2014).

5.1.3 Chronic Lymphocytic Leukemia

In CLL, the WBCs do not work properly and their count increases. This type of cancer is most common in adults. CLL symptoms include weight loss, fever, fatigue, and weakness (Oostindjer et al., 2014).

5.1.4 Chronic Myeloid Leukemia

CML is a slow-spreading cancer type normally found in middle-aged adults, as shown in Figure 5.2. Normally, the symptoms of CML include anemia, night sweats, and loss of weight. CML develops when the bone marrow produces genetically modified stem cells. This type of cancer is less severe as compared to acute leukemia (Oostindjer et al., 2014).

In the fight against foreign invaders, each type of WBCs has a distinct defensive role to play. However, the neutrophil is a sort of WBC that protects the body from germs and fungus. When an infection attacks, it is the first line of defense (Patil, Patil, & Birajdar, 2021). By attacking and destroying parasites and cancer cells, the eosinophil aids allergic reactions. Furthermore, monocytes enter cells to break down the body's damaged tissues (Patil et al., 2021). When pathogenic organisms penetrate your blood, basophils, which are tiny cells, seem to ring an alarm. They generate molecules that help to regulate the body's immune response,

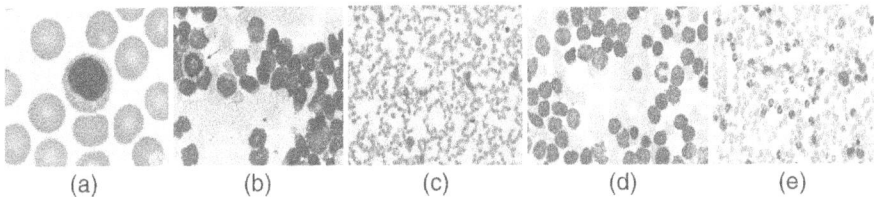

Figure 5.2   Images of leukemia subtypes: (a) Healthy, (b) ALL, (c) AML, (d) CLL, and (e) CML.

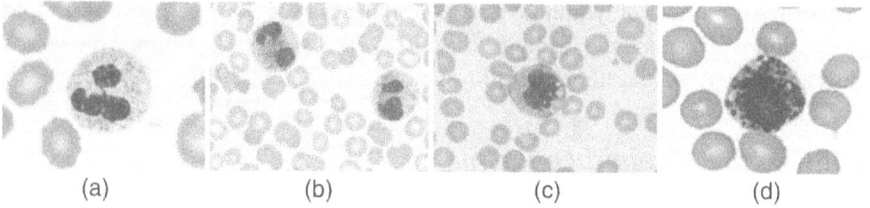

Figure 5.3 Leukocyte types: (a) neutrophil, (b) eosinophil, (c) monocyte, and (d) basophil.

such as histamine, which is an allergic illness. To fight against germs, viruses, and other potentially harmful attackers, lymphocytes produce antibodies (Anwar et al., 2020). These types of WBCs are depicted in Figure 5.3.

5.1.5 Leukemia Diagnosis

The early-stage identification of leukemia from bloodstain images is essential for the patient's recovery. Therefore, hematologists and pathologists typically performed manual detection of leukemia, by observing blood smear images. However, manual methods for blast cell identification require skilled pathologists. These manual methods are time-consuming and provide inaccurate results (Bibi, Sikandar, Ud Din, Almogren, & Ali, 2020). In this chapter, various leukemia diagnosis techniques have been reported, which especially concentrate on the implementation of modern imaging and artificial intelligence (AI) techniques. In the bone marrow, an unusual increase of WBCs is the cause of leukemia. Consequently, a bone marrow needle biopsy may be suggested by the pathologist to verify the kind of leukemia. Some advanced leukemia diagnosis methods and treatments are chemotherapy, radiation therapy, immunophenotyping, etc. Treatment for leukemia is determined by the kind and stage of the disease. There are some treatments to fight against leukemia.

5.1.5.1 Chemotherapy

Chemotherapy is a drug treatment that employs the use of chemicals to kill rapidly multiplying cells in the body. However, these medications can be taken as pills or injected directly into the bloodstream. Chemotherapy is mostly used to medicate cancer because the cancer cells grow rapidly and multiply more speedily than other cells in the body (Bibi et al., 2020).

5.1.5.2 Radiation Therapy

Radiation therapy, also called radiotherapy, uses invisible high-energy beams to eliminate cancerous cells which also inhibit the cancer cells from proliferating and replicating. This radiation is applied to the collection of cancer cells in your body or may be given to the whole body. Moreover, radiation therapy of the entire body is generally a critical step before a bone marrow transplant. This therapy can be applied alone or with chemotherapy, to treat leukemia (Bibi et al., 2020).

5.1.5.3 Immunophenotyping

Immunophenotyping is a test that is used to identify cells, which is based on the marker or antigen on the exterior of the cells. This technique is useful to identify leukemia and the type of leukemia. Immunophenotyping has also been used to distinguish cells from various kinds of groups based on the markers (Das & Dutta, 2020).

5.1.6 Leukemia Imaging Datasets

The publicly available datasets associated with leukemia are analyzed in this section. To train and test the model, several researchers generally utilize and access these publicly available datasets which can be easily downloaded from the repository. These datasets help to test and train a model for the leukemia diagnostic process, which is summarized in this section.

5.1.6.1 ALL-IDB1 Dataset

The ALL-IDB imaging database is a freely available ALL dataset that can be easily downloaded from ALL-IDB dataset (2022) and is depicted in Figure 5.4. The specimens in the ALL-IDB dataset are acquired from M. Tettamanti Research Center, Monza, Italy. This dataset is divided into two categories: ALL-IDB1 and ALL-IDB2, both are focused on image segmentation and classification. However, this dataset consists of healthy and leukemia patients' blood samples. ALL-IDB1 dataset

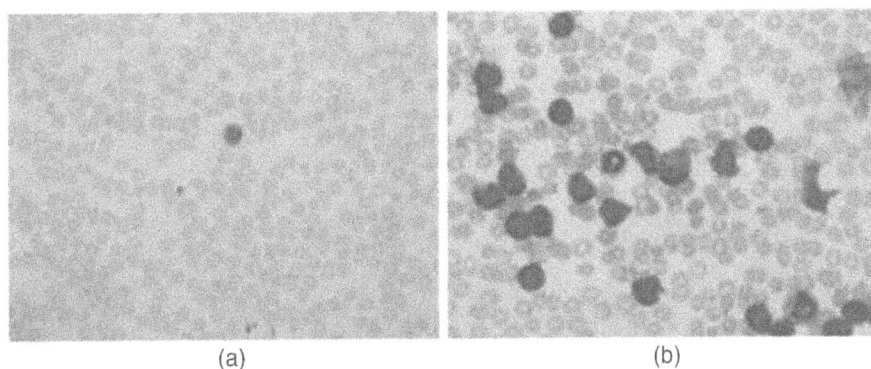

(a)   (b)

Figure 5.4 **ALL_IDB1 dataset. (a) Healthy image. (b) ALL-affected image.**

includes a total of 108 images that are in RGB, of which 49 are malignant images and the remaining 59 are normal images. Images in the ALL-IDB dataset are in JPG format along with 24 bits color depth which was preserved in September 2005. Moreover, it holds about 39,000 blood components, in which leukemia has been detected by the hematologist. The first 33 images have a resolution of $1,712 \times 1,368$, while the rest of the images have $2,592 \times 1,944$ resolution. The images were captured at various microscope magnifications varying between 300 and 500 with hue and brightness differences. This dataset is seized for testing the segmentation capacity and the accuracy of the classification system (Anwar et al., 2020).

5.1.6.2 ALL-IDB2 Dataset

The ALL-IDB2 dataset contains the cropped area of interest images of normal and blast cells. This dataset is made up of 260 images of which 130 are normal images and the remaining 130 are leukemia-affected images. Besides, all the images are in TIF format that contains 257×257 resolution. It is a freely available dataset shown in Figure 5.5. Its purpose is to evaluate the classification system's performance (Anwar et al., 2020).

5.1.6.3 American Society of Hematology (ASH) Image Bank

ASH image bank (ASH Image Bank, 2021) is an open-source imaging database. This dataset consists of a complete library of images associated with a vast range of hematological topics which is downloaded from. This newly rebuilt dataset was launched in March 2016 and includes 2,100 images that are shown in Figure 5.6.

The use of an automated system is always necessary to diagnose leukemia properly. The study's primary goal is to provide a review of the attainment of researchers to summarize the previous finding for the identification and classification of leukemia. However, various machine learning (ML) and deep learning (DL) approaches

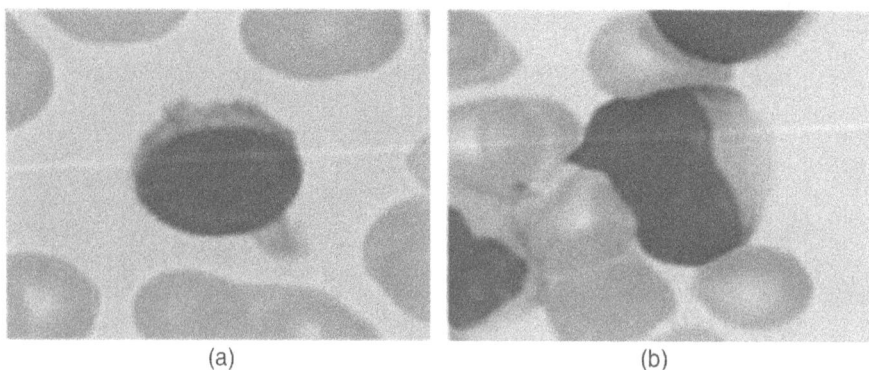

(a)   (b)

Figure 5.5   ALL_IDB2 dataset. (a) Healthy image. (b) ALL-affected image.

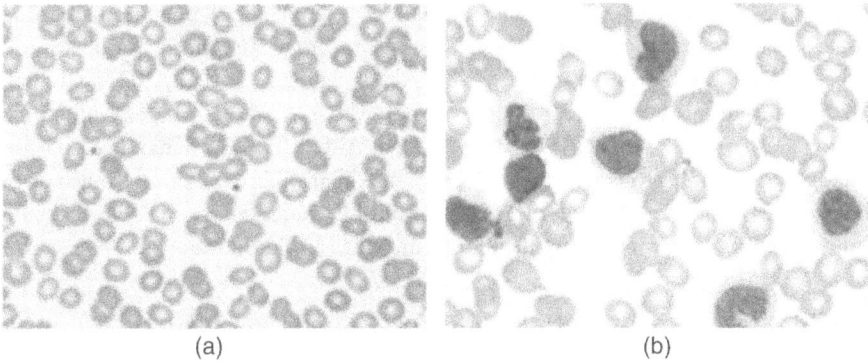

Figure 5.6   ASH Image Bank dataset. (a) Healthy image. (b) ALL-affected image.

and techniques have been used in past research to identify leukemia, which is discussed below.

The remaining sections of this chapter are organized as follows: Section 5.2 describes a comprehensive review of the literature. Section 5.3 describes a detailed discussion of the review and presents the study findings and gaps. Finally, Section 5.4 concludes the chapter.

5.2 Literature Review

In this section, several algorithms for leukemia detection are briefly discussed. In the subsequent section, recently ML and DL articles have been compiled to diagnose leukemia using microscopic images.

5.2.1 AI

AI is a branch of computer system. It is concerned with the creation of computer algorithms to mimic the way that human beings learn to predict more accurate results. AI usually focuses on creating smart machines that can perform tasks that normally require human intelligence (Mughal, Muhammad, Sharif, Rehman, & Saba, 2018). Generally, AI works on the large, labeled training dataset, analyzing the data patterns and utilizing these patterns for future prediction. The advanced AI techniques are ML and DL. AI is rapidly becoming a seamless part of our everyday life. Moreover, there are ongoing initiatives in the realms of medical science and healthcare to incorporate advancements in AI for immediate medical diagnosis and care (Larabi-Marie-Sainte, Aburahmah, Almohaini, & Saba, 2019).

The detection and diagnosis of retinal diseases such as hypertensive retinopathy (Akbar, Hassan, Akram, Yasin, & Basit, 2017), papilledema (Saba, Akbar, Kolivand, & Ali Bahaj, 2021), brain tumor (Gull, Akbar, & Safdar, 2021), glaucoma (Akbar, Hassan, Shoukat, Alyami, & Bahaj, 2022; Shoukat, Akbar, Hassan, Rehman, & Ayesha, 2021), melanoma (Safdar, Akbar, & Gull, 2021), leukemia (Ain, Akbar, Gull,

Hussain, & Ayesha, 2022; Ain, Akbar, Hassan, & Naaqvi, 2022), pneumonia (Urooj, Akbar, Hassan, Firdous, & Bashir, 2022), skin cancer (Khan, Sharif, Raza, Anjum, Saba, & Shad, 2022), breast cancer (Abid, Akbar, Hassan, & Gull, 2022; Mughal, Sharif, Muhammad, & Saba, 2018), liver (Abid, Akbar, Abid, Hassan, & Gull, 2023; Naaqvi, Akbar, Hassan, & Ain, 2022; Naaqvi, Akbar, Hassan, Khalid, & Bashir, 2022), and central serous retinopathy (Hassan, Akbar, Rehman, Saba, Kolivand, & Bahaj, 2021) can be performed through ML and DL methodologies using OCT and fundus images (Muhsin, Rehman, Altameem, Saba, & Uddin, 2014).

5.2.1.1 Conventional ML-based Leukemia Detection

ML is a branch of AI. It means "machine to learn" and the machine learns by its experience and mistakes. ML is subcategorized into supervised learning, unsupervised learning, and reinforcement learning (Supardi et al., 2012). The machine uses labeled datasets in supervised learning. However, these datasets are designed to supervise the programs and algorithms to classify the data and help predict outcomes precisely. The training stage keeps repeated until the model contains an absolute degree of accuracy. The various examples of supervised learning are KNN, decision tree, random forest, logistic regression, etc. Following that, in unsupervised learning, ML algorithms used unlabeled datasets to analyze and cluster the data. These algorithms work on their own to locate the hidden patterns, without human involvement. The Apriori algorithm and K-means are examples of unsupervised learning. Similarly, reinforcement learning is a type of ML that consists of taking a sequence of decisions to gain maximum reward. Normally, it is concerned with how software agents should take action in a scenario and learn with trial-and-error experimentation (Sadler, 2015). An example of reinforcement learning is Markov decision process. Figure 5.7 depicts a ML model to classify leukemia.

This section provides a complete contemplation based on the recent study that aims to engage the conventional methods in blood cancer. Various tedious methods are still used to diagnose blood cancer.

Abdeldaim et al. (2018) coined a system to recognize the ALL from the blood-stain images. WBCs were segmented using the suggested approach, which included RGB to CMYK color conversion, histogram equalization, and the Zack algorithm. Some features including texture, color, and shape were removed. To reduce the gap between feature values, three normalization techniques (min–max, gray-scaling,

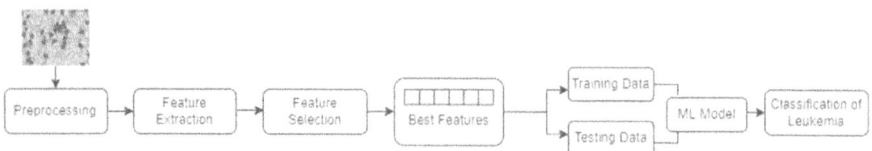

Figure 5.7 Machine learning model of leukemia classification.

and *z*-score) were applied. Finally, various classifiers were used for validation. ALL-IDB2 dataset was used having 260 images and achieved 96.01% classification correctness by the KNN classifier.

Kumar, Mishra, and Asthana (2018) presented an automatic image-based algorithm for the identification of acute leukemia. Manually detecting cancer was tedious and time-consuming while computerized methods are concise and provide accurate clinical results. However, the proposed algorithm consists of various steps like image preprocessing for noise removal in microscopic images, image segmentation, extraction of features, and then image classification. The suggested system was tested with closest neighbor (KNN) and naive Bayes classifiers on 60 samples from multiple datasets resulting in an accuracy of 92.8%.

Dasariraju, Huo, and McCalla (2020) presented a ML method to recognize and segment the abnormal WBCs to diagnose the AML from the images. Dataset was obtained from the repository of the Cancer Imaging Archive, which is a publicly available database for cancer research. Conversion of the image into LAB format, multi-Otsu's thresholding, and morphological dilation were applied to attain nucleus and cytoplasm for the segmentation process. A total of 16 features were extracted, and 2 new features, nucleus and cytoplasm ratio (N:C ratio), were also extracted with Gini importance. Finally, for the classification of immature leukocytes, a random forest classifier was applied that yielded accuracy of 92.99%.

Das and Dutta (2020) proposed a Gini index–based fuzzy naive Bayes (GFNB) classifier for automatic detection of leukemia. The input multi-cell blood-stained images were preprocessed for the accurate classification of leukemia. The preprocessed images were segmented through the updating thresholding approach that extracts texture features. GFNB classifier recognizes blasting images and also counts blast cells for identifying the presence of leukemia. A publicly accessible dataset named ALL-IDB1 was utilized that contains 108 images and achieved 95% accuracy.

Bodzas, Kodytek, and Zidek (2020) presented a ML framework to automatically diagnose the ALL from microscopic blood smear images. The proposed system presents an extensive preprocessing method that depends on the arithmetic operation to appreciate the contrast of the image. Furthermore, to remove the surrounding artifacts of the blood, a three-phase filtration algorithm was implemented. A total of 16 features, of which 9 had morphological characteristics, while the other 7 had statistical characteristics, were extracted. Finally, two classifiers, SVM and ANN, were applied for the classification purpose. The ANN achieved the best results of 100% and 97.52% sensitivity and accuracy, respectively. A dataset of 31 blood samples was used, sponsored by the Department of Haemato-oncology at the University Hospital Ostrava.

Ranjitha and Duth (2021) proposed architecture to segment the WBCs from the blood images. The blood images were initially preprocessed using RGB color space. Following that, the *K*-means categorization algorithm was applied for image segmentation. Finally, some features such as average, minimum, and maximum intensity were extracted. Dataset was acquired from the Kaggle repository and yielded 90% accuracy.

Ramya and Lakshmi (2022) presented a fractional black widow-based neural network (FBW-NN) to diagnose the AML from the blood images. First, in the preprocessing stage, a median filter was utilized to remove the noise. Then, adaptive fuzzy entropy (AFE) was carried out for segmentation, and statistical and image-level features were extricated. Moreover, FBW-NN was applied for the classification of AML. For the experimentation, two AML datasets, AML morphology and CPTAC dataset, were used. The presented network was implemented in MATLAB and achieved 95.56% accuracy.

Table 5.1 summarizes the leukemia detection techniques and algorithms that are arranged in ascending order. This table gives readers a quick overview of leukemia detection technology.

Table 5.1   Previous Studies for Leukemia Detection through Conventional ML

Author(s)	Area of Application	Technique(s)	Classifier(s)	Dataset(s)	Accuracy (%)
Abdeldaim et al., 2018	ALL	Zack algorithm	*K*-NN	ALL-IDB2	96.01%
Kumar et al., 2018	Acute leukemia	*K*-means	*K*-NN and naive Bayes	Dr. RML Awadh Hospital, Lucknow	92.8%
Dasariraju et al., 2020	Identify the AML	LAB format, multi-Otsu's thresholding, and morphological dilation	Random forest	The Cancer Imaging Archive	92.99%.
Das et al., 2020	Leukemia classification	Thresholding	GFNB classifier	ALL-IDBI	95.91%
Bodzas et al., 2020	ALL	Three-phase filtration algorithm	SVM and ANN	Department of Haemato-oncology at University Hospital Ostrava	96.72% & 97.52%
Ranjitha et al., 2021	WBCs classification	*k*-Means	*k*-Means algorithm	Kaggle repository	90%
Ramya et al., 2022	AML	Adaptive fuzzy entropy (AFE)	Fractional black widow-based Neural Network (FBW-NN)	AML morphology and CPTAC dataset	95.56%

5.2.2 Leukemia Detection Using Artificial Neural Network (ANN)

An ANN is a part of supervised learning that resembles the human brain, which is associated with plenty of neurons. Neurons are message-carrier that are human-inspired systems and they try to work like the human brain. In addition, ANN consists of input, output, and hidden layers which are connected with weighted connections (Khan, Sajjad, Hussain, Ullah, & Imran, 2020). The value (weight) of a connection is adjusted to learn a neural network. The based-on weights output layer produced results. A neural network contains training and testing phases, the training phase is used for learning of network while the testing phase is used to calculate the correctness of the classifier. Many studies are proposed in this literature that used ANN to diagnose leukemia and its subtypes from the blood smear image.

5.2.2.1 DL

DL is a ML subclass that works with neural networks. These neural networks are dependent on the formation of the human brain and attempt to mimic the human brain. In the most recent survey, DL algorithmic programs are applied in the domain of voice recognition (Sabzi Shahrebabaki, Imran, Olfati, & Svendsen, 2019), natural language processing (Kastrati, Imran, & Yayilgan, 2019), and image recognition (Altaf, Islam, Akhtar, & Janjua, 2019) without human interference. Typically, DL is used where feature extraction is not performed by human engineers but discovered through a learning process. DL demonstrated satisfactory performance to design an end-to-end network using CNN (Sajjad, Zahir, Ullah, Akhtar, & Muhammad, 2020). Many people prefer to employ DL techniques, particularly convolutional networks, to analyze the results. To examine a significant amount of data, DL methods are acceptable where human-like acumen is required. Furthermore, quality knowledge is necessary to extricate the best features from the vast data (Haskins, Kruger, & Yan, 2020). In medical imaging, convolutional neural networks (CNNs) are commonly employed (Lundervold & Lundervold, 2019).

5.2.2.2 CNN

The CNN or ConVNet is a framework of DL, mostly applied to examine visual imagery (Latif et al., 2019). Convolutional layers, pooling, and a fully connected layer all are part of the CNN paradigm. As with any other ANN, gradient descent and backpropagation are used to train it. At the output nodes, a SoftMax function is used to classify leukemia (Khan et al., 2020).

Rehman et al. (2018) coined a sober method to identify acute lymphoblastic leukemia (ALL) including its subtypes. Initially, separation of lymphoblast from the bone marrow images through thresholding approach. AlexNet was specifically used for the classification. For the evaluation, a total of 330 images were used. The obtained outcomes were collated with further classifiers such as KNN, naive Bayes, and SVM. Exploratory results disclose that this technique achieved 97.78% accuracy.

Wang et al. (2018) presented a method PatternNet-fused ensemble of convolutional neural network (PECNN) for the detection and categorization of WBCs. The presented ensemble approach used PatternNet, which was based on fusing results of the multiple CNNs. For experimentation, several data values of 410 images were used, assembled from personal GitHub. This method yielded an accuracy of 99.37%. PECNN outperformed in the middle of noisy data.

Mohamed et al. (2018) presented an automated classification system of leukocytes and their subtypes. The proposed system started with the segmentation process that converts input blood smear images into RGB colors. Then different features, including morphological, texture, statical, and size ratio, were extracted. Finally, random forest classifer (RFC) was applied to classify the WBCs and their different types. A dataset of 105 blood images was used and achieved 94.3% of classification accuracy.

Jha and Dutta (2019) developed a hybrid method for identifying leukemia from images of bloodstains. In this model, blood smear images were preprocessed through resizing, and then Mutual Information (MI) was performed for the segmentation that integrates the active contour model and fuzzy C-means (FCM). Some statistical images were taken out and given to Chronological-Sine, Cosine-Algorithm (SCA) based on deep convolutional neural network for classifying leukemia. Blood slight pictures were contemplated from the (ALL-IDB2) database for the experimentation having an accuracy of 98.7%.

Kumar et al. (2020) exhibit a vigorous mechanism for classifying multiple myeloma (MM) and ALL using the SN-AM dataset. Multiple myeloma is a malignancy that collects the cancer prison (cells) in the bone (marrow) instead of delivering them in the blood circulation flow. This study proposed dense convolutional neural network (DCNN) framework, this model works on cell images; it preprocesses the image at the early stage and then the best features were extracted. A dataset of 424 images was used for experimentation. The proposed model yielded an overall accuracy of 97.2%.

Kasani et al. (Kasani, Park, & Jang, 2020) suggested a DL-aggregated model that was capable of classifying ALL at the early stage. Different data intensification techniques, for instance, vertical flips, horizontal, contrast adjustment, and brightness correction, were applied to expand the dataset. Implementation of this model consists of transfer learning, hyper-parameter, and ensemble techniques to extract the more invidious feature from a dataset. After the dataset preprocessing, various professional CNN architectures were employed such as inception V3, AlexNet, DenseNet201, VGGNet-16, VGGNet19, Xception, MobileNet, ShuffleNet, and two NASNet models. The proposed ensemble model yielded 96.58% overall accuracy, then the individual architecture. This paper experimentally verified that NASNet large and VGG19 are the most effective models for all learners.

Anwar et al. (2020) suggested a CNN-based model for the early detection of ALL. The proposed CNN architecture consists of a total of ten layers. The dataset was achieved from the ALL-IDB1 and ALL- IDB2, a total of 368 uncleansed blood images, which had previously been classified as blast or non-blast cells. After performing several data expansion techniques (increase the dataset), the dataset size now contains 736 total images for a healthier training process and reduced overtraining. This CNN model eliminated any segmentation or feature extraction techniques, and it works efficiently on unprocessed data having 99.5% overall accuracy. This model will be helpful for pathologists in diagnosing ALL.

Bibi et al. (2020) suggested a framework to identify leukemia quickly and efficiently, consisting of the Internet of Medical Things (IoMT). To identify leukemia and its subtypes, the model used dense convolutional neural network (DenseNet-121) and residual convolutional neural network (ResNet-34). The designed IoMT system includes medical gadgets linked to network components with the support of cloud computing. A blood smear image was uploaded on the leukemia cloud and applied data augmentation techniques, DenseNet-121 and ResNet-34, that operate on many images. After identification, the results were sent to healthcare which could save the patient and physician time. ASH image bank and ALL-IDB datasets were used for the evaluation. The proposed framework achieved 99.56% and 99.91% average accuracy for ResNet-34 and DenseNet-121, respectively.

Sahlol, Kollmannsberger, and Ewees (2020) presented a hybrid approach to diagnosing ALL. A powerful CNN architecture named VGGNet was employed for feature extraction from WBCs and then extracted features were filtered using the statistically enhanced salp swarm algorithm (SESSA). SESSA extracts only applicable features and removes noisy and irrelevant features. The proposed approach achieves high accuracy and reduces complexity as well. The SESSA selected only 1 K from 25 K feature numbers while improving the performance simultaneously. ALL-IDB2 and C-NMC datasets were used for the evaluation. The proposed models achieved 96.11% and 87.9% classification accuracy, respectively.

Sakthiraj (2021) presented an IoMT-based hybrid convolutional neural network with Interactive Autodidactic nSchool (HCNN-IAS) technique. However, to reduce noise, overfitting, and to enlarge the datasets, various data transformation approaches were employed. Following that, the IAS method was used to extract features, fuse them, and classify them. First, local and global features were extricated from the leukemia datasets. Then, to fuse the extracted features, a self-attention strategy was used. Finally, using the SoftMax layer of HCNN, the classification of leukemia and its subgroups was completed. The ASH image bank dataset was used for the experimentation and achieved 99% classification accuracy.

Khandekar, Shastry, Jaishankar, Faust, and Sampathila (2021) proposed a You Only Look Once (YOLOv4) object detection algorithm to help to diagnose the ALL. YOLOv4 is a CNN-based architecture that contains four main parts: input, neckbone, neck, and dense prediction. Experimentation was carried out using two datasets: ALL-IDB1 having 108 images and C_NMC_2019 containing 10,661 images. The presented framework obtained 96.06% and 98.7% classification accuracy for ALL-IDB1 and C_NMC_2019 datasets, respectively.

Boldú, Merino, Acevedo, Molina, and Rodellar (2021) suggested a CNN-based fine-tuning model named ALNet to diagnose acute leukemia and its subtypes using blood images. This technique is based on two modules: the first module is used to differentiate the abnormal promyelocytes from other mononuclear blood cell images based on a VGG16. The second module consists of VGG19 to diagnose myeloid blasts and B-lymphoblasts. A total of 731 blood images were acquired from CellaVision DM96. The proposed model achieved 94.2% accuracy for leukemia detection and 89.5% accuracy for subtypes of leukemia.

Amin et al. (2021) proposed an integrated model for the classification of WBCs. First, RGB images were converted into HSV to find the best color space. Then, global thresholding was applied for the segmentation process. Different CNN models were applied to extricate the deep features and for classification. Then, depending on the best scores, a non-dominated sorting genetic algorithm (NSGA) was applied to select the best feature. ALL-IDB1, ALL-IDB2, and LISC datasets were used for experimentation. ALL-IDB1 dataset achieved higher accuracy of 0.9907 using the decision tree (DT) classifier.

Ullah et al. (2021) developed a CNN-based attention model named efficient channel attention (ECA) to classify ALL and healthy images. In the preprocessing phase, input images were resized, and extracted the RGB color values. Then, various data augmentation approaches were applied to increase the dataset size. For the classification, a CNN model named VGG16 based on ECA was applied. The proposed model used C-NMC 2019 dataset that contain 10,661 cell images and yielded 91.1% ALL and healthy cell classification accuracy.

Shaheen et al. (2021) presented an Alex-Net-based identification framework for recognizing AML, using microscopic bloodstain images. Moreover, AlexNet's performance was compared to that of a LeNet-5-based model. First, in the preprocessing phase, the dataset was resized into a 256×256 resolution. Then, the architecture of AlexNet was applied, which consists of five convolutional layers, three maximum pooling, and three FC layers. The experimentation was performed on 4,000 blood samples, provided by the tertiary care hospital of Peshawar, Pakistan. Experimentation result shows that AlexNet yielded 98.58% classification accuracy.

Abas, Abdulazeez, and Zeebaree (2022) presented a CAD3 framework that consists of three models. The first model utilized YOLOv2 layers for the WBCs detection. After the detection of WBCs, the second model was applied that contained a CNN model for the WBCs classification. The suggested CNN model consists of three convolutional layers, three max-pooling layers, and two fully connected layers. Lastly, another CNN model was applied for the WBCs visualization which is the third model of CAD3. ALL-IDB1 and BCCD dataset was utilized which achieved 94.3% leukocytes classification accuracy.

Elhassan, Rahim, Swee, Hashim, and Aljurf (2022) developed a hybrid feature extrication model to extract the WBCs to diagnose the AML from the blood images. In the first stage, a CMYK-moment localization technique was applied to extricate the region of interest (ROI). Then, with the help of feature fusion, 2D convolutional layers were utilized to extricate the features. Different classifiers were applied to measure the accuracy. By using two datasets, AML cytomorphology and CellaVision DM96, the SVM classifier achieved the best accuracies of 97.57% and 96.41%, respectively.

Ansari, Navin, Sangar, Gharamaleki, and Danishvar (2023) presented a customized DL-based model to diagnose ALL and AML using monocytes and lymphocytes images. A private dataset collected from 44 patients, including 184 ALL images and 469 images of AML, was used. The images were resized into 224×224 and converted to grayscale in preprocessing phase. Besides, the dataset was augmented employing various data transformation approaches. The customized DL model comprised of different CNN layers was utilized to classify acute leukemia. The designed framework yielded 99% accuracy using private dataset.

Manescu et al. (2023) designed a DL-based model named MILLIE to classify acute promyelocytic leukemia (APL), normal, and AML images from peripheral blood smears. Two publicly accessible benchmarks named ALL-IDB1 and ASH datasets were used containing 449 images. Initially, images were transformed into HSV and Otsu's thresholding was applied for segmentation. The designed MILLIE model containing different CNN layers was used to classify the normal, APL, and AML images and obtained AUC of (0.94 ± 0.04).

Ahmad et al. (2023) proposed a customized DL model to classify WBC subtypes from blood images. A publicly available dataset having 5,000 images was used for leukocytes categorization. In the preprocessing step, enhancement, resize, and augmentation were performed. Two CNN models DenseNet201 and DarkNet53 were employed for feature extraction. The fused features were selected through quantum inspired evolutionary algorithm (QIEA). After that, neural network was selected for classification purposes. The presented model yielded highest accuracy of 99.8%, 0.997 of precision, F1 score of 0.998, 0.995 of sensitivity, and 0.998 of sensitivity.

5.3 Discussion

After the detailed study of 44 different relevant articles, Section 5.2 glanced at various leukemia detection techniques and algorithms. Therefore, this section demonstrates a comparative analysis of several ML and DL algorithms to identify leukemia. There were essentially two kinds of this approach: (a) conventional ML-based leukemia detection and (b) DL-based leukemia detection. The key information of pertinent publications about both categories has been illustrated in Tables 5.1 and 5.2. This information includes the author's name, area of application, segmentation techniques, classifiers, datasets name, and results. Most of the studies available in this

Table 5.2   Previous Studies for Leukemia Detection through DL

Authors	Area of Application	Techniques	Datasets	Results
Rehman et al. (2018)	ALL	Threshold method, AlexNet	Amreek Clinical Laboratory Swat KP Pakistan	97.78% of classification accuracy
Wang et al. (2018)	WBCs classification	PECNN	GitHub	99.37% accuracy
Mohamed et al. (2018)	WBCs classification	Random forest classifier	Medical Image and Signal Processing Research Center (MISP)	94.3% classification accuracy
Jha and Dutta (2019)	ALL	SCA-based DL CNN model	ALL-IDB2	98.7% classification accuracy, 98% TPR, and 98% TNR
Kumar et al. (2020)	ALL and multiple myeloma (MM)	Optimized CNN model	SN-AM	97.25%, 100%, 93.97%, 95.19%, and 96.89% accuracy, precision, recall, specificity, and F1 score, respectively
Kasani et al. (2020)	ALL	CNN (Ensemble of NASNetLarge and VGG19)	SBI-Lab	96.58% overall accuracy, 96.94% precision, 91.75% recall, and 94.67% F1 score
Anwar et al. (2020)	ALL	CNN	ALL-IDB and ALL-IDB2	99.5% accuracy
Bibi et al. (2020)	Leukemia subtypes identification	ResNet-34 and DenseNet-121	ALL-IDB and ASH image bank	99.56% and 99.91% accuracy on ResNet-34 and DenseNet-121
Sahlol et al. (2020)	WBCs classification	VGGNET, SESSA, and SVM	ALL-IDB2 and C-NMC-2019	96.11% and 87.9% accuracy using both datasets

(Continued)

Table 5.2   (Continued)

Authors	Area of Application	Techniques	Datasets	Results
Sakthiraj (2021)	Leukemia and its subtypes	CNN	ASH image bank	99% accuracy
Khandekar et al. (2021)	ALL	CNN-based model	ALL-IDB1 & C_NMC_2019	96.06% accuracy and 98.7% accuracy
Boldu et al. (2021)	Leukemia and subtypes	CNN	CellaVision DM96	94.2% (leukemia) 89.5% (leukemia subtypes)
Amin et al. (2021)	WBCs classification	Decision tree	ALL-IDB1, ALL-IDB2, and LISC	0.9992% accuracy
Ullah et al. (2021)	ALL classification	VGG16 with Efficient Channel Attention (ECA)	C_NMC_ 2019	0.931%, 0.906%, 0.957%, 0.957%, and 0.930% accuracy, recall, specificity, precision, and F1 score, respectively, in fold-1 and 91.1% average accuracy with 0.013 STD
Shaheen et al. (2021)	AML	CNN (AlexNet)	Tertiary care hospital of Peshawar	98.58% accuracy and 87.4% precision
Abas et al. (2022)	WBCs classification	CNN model	ALL-IDB1 and BCCD	94.3% accuracy and 96% precision
Elhassan et al. (2022)	WBCs and AML	SVM	AML cytomorphology and CellaVision DM96	97.57% accuracy and 96.41% sensitivity
Ansari et al. (2023)	ALL and AML detection	Customized CNN model	Private dataset	99% accuracy

(Continued)

Table 5.2 (Continued)

Authors	Area of Application	Techniques	Datasets	Results
Manescu et al. (2023)	Classify normal, ALL, and AML images	CNN-based MILLIE model	ALL-IDB1 and ASH dataset	AUC of (0.94 ± 0.04)
Ahmad et al. (2023)	WBCs subtypes	Neural network	Publicly available dataset	99.8% accuracy, 0.997% precision, 0.998 F1 score, 0.995% and 0.998% sensitivity

literature are concerned with the automatic detection of leukemia, acute leukemia, WBCs identification, and AML. However, just a few studies are being used to diagnose the other types of leukemia using image processing approaches. About 42% of the work available in this study is related to diagnosing ALL. Among that, 29% of the available research is to identify WBCs and 18% of literature has been used to identify the presence of leukemia. Moreover, around 11% of data is also added in this literature to help diagnose AML from the blood microscopic images. Hence, the area-wise division of existing research. On the other hand, about 43% of the ALL-IDB dataset and 35% of other datasets like ASH image bank, C-NM-C-2019, etc. have been used in this study. Besides, it can be observed that about 22% of private datasets have been used, as depicted in Figure 5.8.

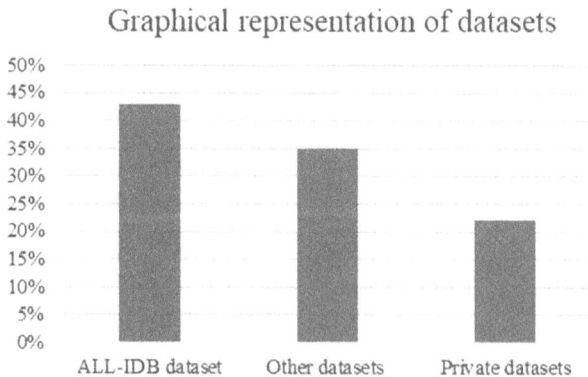

Figure 5.8 Graphical representation of used datasets.

The AI methods used in this chapter are premised on ML and DL perspectives to identify the presence of leukemia and different types of leukemia from bloodstain images. Supervised learning, unsupervised learning, and reinforcement learning are the three subcategories of ML. From a cautious inspection, it can be decided that the implementation of the ML technique has achieved good outcomes in terms of accuracy to identify leukemia. The DL technique, on the other hand, produces entirely advantageous results for detecting leukemia through image analysis. DL techniques yield superior results as compared to classical ML techniques on provided dataset. The aforementioned methods were proven to be faster, more efficient, and yielded the best accuracies and analysis as compared to manual methods.

For leukemia diagnosis, state-of-the-art approaches used a variety of classifiers. The distribution of various classifiers employed in the literature is depicted in Figure 5.9. However, in the ML category, about 24% of the SVM classifier has been employed for classification purposes. SVM classifier achieved a higher classification accuracy of 98.6% using a private dataset named HMC hospital. Furthermore, the application of DL approaches such as CNNs has been 42% used in this review. In DL, CNNs architecture named DenseNet-121 attained 99.91% classification accuracy by using ASH image bank and ALL-IDB datasets. To detect and classify leukemia and other blood cells, most of the researchers used two quite popular ALL datasets: ALL-IDB1 and ALL-IDB2 datasets. About 22% of ML/DL methods were trained and evaluated on private datasets which are not publicly available. Due to the lack of large, labeled datasets, traditional DL models are ineffectual to attain marvelous performance. This raises serious

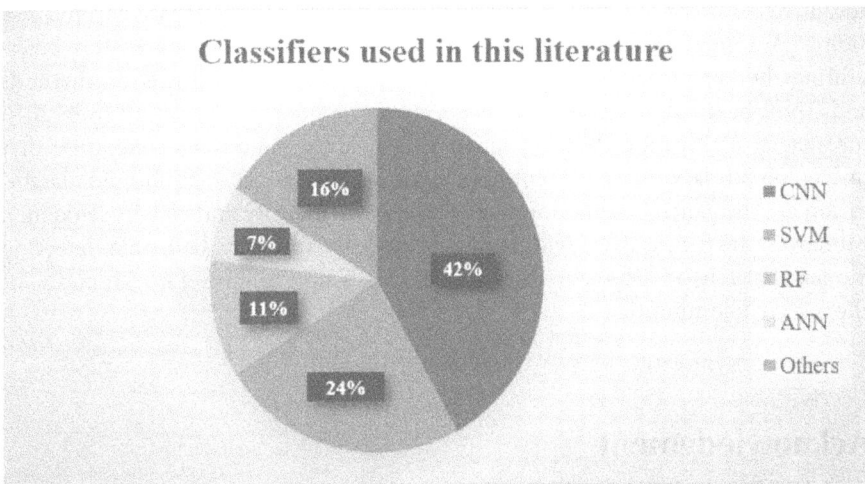

Figure 5.9 Various classifiers used in this study or comparison of classifiers.

concerns about their sincerity and authenticity. As a result, to train and test DL models, the research team should have access to more public datasets. This action will empower the research community to use the datasets freely and standardize the models for the detection of leukemia.

5.4 Conclusion

Generally, leukemia was manually examined by microscopic images of blood with the help of experienced hematologists and oncologists. However, this manual approach is tedious and error-prone. With technological advancements, leukemia may now be detected automatically through numerous AI models. Hence, the most recent technology depends on AI-based models, such as ML and DL. These methods are used to produce precise detection models that are developed and evaluated on legacy databases. After the training and testing phase, the researchers and scientists employ these models to automatically detect and classify leukemia. In recent years, these AI-based models are used in various economically available products and are becoming more precise and authentic.

A detailed state-of-the-art review has been offered in this literature to detect leukemia using AI algorithms and techniques. This chapter presents multiple segmenting, feature extraction, and classification techniques to detect leukemia from bloodstain images efficiently. In this study, DL methods outperformed ML methods. A CNN-based DenseNet-121 algorithm introduced by Bibi et al. (2020) depicts promising performance with 99.91% classification accuracy. However, there are many studies to detect ALL and AML, but only a very few are for chronic detection. Therefore, there is a scope for researchers to develop automated systems to aid hematologists to recognize and segregate chronic leukemia. Automatic methods to analyze the bloodstain images as well as determining the type of leukemia took a drive after 2010. The clustering methods and ANN-based algorithms have also been noticed during the period from 2016 for image classification. We concluded after reading the different literature that microscopic image enhancement, segmentation, feature extraction, and classification are the general methodology that is used to identify and classify leukemia. Moreover, the future scope will be to develop fully accessible leukemia-detecting models that rely on DL techniques that are easily accessible and user-friendly for the research community.

Acknowledgment

This work was supported by the Riphah Artificial Intelligence Research (RAIR) Lab, Riphah International University, Faisalabad Campus, Pakistan.

References

Abas, S. M., Abdulazeez, A. M., & Zeebaree, D. Q. (2022). A YOLO and convolutional neural network for the detection and classification of leukocytes in leukemia. *Indonesian Journal of Electrical Engineering Computer Science*, 25(1), 200–213.

Abdeldaim, A. M., Sahlol, A. T., Elhoseny, M., & Hassanien, A. E. (2018). Computer-aided acute lymphoblastic leukemia diagnosis system based on image analysis. In *Advances in Soft Computing and Machine Learning in Image Processing* (pp. 131–147). Springer.

Abid, M., Akbar, S., Abid, S., Hassan, S. A., & Gull, S. (2023, February). Detection of lungs cancer through computed tomographic images using deep learning. In *2023 4th International Conference on Advancements in Computational Sciences (ICACS)* (pp. 1–6). IEEE.

Abid, S., Akbar, S., Hassan, S. A., & Gull, S. (2022, October). Automatic detection of breast cancer through mammogram images. In *2022 International Conference on IT and Industrial Technologies (ICIT)* (pp. 1–7). IEEE.

Ahmad, R., Awais, M., Kausar, N., Tariq, U., Cha, J.-H., & Balili, J. (2023). Leukocytes classification for leukemia detection using quantum inspired deep feature selection. *Cancers*, 15(9), 2507.

Ain, Q. U., Akbar, S., Gull, S., Hussain, M., & Ayesha, N. (2022). Leukemia detection using machine and deep learning through microscopic images: A review. In Saba, T., Rehman, A., Roy, S. (Eds.), *Prognostic Models in Healthcare: AI and Statistical Approaches* (pp. 261–291). Springer, Singapore.

Ain, Q. U., Akbar, S., Hassan, S. A., & Naavi, Z. (2022, May). Diagnosis of leukemia disease through deep learning using microscopic images. In *2022 2nd International Conference on Digital Futures and Transformative Technologies (ICoDT2)* (pp. 1–6). IEEE.

Akbar, S., Hassan, T., Akram, M. U., Yasin, U. U., & Basit, I. (2017). AVRDB: Annotated dataset for vessel segmentation and calculation of arteriovenous ratio. In *Proceedings of the International Conference on Image Processing, Computer Vision, and Pattern Recognition (IPCV)* (pp. 129–134). The Steering Committee of the World Congress in Computer Science, Computer Engineering and Applied Computing (WorldComp).

Akbar, S., Hassan, S. A., Shoukat, A., Alyami, J., & Bahaj, S. A. (2022). Detection of microscopic glaucoma through fundus images using deep transfer learning approach. *Microscopy Research and Technique*, 85(6), 2259–2276.

ALL-IDB dataset. (2022). Retrieved from https://www.kaggle.com/datasets/priyaadharshini vs062/leukemia-dataset

Altaf, F., Islam, S. M., Akhtar, N., & Janjua, N. (2019). Going deep in medical image analysis: Concepts, methods, challenges, and future directions. *IEEE Access*, 7, 99540–99572.

Amin, J., Sharif, M., Anjum, M. A., Yasmin, M., Khattak, K. I., Kadry, S., & Seo, S. (2021). An integrated design based on dual thresholding and features optimization for white blood cells detection. *IEEE Access*, 9, 151421–151433.

Ansari, S., Navin, A. H., Sangar, A. B., Gharamaleki, J. V., & Danishvar, S. (2023). A customized efficient deep learning model for the diagnosis of acute leukemia cells based on lymphocyte and monocyte images. *Electronics*, 12(2), 322.

Anwar, S., & Alam, A. (2020). A convolutional neural network–based learning approach to acute lymphoblastic leukaemia detection with automated feature extraction. *Medical Biological Engineering Computing*, 58(12), 3113–3121.

ASH Image Bank. (2021). Retrieved from http://imagebank.hematology.org/searchresu lt#?cludoquery=leukemia&cludopage=2&cludorefurl=http%3A%2F%2Fimageb ank.hematology.org%2F&cludorefpt=ImageBank%20%7C%20Home%20%7C% 20Regular%20Bank&cludoinputtype=standard

Bibi, N., Sikandar, M., Ud Din, I., Almogren, A., & Ali, S. (2020). IoMT-based automated detection and classification of leukemia using deep learning. *Journal of Healthcare Engineering, 2020*, 6648574.

Bodzas, A., Kodytek, P., & Zidek, J. (2020). Automated detection of acute lymphoblastic leukemia from microscopic images based on human visual perception. *Frontiers in Bioengineering and Biotechnology, 58*, 1005.

Boldú, L., Merino, A., Acevedo, A., Molina, A., & Rodellar, J. (2021). A deep learning model (ALNet) for the diagnosis of acute leukaemia lineage using peripheral blood cell images. *Computer Methods Programs in Biomedicine, 202*, 105999.

Chen, L., Li, S., Bai, Q., Yang, J., Jiang, S., & Miao, Y. (2021). Review of image classification algorithms based on convolutional neural networks. *Remote Sensing, 13*(22), 4712.

Das, B. K., & Dutta, H. S. (2020). GFNB: Gini index–based fuzzy naive Bayes and blast cell segmentation for leukemia detection using multi-cell blood smear images. *Medical & Biological Engineering & Computing, 58*(11), 2789–2803.

Dasariraju, S., Huo, M., & McCalla, S. (2020). Detection and classification of immature leukocytes for diagnosis of acute myeloid leukemia using random forest algorithm. *Bioengineering, 7*(4), 120.

Elhassan, T. A. M., Rahim, M. S. M., Swee, T. T., Hashim, S. Z. M., & Aljurf, M. (2022). Feature extraction of white blood cells using CMYK-moment localization and deep learning in acute myeloid leukemia blood smear microscopic images. *IEEE Access, 10*, 16577–16591.

Felman, A. (2024). How does blood work, and what problems can occur? Retrieved from https://www.medicalnewstoday.com/articles/196001#structure

Gull, S., Akbar, S., & Safdar, K. (2021, December). An interactive deep learning approach for brain tumor detection through 3D magnetic resonance images. In *2021 International Conference on Frontiers of Information Technology (FIT)* (pp. 114–119). IEEE.

Haskins, G., Kruger, U., & Yan, P. (2020). Deep learning in medical image registration: A survey. *Machine Vision Applications, 31*(1), 1–18.

Hassan, S. A., Akbar, S., Rehman, A., Saba, T., Kolivand, H., & Bahaj, S. A. (2021). Recent developments in detection of central serous retinopathy through imaging and artificial intelligence techniques: A review. *IEEE Access, 9*, 168731–168748.

Howard, A. G. (2013). Some improvements on deep convolutional neural network based image classification. arXiv:1312.5402.

Jha, K. K., & Dutta, H. S. (2019). Mutual information based hybrid model and deep learning for acute lymphocytic leukemia detection in single cell blood smear images. *Computer Methods Programs in Biomedicine, 179*, 104987.

Kasani, P. H., Park, S. W., & Jang, J.-W. (2020). An aggregated-based deep learning method for leukemic B-lymphoblast classification. *Diagnostics, 10*(12), 1064.

Kastrati, Z., Imran, A. S., & Yayilgan, S. Y. (2019). The impact of deep learning on document classification using semantically rich representations. *Information Processing Management, 56*(5), 1618–1632.

Kessenbrock, K., Plaks, V., & Werb, Z. J. C. (2010). Matrix metalloproteinases: Regulators of the tumor microenvironment. *Cell, 141*(1), 52–67.

Khan, M. A., Sharif, M. I., Raza, M., Anjum, A., Saba, T., & Shad, S. A. (2022). Skin lesion segmentation and classification: A unified framework of deep neural network features fusion and selection. *Expert Systems, 39*(7), e12497.

Khan, S., Sajjad, M., Hussain, T., Ullah, A., & Imran, A. S. (2020). A review on traditional machine learning and deep learning models for WBCs classification in blood smear images. *IEEE Access, 9*, 10657–10673.

Khandekar, R., Shastry, P., Jaishankar, S., Faust, O., & Sampathila, N. (2021). Automated blast cell detection for acute lymphoblastic leukemia diagnosis. *Biomedical Signal Processing Control, 68,* 102690.

Kumar, D., Jain, N., Khurana, A., Mittal, S., Satapathy, S. C., Senkerik, R., & Hemanth, J. D. (2020). Automatic detection of white blood cancer from bone marrow microscopic images using convolutional neural networks. *IEEE Access, 8,* 142521–142531.

Kumar, S., Mishra, S., & Asthana, P. (2018). Automated detection of acute leukemia using *k*-mean clustering algorithm. In Advances in Computer and Computational Sciences (pp. 655–670). Springer.

Larabi-Marie-Sainte, S., Aburahmah, L., Almohaini, R., & Saba, T. (2019). Current techniques for diabetes prediction: Review and case study. *Applied Sciences, 9*(21), 4604.

Latif, A., Rasheed, A., Sajid, U., Ahmed, J., Ali, N., Ratyal, N. I., & Khalil, T. (2019). Content-based image retrieval and feature extraction: A comprehensive review. *Mathematical Problems in Engineering, 2019.* https://doi.org/10.1155/2019/9658350

Lundervold, A. S., & Lundervold, A. (2019). An overview of deep learning in medical imaging focusing on MRI. *Zeitschrift für Medizinische Physik, 29*(2), 102–127.

Manescu, P., Narayanan, P., Bendkowski, C., Elmi, M., Claveau, R., Pawar, V., & Fernandez-Reyes, D. (2023). Detection of acute promyelocytic leukemia in peripheral blood and bone marrow with annotation-free deep learning. *Scientific Reports, 13*(1), 2562.

Mohamed, H., Omar, R., Saeed, N., Essam, A., Ayman, N., Mohiy, T., & AbdelRaouf, A. (2018). Automated detection of white blood cells cancer diseases. Paper presented at the *2018 First International Workshop on Deep and Representation Learning (IWDRL).*

Mughal, B., Muhammad, N., Sharif, M., Rehman, A., & Saba, T. (2018). Removal of pectoral muscle based on topographic map and shape-shifting silhouette. *BMC Cancer, 18,* 1–14.

Mughal, B., Sharif, M., Muhammad, N., & Saba, T. (2018). A novel classification scheme to decline the mortality rate among women due to breast tumor. *Microscopy Research and Technique, 81*(2), 171–180.

Muhsin, Z. F., Rehman, A., Altameem, A., Saba, T., & Uddin, M. (2014). Improved quadtree image segmentation approach to region information. *The Imaging Science Journal, 62*(1), 56–62.

Naaqvi, Z., Akbar, S., Hassan, S. A., & Ain, Q. U. (2022, May). Detection of liver cancer through computed tomography images using deep convolutional neural networks. In *2022 2nd International Conference on Digital Futures and Transformative Technologies (ICoDT2)* (pp. 1–6). IEEE.

Naaqvi, Z., Akbar, S., Hassan, S. A., Khalid, A., & Bashir, M. J. (2022). Automatic detection of liver cancer using artificial intelligence and imaging techniques: A review. In: Saba, T., Rehman, A., Roy, S. (Eds.), *Prognostic Models in Healthcare: AI and Statistical Approaches* (pp. 315–345). Springer, Singapore.

Oostindjer, M., Alexander, J., Amdam, G. V., Andersen, G., Bryan, N. S., Chen, D., & Haug, A. (2014). The role of red and processed meat in colorectal cancer development: A perspective. *Meat Science, 97*(4), 583–596.

Patil, A., Patil, M., & Birajdar, G. J. (2021). White blood cells image classification using deep learning with canonical correlation analysis. *IRBM, 42*(5), 378–389.

Ramya, V. J., & Lakshmi, S. (2022). Acute myelogenous leukemia detection using optimal neural network based on fractional black-widow model. *Signal, Image Video Processing, 16*(1), 229–238.

Ranjitha, P., & Duth, S. (2021). *Detection of blood cancer-leukemia using K-means algorithm.* In 2021 5th International Conference on Intelligent Computing and Control Systems (ICICCS). IEEE, Madurai.

Rehman, A., Abbas, N., Saba, T., Rahman, S. I. u., Mehmood, Z., & Kolivand, H. (2018). Classification of acute lymphoblastic leukemia using deep learning. *Microscopy Research and Technique, 81*(11), 1310–1317.

Saba, T., Akbar, S., Kolivand, H., & Ali Bahaj, S. (2021). Automatic detection of papill-edema through fundus retinal images using deep learning. *Microscopy Research and Technique, 84*(12), 3066–3077.

Sabzi Shahrebabaki, A., Imran, A. S., Olfati, N., & Svendsen, T. (2019). A comparative study of deep learning techniques on frame-level speech data classification. *Circuits, Systems, Signal Processing, 38*(8), 3501–3520.

Sadler, J. E. (2015). What's new in the diagnosis and pathophysiology of thrombotic thrombocytopenic purpura. *Hematology 2014, the American Society of Hematology Education Program Book, 2015*(1), 631–636.

Safdar, K., Akbar, S., & Gull, S. (2021, December). An automated deep learning based ensemble approach for malignant melanoma detection using dermoscopy images. In *2021 International Conference on Frontiers of Information Technology (FIT)* (pp. 206–211). IEEE.

Sahlol, A. T., Kollmannsberger, P., & Ewees, A. A. (2020). Efficient classification of white blood cell leukemia with improved swarm optimization of deep features. *Scientific Reports, 10*(1), 1–11.

Sajjad, M., Zahir, S., Ullah, A., Akhtar, Z., & Muhammad, K. (2020). Human behavior understanding in big multimedia data using CNN based facial expression recognition. *Mobile Networks Applications, 25*(4), 1611–1621.

Sakthiraj, F. S. K. (2021). Autonomous leukemia detection scheme based on hybrid convolutional neural network model using learning algorithm. *Wireless Personal Communication, 126*(3), 2191–2206.

Shaheen, M., Khan, R., Biswal, R., Ullah, M., Khan, A., Uddin, M. I., & Waheed, A. (2021). Acute myeloid leukemia (AML) detection using AlexNet model. *Complexity, 2021*.

Shoukat, A., Akbar, S., Hassan, S. A. E., Rehman, A., & Ayesha, N. (2021, December). An automated deep learning approach to diagnose glaucoma using retinal fundus images. In *2021 International Conference on Frontiers of Information Technology (FIT)* (pp. 120–125). IEEE.

Supardi, N., Mashor, M., Harun, N., Bakri, F., & Hassan, R. (2012). Classification of blasts in acute leukemia blood samples using k-nearest neighbour. In 2012 IEEE 8th International Colloquium on Signal Processing and its Applications (pp. 461–465). IEEE, Malacca, Malaysia. doi: 10.1109/CSPA.2012.6194769

Ullah, W., Ullah, A., Haq, I. U., Muhammad, K., Sajjad, M., & Baik, S. W. (2021). CNN features with bi-directional LSTM for real-time anomaly detection in surveillance networks. *Multimedia Tools Applications, 80*(11), 16979–16995.

Urooj, F., Akbar, S., Hassan, S. A., Firdous, S., & Bashir, M. J. (2022). Computer-aided diagnosis of pneumothorax through X-ray images using deep learning: A review. In Saba, T., Rehman, A., Roy, S. (Eds.), *Prognostic Models in Healthcare: AI and Statistical Approaches* (pp. 403–432). Springer, Singapore.

Wang, J. L., Li, A. Y., Huang, M., Ibrahim, A. K., Zhuang, H., & Ali, A. M. (2018). *Classification of white blood cells with PatternNet-fused ensemble of convolutional neural networks (PECNN)*. In 2018 IEEE International Symposium on Signal Processing and Information Technology (ISSPIT). Springer, Louisville, KY.

Chapter 6

Improvement Alzheimer's Segmentation by VGG16 and U-Net Autoencoder Techniques

Karrar A. Kadhim[1], Farhan Mohamed[1], and Ghalib Ahmed Salman[2]

[1]*Department of Emerging Computing, Faculty of Computing, Universiti Teknologi Malaysia, Johor Bahru, Malaysia*

[2]*Department of Computer Science, Middle Technical University, Baghdad, Iraq*

6.1 Introduction

Alzheimer's is a progressive and irreversible neurological disorder primarily affecting the brain's cognitive functions, memory, and behavior. It is the most common cause of dementia, a syndrome characterized by a decline in cognitive abilities that interferes with daily functioning and quality of life. Alzheimer's disease (AD) primarily affects older individuals, with the risk increasing significantly with age (Adzhar et al., 2022; Fahad et al., 2018). As the global population ages, the prevalence of AD has been rising, making it a critical concern for healthcare systems and society (Lin et al., 2023). By this degeneration, brain move from one stage to another, this process of moving is called conversion or progression. Generally, AD converts in three stages. The first stage is clinical normal (CN), where the subject

DOI: 10.1201/9781032626345-6

does not show signs of objective cognitive. The next stage is mild cognitive impairment (MCI) (Husham et al., 2016). Subject with MCI is at the risk of converting to AD. It has been reported that 7% of subjects with MCI convert to AD each year (Scharre et al., 2021). Subjects with MCI can be divided into two subclasses, depending on the progression of the disease. Subjects with MCI who later convert to AD are considered to progressive MCI (pMCI), whereas subjects who have stable MCI are considered to stable MCI (sMCI). One important research field that researchers are following is how to differentiate between sMCI and pMCI in order to identify MCI patients who are at high risk of converting to AD, so early detection of this group of patients may help clinicians to effectively treat the condition (Iftikhar et al., 2017).

The development of AD has been investigated by large amount of research. The main goal of this chapter is to discover AD development over time and to understand the related abnormalities that take place in the brain. Also, this chapter studied the patterns of progression of multiple factors. Understanding these abnormalities and progression factors is necessary for selecting features for predicting AD progression (Heesterbeek et al., 2020). AD-related pathologies appear many years before clinical onset of the disease (Jabeen et al., 2018; Salvatore et al., 2015). This means that the AD pathology develops while the individual is still cognitive.

In this study, a comprehensive methodology is presented to enhance the localization and classification of AD. The approach begins with rigorous preprocessing, including data augmentation and the utilization of advanced neural architectures to optimize data quality. To improve classification accuracy, the Visual Geometry Group 16 (VGG16) architecture is tailored, and the data is carefully divided into distinct subsets: 70% for testing, 20% for training, and 10% for validation. A pivotal contribution is the development of a U-Net Autoencoder model dedicated to MRI segmentation, enabling precise localization of affected brain regions, a crucial factor in AD diagnosis. The comprehensive evaluation incorporates standard measurements for classification performance, such as accuracy, sensitivity, and specificity, and a comparative analysis assessing segmentation performance through the average voxel/volume estimation error%. Utilizing datasets from the Alzheimer's Disease Neuroimaging Initiative (ADNI), robustness and comprehensiveness are ensured. This multifaceted methodology aims to advance the understanding and diagnosis of AD through improved localization and classification techniques (Jamal et al., 2017; Javed et al., 2020).

6.2 Related Works

Various techniques have been proposed for the localization of brain structures, falling into several categories, including manual methods, spatial relation-based methods, atlas-based methods, statistical shape model–based approaches, and deep learning–based detection strategies (Basher et al., 2019) (Nawaz et al., 2021).

Manual localization relies heavily on operators' expertise, often requiring a radiologist's skills, which can be quite time-consuming and costly (Khan et al., 2022; Magadza and Viriri, 2021). Spatial relation–based methods, conversely, employ predefined rules, such as fuzzy sets, to determine localization (Pedrycz and Wang, 2015). Atlas-based methods offer automated localization but necessitate an atlas for extrapolating information to the target dataset through co-registration procedures (Basher et al., 2020). Although this method can achieve precise automatic localization, it generally demands significant computational time and data resources (Basher et al., 2019). As a result, researchers have begun to explore alternative approaches like statistical shape model–based methods, which can predict shape variations within a training population (Allahdadian et al., 2019; Larabi-Marie-Sainte et al., 2019; Peiffer et al., 2022). This approach identifies and parameterizes the mean approximate shape from all shapes within the training data. Utilizing this mean shape, statistical shape model–based methods determine the approximate position of the targeted anatomy (Guezou-Philippe et al., 2023; Mughal et al., 2018a, b).

Basher et al. (2019) introduced an approach that combines a Hough voting method with a convolutional neural network (CNN) to automate the localization of brain anatomical structures, particularly the hippocampus. These models harnessed a deep CNN to compute displacement vectors, capitalizing on the Hough voting strategy across multiple three-viewpoint patch samples. These displacement vectors were incorporated into the sample positions to estimate the target location. In order to learn efficiently from the samples, a dual local and global strategy was employed. This involved training multiple local models to extract patches from the vicinity of the hippocampus location and then combining them to make a localized prediction. Furthermore, Basher et al. (2020), introduced a deep learning–driven approach for quantitatively assessing the discrete volume of the hippocampus within volumetric MRI scans, eliminating the need for prior segmentation. Their method involved the development of a 2D CNN model utilizing three-channel 2D patches to predict the quantity of voxels associated with the hippocampus. The estimated count of hippocampal voxels was subsequently multiplied by the voxel volume to calculate the discrete volume of the hippocampus. Lian et al. (2018) introduced a hierarchical-fully convolutional network (H-FCN) to accurately identify discriminative local patches and regions within whole-brain structural MRI data. They subsequently learn and fuse multiscale feature representations to construct hierarchical classification models for AD diagnosis. Simoes et al. (2014) proposed a novel method that circumvents the need for specific brain region segmentation or nonlinear alignment to a template. Their approach conducts 3D texture analysis using local binary patterns computed from local image patches throughout the entire brain. These texture patterns are then combined within a classifier ensemble. This innovative approach eliminates the necessity for segmenting specific brain structures and nonlinear registration to a template, making it a promising option for clinical implementation, particularly in the early diagnosis of AD (Saba et al., 2012).

Duarte et al.'s (2022) various CNN architectures, including 2D, 2.5D, and 3D U-shaped convolutional neural networks (U-Net CNNs), were deployed to conduct semantic segmentation on FLAIR images. These models underwent evaluation using brain volumes sourced from 186 individuals. The results were systematically analyzed both across the entire brain and by specific brain regions, such as the frontal, occipital, parietal, temporal lobes, and the insula, to pinpoint disparities in their performance.

Simoes et al. (2014) introduced a method referred to as "LBP-TOP + cohort," which was employed to analyze the discriminative brain regions between a cohort of normal control subjects and a group of AD patients. They conducted 3D texture analysis using local binary patterns computed at local image patches across the entire brain, which were then amalgamated within a classifier ensemble. This approach achieved its objectives without necessitating the segmentation of specific brain structures or the execution of nonlinear registration to a template. These attributes indicate that this method holds promise for clinical implementation and has the potential to aid in the early diagnosis of AD. To provide a comprehensive overview of the key segmentation techniques, their respective advantages and limitations, the authors have thoughtfully summarized them in Table 6.1.

Although all previous studies achieved good results in classifying AD, researchers were able to segment the hippocampus to obtain the best results in detecting and determining the stage of the disease. However, interest in localizing brain regions and comparing them is still important to obtain information on the extent to which vital factors are affected. In this chapter, the primary focus was on assessing

Table 6.1 A Concise Overview of the Primary Segmentation Methods along with Their Associated Strengths and Weaknesses

Literature	Techniques	Advantages	Limitation
Simoes et al. (2014)	LBP-TOP + cohort	The ability to diagnose AD without relying on specific brain structure segmentation. This method does not require a priori segmentation of brain structures. This simplifies the preprocessing pipeline	The study's findings are based on a specific dataset that includes very mild-to-mild AD subjects and healthy elderly controls. potentially limiting the generalizability of the results. A clinical validation on larger and more diverse datasets is needed to confirm its effectiveness and reliability

(Continued)

Table 6.1 (Continued)

Literature	Techniques	Advantages	Limitation
Lian et al. (2018)	Hierarchical FCN + automatic discriminative localization	H-FCN to identify discriminative local patches and regions, automatically learn high-nonlinear feature representations	The structural alterations resulting from dementia can exhibit variations in different brain regions. Hence, it is imperative to enhance this approach by incorporating multiscale image patches. The location proposal module is currently separated from the subsequent network. To improve the system, there is a need to integrate this crucial module seamlessly, enabling it to automatically and precisely generate location proposals tailored to individual subjects
Basher et al. (2019)	Hough voting + CNN	Combines a Hough voting technique with a CNN to autonomously identify brain anatomical structures. Calculated displacement vectors by the Hough voting strategy	The combination of Hough voting, and CNNs introduces added complexity to the model. This complexity may lead to longer training times and increased memory usage. The scalability of the proposed approach to handle larger and more diverse datasets is not explicitly discussed. Adapting the model to different datasets may require additional adjustments and optimizations
Duarte et al. (2022)	2D, 2.5D, and 3D + U-Net CNNs	The accuracy of predicted white matter hyperintensity (WMH) volumes on the test data was notably high when compared to manual segmentation	The limited dataset selection may restrict the model's ability to generalize to a broader population or other imaging datasets. Structural alterations caused by dementia can exhibit variations in various regions of the brain, including white matter

the precision of the U-Net localization technique through automated localization employing the U-Net Autoencoder. This diagnosis enables to determine the stage of the disease with high accuracy, in addition to identifying the most damaged area, which affects vital factors such as memory, movement, speech, etc. Another observation made is that still the big challenge that the researchers are facing is predicting the conversion from MCI to AD due the heterogeneity of MCI; however, a good classification accuracy has been noticed in some works when the goal is to classify the CN from AD.

6.3 Material and Methods

The primary objectives of this chapter are to comprehensively investigate and present innovative methods for the classification and segmentation of AD. The chapter presents an algorithm designed to segment and visualize variations in symmetry between the right and left hemispheres of the brain, while also generating features that represent these asymmetries. This chapter aims to investigate an improved method for accurately classifying and segmenting AD using neuroimaging data. The chapter presents cutting-edge approaches, discusses their practical implications, and identifies future research directions. Brain anatomical structures exhibit significant variations related to phenotypes, age, gender, and disease. Consequently, applying a single segmentation method across all phenotypic categories poses a challenge, as it may not consistently deliver reliable results.

6.3.1 Data of ADNI

The trained model, we developed was employed to analyze data from the ADNI database. Its primary purpose was to model the classification and features extraction, addressing the complexity of a multistep prediction problem. The study's conclusion affirmed that the proposed model surpassed the performance of the baseline models. The resultant dataset (6,280 samples) was randomly partitioned into training, testing, and validation sets. The training set consisted of 70% of the data (4,396 samples), the testing set comprised 20% (1,256 samples), and the validation set contained the remaining 10% (628 samples).

6.3.2 Data Preprocessing

Preceding the input of data into the VGG16 model, an array of meticulous preprocessing procedures was executed, enhancing the dataset's quality and diversity. Inclusive within these preprocessing protocols, we employed a spectrum of data augmentation strategies, encompassing techniques such as controlled zooming and calibrated brightness adjustments. The deliberate application of these augmentations introduced controlled variabilities, thereby conferring adaptability to the model across a spectrum of real-world scenarios and fluctuating lighting conditions. This augmented dataset significantly enriched the model's learning capacity, reinforcing its ability to discern intricate patterns and subtle variances.

6.3.2.1 Optimization SGD with Momentum

In pursuit of practical learning and convergence, we harnessed the potency of the stochastic gradient descent (SGD) optimization algorithm complemented by momentum. This strategic fusion of optimization techniques facilitated swift convergence by seamlessly integrating the momentum amassed from prior iterations. Such amalgamation empowered the model to transcend local minima and navigate the solution space flexibly. The synchronized interplay between SGD and momentum synergistically honed the model's parameter updates, culminating in an elevated aptitude for capturing intricate patterns intrinsic to AD.

6.3.2.2 Model Training and Evaluation

The robust training of our classification model was conducted meticulously, employing the augmented and meticulously preprocessed dataset. With meticulous attention to detail, we judiciously partitioned the dataset into distinct subsets, comprising training, testing, and validation segments. This strategic partitioning allowed us to refine the model's performance optimization and subsequent evaluation. Through an iterative process of backpropagation, the model diligently imbibed the capacity to discern between instances of AD and healthy subjects (Duan et al., 2023). Gradually, the model fine-tuned its parameters, progressively elevating its accuracy quotient to optimal levels.

6.3.3 Classification Approach by VGG-16

A fundamental goal of the study was to classify instances of AD, intending to distinguish patterns and differences between healthy individuals and those afflicted by the disease. In pursuit of precise classification, we adopted an advanced strategy centered around utilizing the VGG16 neural network architecture.

Central to the classification methodology is utilizing the VGG16 architecture, a well-regarded framework renowned for its prowess in image classification endeavors. Distinctive for its deep convolutional layer hierarchy, interleaved with pooling and fully connected layers, VGG16 excels in extracting intricate features embedded within images (Akiyama et al., 2020). Exploiting its inherent ability to learn progressive hierarchies of features – ranging from fundamental edges to intricate high-level patterns – we harnessed VGG16's capacity to meticulously discriminate

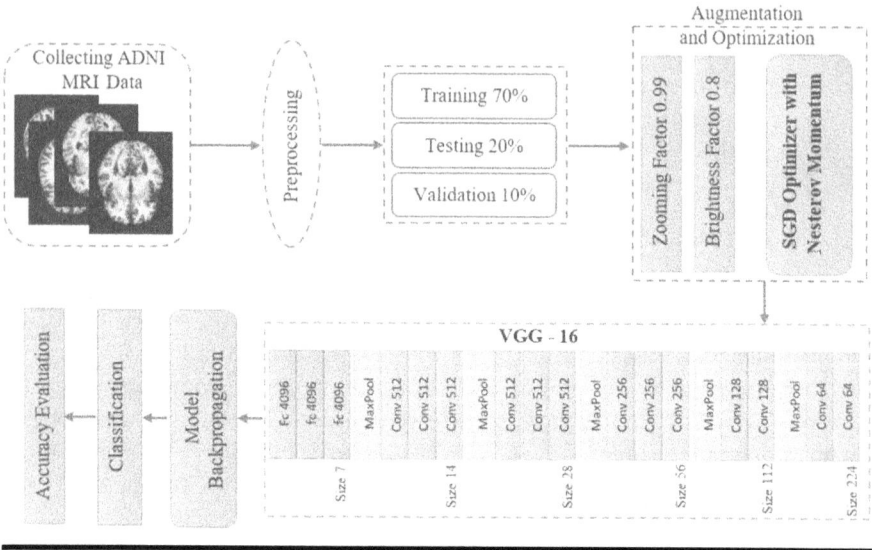

Figure 6.1   A classification mechanism using the VGG16 algorithm.

between instances of AD and healthy subjects. This approach was complemented by a combination of data preprocessing, augmentation, and optimization techniques to ensure the accuracy of our results. The classification stage was divided into four sections. The first is collecting datasets from ADNI (https://adni.loni. usc.edu/data-samples/adni-data/), and then divide the data into 70% for training, 20% testing, and 10% validation. The second stage is to increase and improve the data. This is done by using image zooming and brightness factors. Then the images are improved using the SGD Optimizer with Nesterov Momentum to obtain new data. In the third stage, the VGG16 model is applied, which represents training the convolutional layers. Finally, the testing stage and calculate the accuracy of the training and testing results (refer to Figure 6.1).

6.3.4 Segmentation and Localization Methods by U-Net Autoencoder

In this chapter, the focus rests on hippocampus segmentation, the intricate process of pinpointing, and outlining the contours of hippocampal structures within cerebral images (Liu et al., 2020). This meticulous procedure assumes paramount significance in diverse medical contexts, including the realms of neuroimaging investigation and the diagnostic landscape of neurological afflictions Hussain et al. (2020). The hippocampus localization strategy consists of a set of steps. The

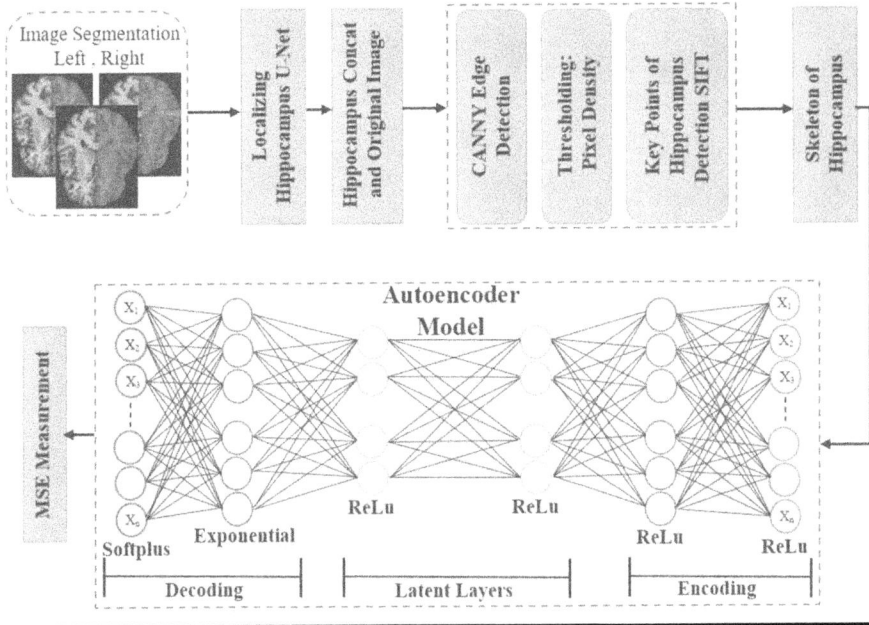

Figure 6.2   The hippocampus localization strategy.

original image is divided into two parts (right and left), and then the hippocampus is localized for each part using U-net. The hippocampus is visualized by merging it and comparing it with the original image. Edge detection for original image by CANNY edge apply thresholding for pixel density and convert it into a mask for image using SIFT to obtain the key points of hippocampus. A skeleton is applied to the hippocampus to obtain the thickness of the extracted edges. Encoding and decoding are applied to reduce the data size and increase the data accuracy, respectively. Finally, the autoencoder model is applied to obtain the results and evaluate it (see Figure 6.2).

The autoencoder–decoder framework, under its ability to capture intricate features, patterns, and relationships, served as an integral tool throughout the comprehensive analysis pipeline (Kang et al., 2022). The encoded representations facilitated a rich understanding of hippocampal structures, enabling enhanced visualization and analysis. The decoder played a crucial role in transforming these encoded representations back into meaningful visualizations that aid researchers and medical professionals in gaining insights into the structural characteristics and abnormalities of the hippocampus. This integration of deep learning and image processing techniques improved visualization and paved the way for more accurate and informative analysis of brain MRI data. Structure of autoencoder framework method is shown in Figure 6.3.

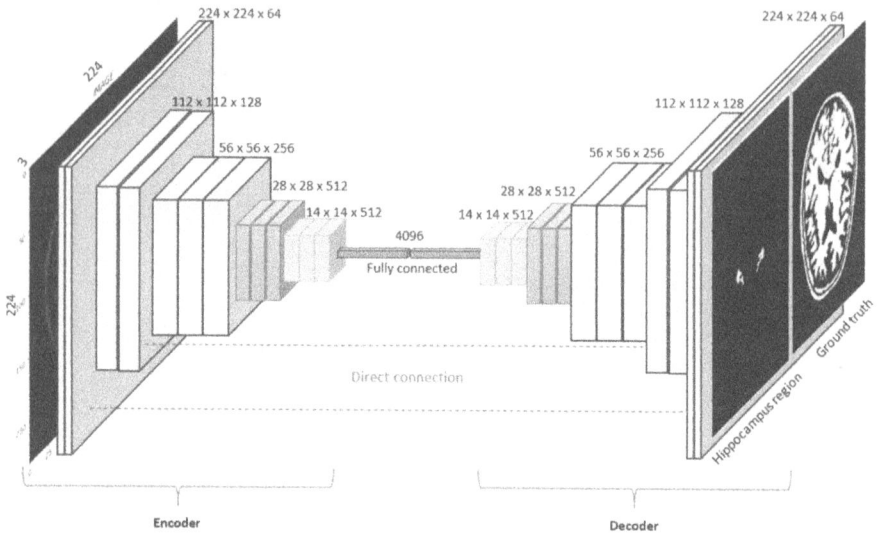

Figure 6.3   Structural autoencoder method to localize the hippocampus.

6.4 Results and Discission

Through the synergistic interplay of the VGG16 architecture, data preprocessing, augmentation, and optimized training, our classification methodology yielded a robust model capable of accurate discrimination between AD and healthy cases. The integration of advanced techniques and comprehensive evaluation metrics showcased the potential of our approach in advancing early detection and diagnosis in AD research. The performance of the classification model was assessed using standard metrics such as accuracy, specificity, and sensitivity (Muhsin et al., 2014; Naz et al., 2019; Tharwat, 2020; Yousaf et al., 2019). These metrics provided a comprehensive understanding of the model's ability to correctly classify cases and its capacity to minimize false positives and negatives. The evaluation criteria serve as a fundamental component for appraising the classification and segmentation methods, playing a pivotal role in the development and enhancement of classification models (Rehman, 2023).

$$\text{Accuracy} = \frac{\text{TP} + \text{TN}}{\text{TP} + \text{FP} + \text{FN} + \text{TN}} \qquad (6.1)$$

These measuring parameters are integral for assessing the performance of classification models in various fields, such as machine learning, statistics, and medical diagnostics.

Sensitivity, also known as recall, holds significance in situations where the focus is on identifying positive outcomes, and the cost of a false positive is relatively low.

In such cases, the objective is to detect as many true positives as possible, even if it means accepting a few false positives (Saba and Rehman, 2013). For instance, when predicting whether a patient has AD or not, it is crucial to have a high sensitivity. This ensures that as many actual positive cases (patients with AD) as possible are identified, even if it results in classifying a few patients who do not have AD as positive cases. The emphasis is on minimizing the chances of missing true positive cases.

$$\text{Sensitivity} = \frac{\text{TP}}{\text{TP} + \text{FN}} \tag{6.2}$$

Specificity is a metric that represents the ratio of true negatives to all negative outcomes (Saba and Rehman, 2013). It becomes particularly important when the focus is on ensuring the accuracy of the negative rate, and there are significant consequences or costs associated with a positive outcome. In situations where avoiding false positives is crucial, and the cost of incorrectly classifying a negative case as positive is high, specificity plays a pivotal role in assessing the model's performance.

$$\text{Specificity} = \frac{\text{TN}}{\text{TN} + \text{FP}} \tag{6.3}$$

The mean squared error (MSE) is a metric commonly used for assessing the accuracy of image reconstruction or regression tasks (Saba et al., 2018a,b). MSE calculates the average squared difference between the predicted values and the ground truth across all pixels (Sadad et al., 2021). In the context of segmentation, the goal is to identify and delineate regions of interest.

$$\text{MSE} = \frac{1}{N} \sum_{i=1}^{N} \left(I_{\text{predicted}}(i) - I_{\text{ground truth}}(i) \right)^2 \tag{6.4}$$

The latent space representations of the hippocampal images underwent a transformation using the autoencoder–decoder network. This transformation aimed to enhance the representation while preserving essential structural information. The network learned to minimize the reconstruction loss, ensuring the transformed representations remained faithful to the original images. The average percentage error is a measure of the average difference between predicted and actual values as a percentage of the actual values. The standard deviation of percentage errors provides information about the variability or spread of these errors. The average percentage error is calculated as the mean of the percentage errors for each data point. The standard deviation of percentage errors (STD) quantifies the spread or dispersion of the percentage errors.

$$\text{Avg.\% error} = \frac{1}{N} \sum_{i=1}^{N} \left| \frac{\text{Actual}_i - \text{Predicted}_i}{\text{Actual}_i} \right| \times 100 \tag{6.5}$$

$$\text{STD} = \sqrt{\frac{1}{N} \sum_{i=1}^{N} \left(\left| \frac{\text{Actual}_i - \text{Predicted}_i}{\text{Actual}_i} \right| \times 100 - \text{Avg. error} \right)^2} \tag{6.6}$$

Here:

N is the total number of data point.
Actual_i is the actual value for the i data point.
Predicted_i is the predicted value for the i data point.

The Jaccard Index, also known as the Intersection over Union (IoU), is a metric commonly used to evaluate the performance of segmentation algorithms. Jaccard Index quantifies the spatial overlap between the predicted segmentation and the ground truth, providing a measure of segmentation accuracy.

$$\text{Jaccard} = \frac{\text{Intersection}}{\text{Predicted Volume U Ground Truth Volume}} \tag{6.7}$$

Here:

Intersection is the number of correctly classified segmented voxels by algorithm and ground truth.
Predicted Volume is the number of classified segmented voxels by the algorithm.
Ground Truth Volume is the number of classified segmented voxels by ground truth.

6.4.1 Classification Model Performance

The training model was employed to assess accuracy and loss after 25 epochs, with each epoch encompassing 5,000 steps, using a dataset comprising 5,000 images from the AD classification dataset.

Here are the results we have got after doing 25 epochs. The outcomes of the classification achieved through deep learning using the enhanced VGG-16 model performance, which yielded a classification accuracy surpassing 98.6%, exhibits considerable promise in contrast to the findings of prior studies. The model history for classification and confusion matrix is illustrated in Figures 6.4 and 6.5.

The number of models used in the method and the accuracy of the results, which are presented in Table 6.2, show that the results obtained during the research are better than other results. Our method is distinct as the system used data improvement methods by Momentum of SGD and augmented data, which increases accuracy in classification stage.

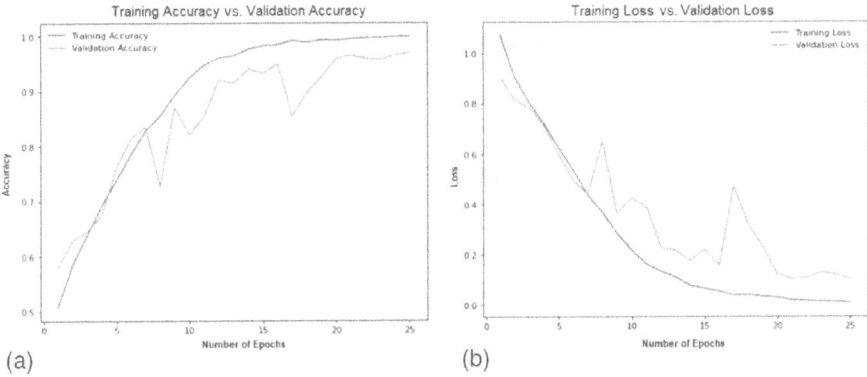

Figure 6.4 **Model history of training and validation per epoch: (a) accuracy, (b) loss.**

The outcomes presented in Table 6.2 indicate that our proposed approach demonstrates favorable outcomes when contrasted with prior investigations in AD classification. Furthermore, it is essential to acknowledge that the variance in the utilized dataset can directly impact result quality.

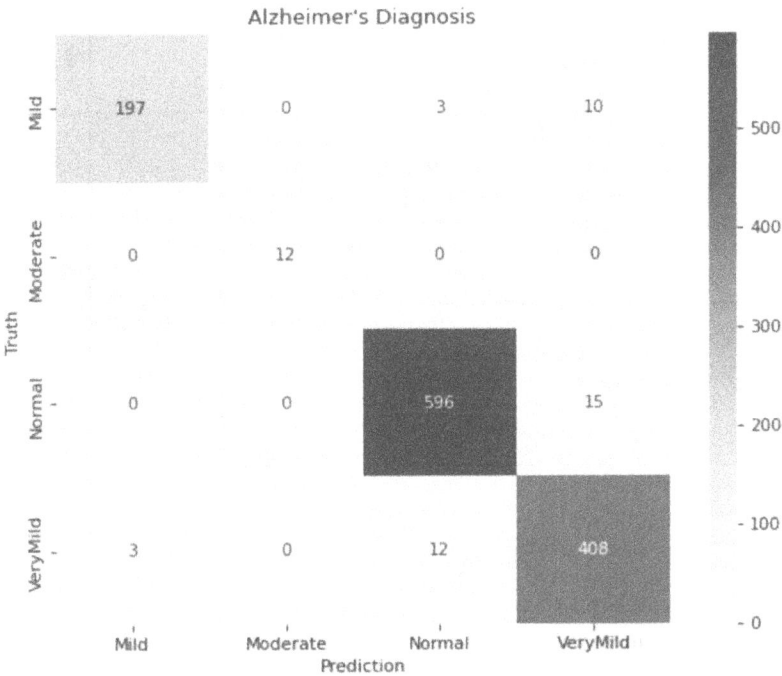

Figure 6.5 **Confusion matrix of VGG16 classification method.**

Table 6.2 A Summary of Explanation of the Most Recent Studies Employing the Baseline MRI Data from ADNI for AD Classification

Literature	Method	Subjects	AD vs. NC vs. pMCI vs. sMCI		
			Accuracy (%)	Sensitivity (%)	Specificity (%)
Lian et al. (2018)	Hierarchical FCN + automatic discriminative localization	1,457 subjects	0.90	0.82	0.97
Simoes et al. (2014)	Local binary patterns three orthogonal projections (LBP-TOP) localizatoin	436 subjects	0.85	0.80	0.91
Liu et al. (2014b)	Conventional classifiers (i.e., linear discriminant analysis, hierarchical SVM, MIL model) + patch-level engineered features	834 subjects	0.92	0.91	0.93
Salvatore et al. (2015)	Conventional classifiers (i.e., LPboosting, SVM) + voxel-level engineered features	509 subjects	0.76	–	–
Liu et al. (2014a)	Stacked autoencoders + region-level engineered features	384 subjects	0.79	0.83	0.87
Liu et al. (2016)	Conventional classifiers (i.e., linear regression, ensemble SVM) + region-level engineered features	459 subjects	0.93	0.95	0.90

(Continued)

Table 6.2   (Continued)

			AD vs. NC vs. pMCI vs. sMCI		
Literature	*Method*	*Subjects*	*Accuracy (%)*	*Sensitivity (%)*	*Specificity (%)*
Korolev et al. (2017)	CNN + hippocampal sMRI	106 subjects	0.85	0.88	0.90
Shi et al. (2017)	Deep polynomial network + region-level engineered features	204 subjects	0.95	0.94	0.96
Proposed method	VGG16 + U-Net Autoencoder	6,280 subjects	0.98	0.95	0.99

6.4.2 *Segmentation and Localization the Hippocampus by U-Net Autoencoder*

Localization and image splitting, the hippocampus, a crucial brain structure associated with memory and spatial navigation, was localized within the brain MRI (Tahir et al., 2019). This was achieved through image processing techniques that highlighted the hippocampal region. Once localized, the image was split into two parts: the left and right hemispheres, each containing one half of the hippocampus. This division facilitated a detailed comparison between the two hemispheres, allowing for the identification of any disparities or abnormalities in the hippocampal structures. localizing the regions of the hippocampus and splitting into left and right hemispheres, and then containing with original image, as shown in Figure 6.6.

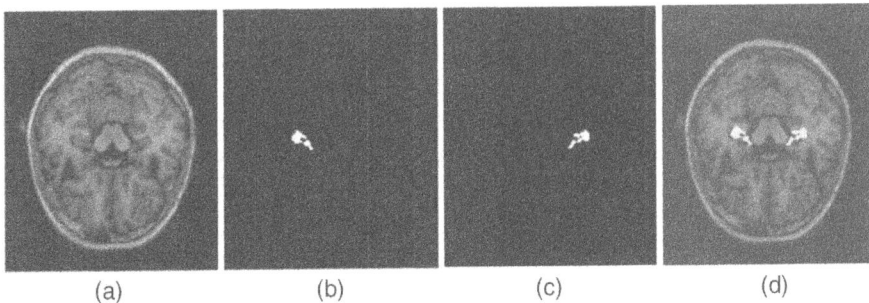

Figure 6.6   Localization of the left and right hippocampus regions. (a) The original image. (b) Left hippocampus region. (c) Right hippocampus region. (d) Visualizing the hippocampus by concatenation with the original image.

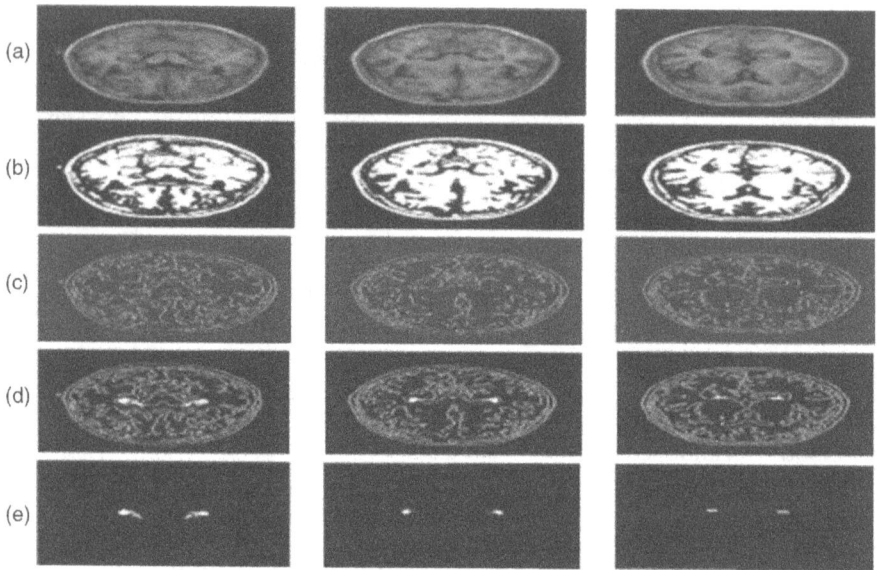

Figure 6.7 Localization and segmentation image with autoencoder U-Net. (a) Original image. (b) Applying the threshold to get the mask of image. (c) Applying Canny edge detection. (d) Visualizing the hippocampus by concatenation with Canny edge detection. (e) Localizing the hippocampus region by U-Net.

The initial stage of hippocampus concatenation involved blending left and right hemisphere images to form a composite representation. The encoder extracted essential features, while the decoder contributed to the reconstruction of the composite image. This process helped enhance the visualization of the hippocampal regions' alignment and symmetry (see Figure 6.7e).

Edge detection and thresholding were facilitated by the latent representations. The decoder assisted in producing thresholder Canny edge-detected images, revealing the edges of hippocampal structures. This visual cue highlighted boundaries, aiding in identifying intricate structural details (see Figure 6.7b and c).

The latent space representations of the hippocampal images underwent a transformation using the autoencoder–decoder network. This transformation aimed to enhance the representation while preserving essential structural information. The network learned to minimize the reconstruction loss, ensuring the transformed representations remained faithful to the original images (see Figure 6.7e). The average voxel/volume estimation error% in a comparative performance analysis is illustrated in Table 6.3.

The localization of the brain into two hemispheres facilitated the identification of the affected region, thereby enhancing our understanding of the most impacted area of the brain. The most important variables are often selected from the left hemisphere of the brain and may suggest that more deterioration has taken place in the left hemisphere than the right hemisphere. The evaluation of segmentation approach achieved 97.3% by Jaccard Index, as seen in Table 6.4.

Table 6.3   Average Voxel/Volume Estimation Error% in a Comparative Performance Analysis

Method	*Avg. %error + STD Left Hippocampus*	*Avg. %error + STD Right Hippocampus*
2D, 2.5D, and 3D U-Net	13.086 + 10.761	17.812 + 14.748
Hough-CNN	4.4027 + 3.4963	4.5211 + 3.7510
LBP-TOP + cohort	29.1 + 1.1	24.5 + 4.2
H-FCN	15.7 ± 2.8	26.6 ± 1.7
Proposed method	2.3698 + 0.0507	3.3906 + 1.0517

Table 6.4   Jaccard Index for Proposed Segmentation Results and Related Works

Reference	*Preprocessing*	*Datasets*	*Method*	*Jaccard Index*
Maruyama et al. (2021)	–	ADNI	SegNet + VGG16	68.2%
Ramya et al. (2022)	2D adaptive bilateral filter	ADNI	Enhanced expectation maximum (EEM) clustering + adaptive histogram (AH) thresholding	80.04%
Rajangam and Palanisamy (2023)	Contour-based brain segmentation (CBBS)	NITRC + ADNI	Automatic segmentation + contouring technique	67%
Proposed method	VGG16 feature map	ADNI	Transfer learning + autoencoder	97.3%

6.5 Discussion

The results of this study underscore the potential of an innovative approach to improving the localization and classification of AD. By meticulously addressing various facets of the research methodology, we sought to enhance the precision and reliability of AD diagnosis. Through a comprehensive process, we delved into the development of a robust pipeline that combines preprocessing, feature engineering, classification, and segmentation techniques, thus aiming to advance the understanding of AD detection.

The tailoring of the Visual Geometry Group 16 (VGG16) architecture is a key element in the classification process. Through this enhancement, we improved the accuracy of AD classification. The decision to split the dataset into testing, training, and validation subsets adheres to the standard best practices in machine learning. This step ensures that our model's generalizability and robustness are rigorously tested, enabling us to trust the model's predictions in real-world scenarios.

This multifaceted methodology advances the understanding and diagnosis of AD by improving the localization and classification techniques. By tackling each stage of the process with precision and innovation, we have demonstrated the potential to make a significant impact in the field of AD research. The integrated approach presented in this study opens the door to more accurate and reliable AD diagnosis, offering potential benefits to individuals, caregivers, and the medical community. However, it is important to acknowledge that while this study has shown promising results, there is room for further research and refinement, and we encourage future investigations in this direction.

6.6 Conclusion

This chapter introduces a fusion approach aimed at enhancing AD classification and localizing the hippocampus, a pivotal factor in disease detection. Our fusion model combines VGG16 and an autoencoder into a unified framework, enabling early AD detection and hippocampus localization.

This approach demonstrated remarkable accuracy in pinpointing the most affected regions of the hippocampus, providing insights into specific areas of impact and their implications for critical physiological factors. The results indicate an impressive classification accuracy of 98.6% and Avg. error STD for hippocampus localization 2.3698 and 3.3906 for left and right hippocampus, respectively, while the Jaccard Index achieved 97.3%. This localization was achieved through a series of preprocessing steps designed to enhance accuracy. By segmenting the hippocampus into two segments and conducting a comparative analysis, we localized the most impacted brain regions. This comprehensive approach holds promise for advancing the understanding and diagnosis of AD, with potential implications for both research and clinical applications.

References

Adzhar, M. A., Manlapaz, D., Singh, D. K. A., & Mesbah, N. 2022. Exercise to improve postural stability in older adults with Alzheimer's disease: A systematic review of randomized control trials. *International Journal of Environmental Research and Public Health, 19*, 10350.

Akiyama, Y., Mikami, T., & Mikuni, N. 2020. Deep learning-based approach for the diagnosis of moyamoya disease. *Journal of Stroke and Cerebrovascular Diseases, 29*, 105322.

Allahdadian, S., Döhler, M., Ventura, C., & Mevel, L. 2019. Towards robust statistical damage localization via model-based sensitivity clustering. *Mechanical Systems and Signal Processing, 134*, 106341.

Basher, A., Choi, K. Y., Lee, J. J., Lee, B., Kim, B. C., Lee, K. H., & Jung, H. Y. 2019. Hippocampus localization using a two-stage ensemble Hough convolutional neural network. *IEEE Access, 7*, 73436–73447.

Basher, A., Kim, B. C., Lee, K. H., & Jung, H. Y. 2020. Automatic localization and discrete volume measurements of hippocampi from MRI data using a convolutional neural network. *IEEE Access, 8*, 91725–91739.

Duan, J., Liu, Y., Wu, H., Wang, J., Chen, L., & Chen, C. 2023. Broad learning for early diagnosis of Alzheimer's disease using FDG-PET of the brain. *Frontiers in Neuroscience, 17*, 1137567.

Duarte, K. T., Gobbi, D. G., Sidhu, A. S., Mccreary, C. R., Saad, F., Das, N., Smith, E. E., & Frayne, R. 2022. Segmenting white matter hyperintensity in Alzheimer's disease using U-Net CNNs. 2022 35th SIBGRAPI Conference on Graphics, Patterns and Images (SIBGRAPI). IEEE, 109–114.

Fahad, H. M., Ghani Khan, M. U., Saba, T., Rehman, A., & Iqbal, S. 2018. Microscopic abnormality classification of cardiac murmurs using ANFIS and HMM. *Microscopy Research and Technique, 81*(5), 449–457.

Guezou-Philippe, A., Dardenne, G., Letissier, H., Yvinou, A., Burdin, V., Stindel, E., & Lefèvre, C. 2023. Anterior pelvic plane estimation for total hip arthroplasty using a joint ultrasound and statistical shape model based approach. *Medical & Biological Engineering & Computing, 61*, 195–204.

Heesterbeek, T. J., Lorés-Motta, L., Hoyng, C. B., Lechanteur, Y. T. E., & Den Hollander, A. I. 2020. Risk factors for progression of age-related macular degeneration. *Ophthalmic and Physiological Optics, 40*, 140–170.

Husham, A., Hazim Alkawaz, M., Saba, T., Rehman, A., & Saleh Alghamdi, J. 2016. Automated nuclei segmentation of malignant using level sets. *Microscopy Research and Technique, 79*(10), 993–997.

Hussain, N., Khan, M. A., Sharif, M., Khan, S. A., Albesher, A. A., Saba, T., & Armaghan, A. 2020. A deep neural network and classical features based scheme for objects recognition: An application for machine inspection. *Multimedia Tools and Applications, 83*(5), 1–23.

Iftikhar, S., Fatima, K., Rehman, A., Almazyad, A. S., & Saba, T. 2017. An evolution based hybrid approach for heart diseases classification and associated risk factors identification. *Biomedical Research, 28*(8), 3451–3455.

Jabeen, S., Mehmood, Z., Mahmood, T., Saba, T., Rehman, A., & Mahmood, M. T. 2018. An effective content-based image retrieval technique for image visuals representation based on the bag-of-visual-words model. *PLoS One, 13*(4), e0194526.

Jamal, A., Hazim Alkawaz, M., Rehman, A., & Saba, T. 2017. Retinal imaging analysis based on vessel detection. *Microscopy Research and Technique, 80*(7), 799–811.

Javed, R., Rahim, M. S. M., Saba, T., & Rehman, A. 2020. A comparative study of features selection for skin lesion detection from dermoscopic images. *Network Modeling Analysis in Health Informatics and Bioinformatics, 9*, 1–13.

Kang, M., Ko, E., & Mersha, T. B. 2022. A roadmap for multi-omics data integration using deep learning. *Briefings in Bioinformatics, 23*, bbab454.

Khan, M. A., Sharif, M. I., Raza, M., Anjum, A., Saba, T., & Shad, S. A. 2022. Skin lesion segmentation and classification: A unified framework of deep neural network features fusion and selection. *Expert Systems, 39*(7), e12497.

Korolev, S., Safiullin, A., Belyaev, M., & Dodonova, Y. 2017. Residual and plain convolutional neural networks for 3D brain MRI classification. 2017 IEEE 14th International Symposium on Biomedical Imaging (ISBI 2017). IEEE, 835–838.

Larabi-Marie-Sainte, S., Aburahmah, L., Almohaini, R., & Saba, T. 2019. Current techniques for diabetes prediction: Review and case study. *Applied Sciences, 9*(21), 4604.

Lian, C., Liu, M., Zhang, J., & Shen, D. 2018. Hierarchical fully convolutional network for joint atrophy localization and Alzheimer's disease diagnosis using structural MRI. *IEEE Transactions on Pattern Analysis and Machine Intelligence, 42*, 880–893.

Lin, Q., Shahid, S., Hone-Blanchet, A., Huang, S., Wu, J., Bisht, A., Loring, D., Goldstein, F., Levey, A., & Crosson, B. 2023. Magnetic resonance evidence of increased iron content in subcortical brain regions in asymptomatic Alzheimer's disease. *Human Brain Mapping, 44*, 3072–3083.

Liu, M., Li, F., Yan, H., Wang, K., Ma, Y., Shen, L., Xu, M., & Initiative, A. S. D. N. 2020. A multi-model deep convolutional neural network for automatic hippocampus segmentation and classification in Alzheimer's disease. *Neuroimage, 208*, 116459.

Liu, M., Zhang, D., & Shen, D. 2016. Relationship induced multi-template learning for diagnosis of Alzheimer's disease and mild cognitive impairment. *IEEE Transactions on Medical Imaging, 35*, 1463–1474.

Liu, S., Liu, S., Cai, W., Che, H., Pujol, S., Kikinis, R., Feng, D., & Fulham, M. J. 2014a. Multimodal neuroimaging feature learning for multiclass diagnosis of Alzheimer's disease. *IEEE Transactions on Biomedical Engineering, 62*, 1132–1140.

Liu, M., Zhang, D., Shen, D., & Alzheimer's Disease Neuroimaging Initiative. 2014b. Hierarchical fusion of features and classifier decisions for Alzheimer's disease diagnosis. *Human Brain Mapping, 35*, 1305–1319.

Magadza, T., & Viriri, S. 2021. Deep learning for brain tumor segmentation: A survey of state-of-the-art. *Journal of Imaging, 7*, 19.

Maruyama, T., Hayashi, N., Sato, Y., Ogura, T., Uehara, M., Ogura, A., Watanabe, H., Kitoh, Y., & Initiative, A. S. D. N. 2021. Simultaneous brain structure segmentation in magnetic resonance images using deep convolutional neural networks. *Radiological Physics and Technology, 14*, 358–365.

Mughal, B., Muhammad, N., Sharif, M., Rehman, A., & Saba, T. 2018a. Removal of pectoral muscle based on topographic map and shape-shifting silhouette. *BMC Cancer, 18*(1), 1–14.

Mughal, B., Sharif, M., Muhammad, N., & Saba, T. 2018b. A novel classification scheme to decline the mortality rate among women due to breast tumor. *Microscopy Research and Technique, 81*(2), 171–180.

Muhsin, Z. F., Rehman, A., Altameem, A., Saba, T., & Uddin, M. 2014. Improved quadtree image segmentation approach to region information. *The Imaging Science Journal, 62*(1), 56–62.

Nawaz, M., Nazir, T., Masood, M., Mehmood, A., Mahum, R., Khan, M. A., Kadry, S., & Thinnukool, O. 2021. Analysis of brain MRI images using improved cornerNet approach. *Diagnostics, 11*, 1856.

Naz, A., Javed, M. U., Javaid, N., Saba, T., Alhussein, M., & Aurangzeb, K. 2019. Short-term electric load and price forecasting using enhanced extreme learning machine optimization in smart grids. *Energies, 12*(5), 866.

Pedrycz, W., & Wang, X. 2015. Designing fuzzy sets with the use of the parametric principle of justifiable granularity. *IEEE Transactions on Fuzzy Systems, 24*, 489–496.

Peiffer, M., Burssens, A., De Mits, S., Heintz, T., Van Waeyenberge, M., Buedts, K., Victor, J., & Audenaert, E. 2022. Statistical shape model-based tibiofibular assessment of syndesmotic ankle lesions using weight-bearing CT. *Journal of Orthopaedic Research®*, *40*, 2873–2884.

Rajangam, S., & Palanisamy, K. 2023. Cerebral cortex segmentation from MR brain images based on contouring technique to detect Alzheimer's disease. *International Journal of Computing and Digital Systems*, *14*, 1–1.

Ramya, J., Maheswari, B. U., Rajakumar, M., & Sonia, R. 2022. Alzheimer's disease segmentation and classification on MRI brain images using enhanced expectation maximization adaptive histogram (EEM-AH) and machine learning. *Information Technology and Control*, *51*, 786–800.

Rehman, A. 2023. Brain stroke prediction through deep learning techniques with ADASYN strategy. 2023 16th International Conference on Developments in eSystems Engineering (DeSE), Istanbul, Turkiye, pp. 679–684.

Saba, T., Al-Zahrani, S., & Rehman, A. 2012. Expert system for offline clinical guidelines and treatment. *Life Science Journal*, *9*(4), 2639–2658.

Saba, T., Bokhari, S. T. F., Sharif, M., Yasmin, M., & Raza, M. 2018a. Fundus image classification methods for the detection of glaucoma: A review. *Microscopy Research and Technique*, *81*(10), 1105–1121.

Saba, T., & Rehman, A. 2013. Effects of artificially intelligent tools on pattern recognition. *International Journal of Machine Learning and Cybernetics*, *4*, 155–162.

Saba, T., Rehman, A., Mehmood, Z., Kolivand, H., & Sharif, M. 2018b. Image enhancement and segmentation techniques for detection of knee joint diseases: A survey. *Current Medical Imaging*, *14*(5), 704–715.

Sadad, T., Rehman, A., Munir, A., Saba, T., Tariq, U., Ayesha, N., & Abbasi, R. 2021. Brain tumor detection and multi-classification using advanced deep learning techniques. *Microscopy Research and Technique*, *84*(6), 1296–1308.

Salvatore, C., Cerasa, A., Battista, P., Gilardi, M. C., Quattrone, A., Castiglioni, I., & Initiative, A. S. D. N. 2015. Magnetic resonance imaging biomarkers for the early diagnosis of Alzheimer's disease: A machine learning approach. *Frontiers in Neuroscience*, *9*, 307.

Scharre, D. W., Nagaraja, H. N., Wheeler, N. C., & Kataki, M. 2021. Self-administered gerocognitive examination: Longitudinal cohort testing for the early detection of dementia conversion. *Alzheimer's Research & Therapy*, *13*, 1–11.

Shi, J., Zheng, X., Li, Y., Zhang, Q., & Ying, S. 2017. Multimodal neuroimaging feature learning with multimodal stacked deep polynomial networks for diagnosis of Alzheimer's disease. *IEEE Journal of Biomedical and Health Informatics*, *22*, 173–183.

Simoes, R., Van Cappellen Van Walsum, A.-M., & Slump, C. H. 2014. Classification and localization of early-stage Alzheimer's disease in magnetic resonance images using a patch-based classifier ensemble. *Neuroradiology*, *56*, 709–721.

Tahir, B., Iqbal, S., Usman Ghani Khan, M., Saba, T., Mehmood, Z., Anjum, A., & Mahmood, T. 2019. Feature enhancement framework for brain tumor segmentation and classification. *Microscopy Research and Technique*, *82*(6), 803–811.

Tharwat, A. 2020. Classification assessment methods. *Applied Computing and Informatics*, *17*, 168–192.

Yousaf, K., Mehmood, Z., Saba, T., Rehman, A., Munshi, A. M., Alharbey, R., & Rashid, M. 2019. Mobile-health applications for the efficient delivery of health care facility to people with dementia (PwD) and support to their carers: A survey. *BioMed Research International*, *2019*, 7151475.

Chapter 7

Skin Cancer Detection and Classification Using Explainable Artificial Intelligence for Unbalanced Data: State of the Art

Ahmad Bilal Farooq, Shahzad Akbar, Qurat ul Ain, Zunaira Naqvi, and Farwa Urooj

Riphah College of Computing, Riphah International University, Faisalabad Campus, Faisalabad, Pakistan

7.1 Introduction

Explainable artificial intelligence–driven technologies are swiftly integrated into everyday routine life. However, many efforts are being made in medical field for real-time diagnosis and treatment. For effective disease detection and diagnosis, machine learning and deep learning techniques in the medical have been utilized to identify multiple diseases, including central serous retinopathy (Hassan, Akbar, & Khan, 2024), papilledema (Akbar et al., 2017), brain tumors (Gull, Akbar, & Naqi, 2023; Gull, Akbar, & Shoukat, 2021; Khan et al., 2023), glaucoma

DOI: 10.1201/9781032626345-7

(Naqi et al., 2023; Shoukat et al., 2023), melanoma (Farooq et al., 2023; Javed, Rahim, Saba, & Rehman, 2020; Safdar, Akbar, & Shoukat, 2021), pneumonia (Ijaz et al., 2023; Urooj, Akbar, Hassan, & Gull, 2023), lungs cancer, Alzheimer's (Ahmad et al., 2021), heart disease (Fahad et al., 2018; Iftikhar et al., 2017), vessel detection (Jamal et al., 2017), breast cancer (Husham et al., 2016), cataract disease (Shirazi, Akbar, Hassan, & Urooj, 2022), and leukemia (Arif et al., 2022).

The human body's most critical and essential part is the skin, which protects us from the harmful environment. However, it is one of the deadliest diseases among all cancers in the present decade. Mostly, skin cancer spreads in the body due to the uncontrolled growth of cells in the human body. Also, the new cells repair the skin when the skin cells are damaged. Another reason for skin cancer is the dangerous ultraviolet rays that come from sun exposure (Zhao et al., 2022).

Moreover, melanoma has been considered the most lethal type of skin cancer among all skin cancer types. The American Cancer Society (ACS) declares that the total number of melanoma cases reported in 2022 in men and women is 99,780 (Raza et al., 2021). The World Health Organization (WHO) reports that 132,000 and 2–3 million victims of melanoma and non-melanoma globally occur, respectively (World Health Organization (WHO), 2021). However, skin cancer is categorized into two types—the first is melanoma, and the second is non-melanoma (Kassani & Kassani, 2019). The types of skin cancer are explained below.

7.1.1 Melanoma

Melanoma has been developed by cells known as melanocytes, which start spreading only when skin melanocytes begin to grow out of control. It appears when the skin is exposed to sunlight, such as the arms, lips, nose, face, hands, etc. Melanoma can be treated only if the disease is detected at an early stage; otherwise, the patient will not survive (Hameed, Shabut, Ghosh, & Hossain, 2020). Furthermore, melanoma can be categorized into various types, which are discussed below.

7.1.1.1 Nodular Melanoma

Nodular melanoma grows quickly compared to the other types of melanoma, and additionally, it grows mostly below the skin. Anyone can have nodular melanoma, such as someone with a family history of people 50 years of age with skin cancer. Symptoms of nodular melanoma are itching, bleeding, and stinging (Thurnhofer-Hemsi & Domínguez, 2021).

7.1.1.2 Lentigo Melanoma

Lentigo melanoma occurs due to overexposure to dangerous sunlight, which contains ultraviolet radiation, and it develops mainly in the neck and head areas.

The main reason for lentigo melanoma is a gene mutation that changes your cells (Toğaçar, Cömert, & Ergen, 2021).

7.1.1.3 Intraocular Melanoma

The main reason for intraocular melanoma is older age and having fair skin. It mainly occurs in the tissues of the eye. Moreover, intraocular melanoma symptoms include dark vision in the iris. After examining the eye, the main cause can be found (Tschandl, Rosendahl, & Kittler, 2018).

7.1.1.4 Acral Lentiginous

Acral lentiginous melanoma mostly occurs in the hands, soles of the feet, and under the nails. It is a dark spot that differentiates between your normal skin and the affected skin color (Basurto-Lozada et al., 2021). Moreover, the symptoms of acral lentiginous include a damaged nail streak and a thick patch that grows on the feet.

7.1.1.5 Mucosal Melanoma

It mainly starts to develop in the mucus area, including the neck and head region, the anus, and the gastrointestinal tract. It is a very rare melanoma type among all melanomas—nearly 1%. The symptoms of mucosal melanoma are not normal, so doctors are still trying to figure out the cause of mucosal melanoma (Vestergaard, Macaskill, Holt, & Menzies, 2008).

7.1.1.6 Desmoplastic Melanoma

Desmoplastic melanoma usually occurs due to genetic disturbances, which form tumors. It has a ratio of only 4%, which is very rare. The affected spots are pink or red in color. Furthermore, it is developed on the face, scalp, neck, and arm (Waheed, Waheed, Zafar, & Riaz, 2017). The graphical representation of melanoma and its types is shown in Figure 7.1.

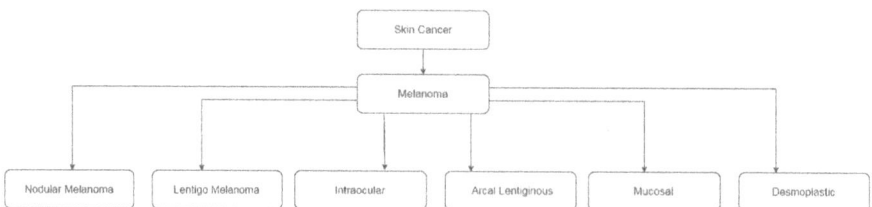

Figure 7.1   Skin cancer melanoma division.

7.1.2 Non-melanoma

The majority of types fall into the non-melanoma category, such as basal cell carcinoma (BCC), squamous cell carcinoma (SCC), and sebaceous gland carcinoma (SGC), and all of these cells are found in the middle layer of the epidermis (Thurnhofer-Hemsi & Domínguez, 2020). Non-melanoma types are easier to treat and diagnose compared to melanoma, which is a hard one. Doctors use biopsy to treat early skin cancer detection, which involves the removal of tissue from suspected skin lesions. Furthermore, medical detection is done to identify whether skin cancer is deadly or not and to discriminate the symptoms, whether it is melanoma or non-melanoma. There are different kinds of non-melanoma types, which are explained below.

7.1.2.1 Bowen's Disease

Bowen's disease has been considered the earliest type of skin cancer that is not life-threatening. Moreover, its symptoms include red, scaly patches on the skin. It is a slowly growing type of skin cancer with a rare chance of becoming dangerous (Wang et al., 2014).

7.1.2.2 Actinic Keratoses

It consists of dry, scaly patches of a different color, such as red or pink, and can vary in size from millimeters to centimeters. Sometimes, the skin can become thick, such as on horns and spikes (Wei, Ding, & Hu, 2020).

7.1.2.3 Squamous Cell Carcinoma

It consists of a rough, crusted surface with a firm pink lump. Sometimes, a spiky horn comes to the surface. Furthermore, the lump is very smooth because, when touched, it may bleed (Schwartz & Schwartz, 1988).

7.1.2.4 Basal Cell Carcinoma

Basal cell carcinoma consists of a small, shiny pink lump with a waxy appearance. The lump can become bigger and rusty, which results in bleeding. Moreover, there has been only a 5% chance of it spreading to other body parts (Wong, Strange, & Lear, 2003). The graphical representation of non-melanoma is shown in Figure 7.2.

Traditionally, imaging data has been collected through the digital camera, which has been used to arrange many images collected from various types of datasets. Sometimes, after collecting images, data is appropriately cleansed, such as noise, hair removal, better contrast, and resizing the images. Furthermore, the processed

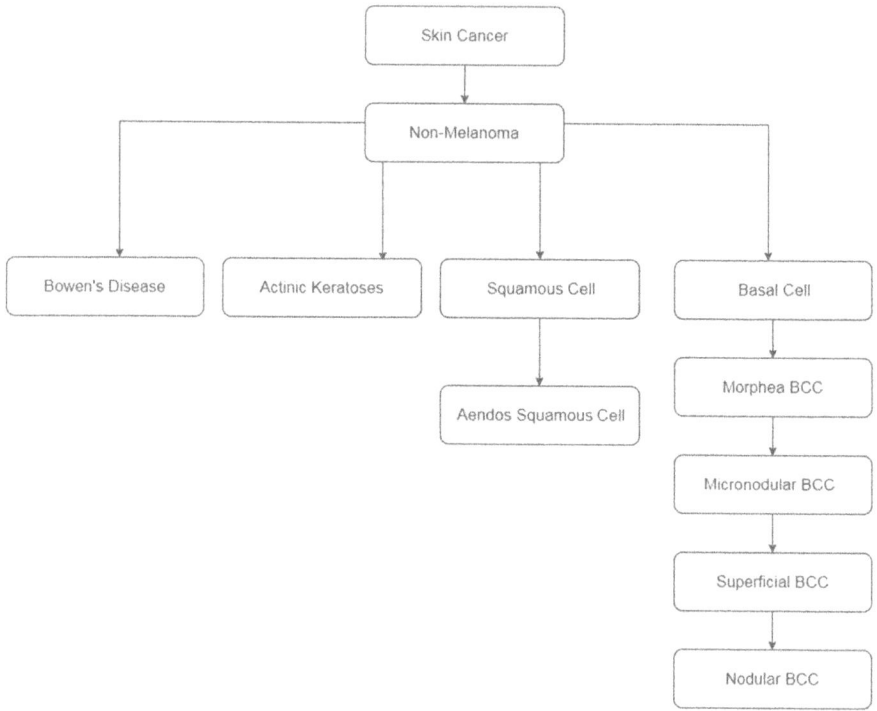

Figure 7.2   Skin cancer non-melanoma division.

data is used in the segmentation process to improve the quality of images. After segmentation, the data is again tested and trained to predict whether it is melanoma or non-melanoma (Sikkandar et al., 2021). Different datasets, such as HAM10000, Dermnet, Atlas Derm, ISIC, and many more, were taken from the Kaggle repository (Ali et al., 2021). In the past decade, deep learning has emerged as a revolutionary field in computer science because it is known as the most realistic subfield of machine learning. Deep learning algorithms perform the same function as the human brain and have been used in various fields, including voice recognition, pattern matching, and bioinformatics. In addition, CNN works in layers such as an input layer, a hidden layer, and an output layer. Furthermore, the main layers of CNN are pooling and fully connected layers, which consist of backpropagation and feed-forward architectures to learn weights available in every connection layer, as shown in Figure 7.3.

The remaining part of this chapter is as follows: Section 7.2 describes existing studies, their working methodologies, the use of datasets, results obtained from the proposed method, and their cons. Section 7.3 elaborates on the discussion of the chapter, for example, what skin is, its types, causes, an overall discussion about their datasets, and the workings of deep learning and machine learning. Section 7.4 finally concludes the chapter.

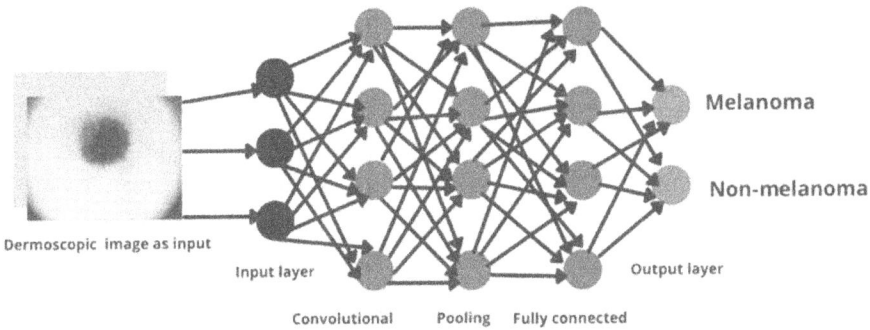

Figure 7.3 **CNN architecture for skin lesion detection and classification.**

7.2 Literature Review

Different types of machine learning and deep learning algorithms have been discussed in this section. Furthermore, the working of algorithms, the accuracies of the proposed methods, specificity, sensitivity, and performance matrices have been elaborated.

Garcia (2021) proposed that ResNet50 be selected for melanoma skin cancer detection. The dataset used by the proposed method contained 27,531 images. The datasets ISIC-2019, PH2 Database, and 7-point were used. The results significantly increased the performance of malignant tumors and benign moles. The proposed method achieved 47.22% Jacquard distance similarity, an F1 score of 0.53%, and a precision of 0.32%. It is one of the best ways to tackle the main challenges in the deep learning medical field.

Thurnhofer-Hemsi and Domínguez (2020) proposed that DenseNet201 be used to detect melanoma skin cancer. For the automatic detection of seven types of skin cancer, transfer learning was applied to CNN to create the two-level classifier. The dataset HAM1000 was used by the proposed method. DenseNet201 achieved 96% accuracy for correct classifications. The simple CNN method performed better than the two-level classifier. The unique class was only required to generate accurate and better results.

Zhang et al. (2020) proposed an optimized CNN for the discrimination of melanoma and non-melanoma. Optimized CNN used a whale optimization algorithm, and other proposed methods were Alex-Net, RESNET, and Inception v3. The dataset was taken from Derma Quest and Dermis, which contained 22,000 images. They used MatLab R2016 software for experimentation, in which the accuracy achieved by the proposed method was 80%.

Pacheco and Krohling (2020) proposed a CNN architecture to detect skin cancer. They were not able to make classification more efficient in SCC and BCC. The dataset contained 1,612 images obtained from the dermatologist Assistant Program (PAD) of melanoma and non-melanoma cells. CNN architectures like ResNet, Google Net, VGG Net, and Mobile Net were utilized. Google Net and Mobile Net achieved

94.48% accuracy, VGG Net obtained 93.37% accuracy, and ResNet achieved 95% accuracy. The aggregation approach would increase its efficiency in SCC and BCC.

Vasconcelos and Vasconcelos (2020) proposed the DCNN technique for melanoma classification. The dataset used by the proposed method was ISIC-2016, and the accuracy achieved by the proposed method was 83%. Its primary purpose is to increase the performance of the proposed method by implementing the RES-NET architecture. The proposed method had the vision of improving the ROI of the lesions.

Thurnhofer-Hemsi and Domínguez (2021) proposed DenseNet201 to detect skin cancer with seven types of moles. The dataset used by the proposed method was HAM10000, which consists of 10,050 images. The proposed technique consists of five neural network states, combining two classifiers, plain and hierarchical. The process of including prediction using probability techniques was a different research line. Data augmentation techniques were applied to achieve better accuracy. The accuracy achieved by the proposed method was 95%.

Ali et al. (2021) proposed a DCNN model for detecting benign and malignant moles. The dataset used by the proposed method was HAM10000. For a better evaluation, the proposed model of DCNN was compared with transfer learning algorithms such as VGG-16, RESNET, and Mobile Net. The accuracy achieved by the proposed method in training was 93.16%, and in testing, it was 91.93%. In the future, the author will work on a large dataset for accurate results.

Jiang, Li, and Jin (2021) proposed DRA Net to detect skin cancer diagnoses with the help of CAD systems. The proposed method's dataset was histopathological images, with 1,167 images. The proposed method achieved better results than traditional models like InceptionV3, ResNet50, and VGG16. The proposed method achieved an accuracy of 86.8%.

Pacheco and Krohling (2021) proposed a Meta-Block algorithm for the classification of skin cancer. The Meta-Block algorithm was compared with Meta Net based on feature extraction. The author used the Metadata process by extracting the relevant images from the dataset. The datasets used by the proposed method were ISIC-2019 and PAD-UFES-20. The proposed method achieved 96% accuracy.

Nida et al. (2022) proposed Retina Net and Conditional Random Field (CRF) to detect melanoma skin cancer and its segmentation. The process was carried out in three steps—the first was preprocessing, the second was melanoma localization, and the last was melanoma segmentation. The datasets used by the proposed method were PH2, ISIC-2017, and ISIC-2018 for melanoma detection. The pixel-level accuracy shown by the proposed method was 94%, with a sensitivity of 93% and a specificity of 97%.

Reis, Turk, Khoshelham, and Kaya (2022) proposed InSiNet, a deep learning technique to diagnose benign and malignant skin cancer moles. The datasets used by the proposed method were HAM10000, ISIC-2018, ISIC-2019, and ISIC-2020. The accuracy and processing time were evaluated using the proposed technique and other machine learning algorithms such as Google Net, Dense Net, ResNet152V2, SVM, and many more. The proposed technique achieved 94.59%, 91.89%, and 90.54% on the ISIC-2018, ISIC-2019, and ISIC-2020 datasets, respectively.

Hurtado and Reales (2021) proposed eight classifiers with different mixtures, such as artificial neural network (ANN), SVM, and KNN, compared with augmentation and without augmentation techniques for the detection of malignant skin cancer. The digital camera captured the images for the dataset. In addition, results were smothered by smooth bootstrapping. The most promising accuracy was given by ANN, which was 87.1%, and later on, it was improved from 84.3%. The computational cost was very slow because it worked directly from the feature vector.

Toğaçar et al. (2021) proposed MobileNetV2 to detect melanoma composed of residual blocks and spiking networks. The dataset for the proposed approach was taken from the ISIC archive, which consisted of 1,800 benign and 1,497 malignant images. In addition, an autoencoder was used to reconstruct the dataset. The accuracy achieved by the proposed approach was 95.27%. For future work, the SNN model would select fewer and fewer features than the current approach.

Zhang (2021) proposed EfficientNet-B6 for the detection and classification of melanoma diagnosis. In addition, the dataset utilized by the proposed method was the ISIC 2020 challenge. The proposed methodology captures the network depth and input resolution in the baseline network. Furthermore, it was expanded by the compound scaling method, which uses compound coefficient ϕ and network depth d. The result generated by the proposed technique was a 91.7 AUC–ROC score. The proposed technique is complex because it utilizes the resources twice to obtain results.

Soenksen et al. (2021) proposed deep convolutional neural network (DCNN) for identifying and classifying melanoma-pigmented skin lesions. The proposed method's dataset was extracted from an online database comprising 38,283 images. The proposed method consisted of three convolutional layers, which extracted the features of single lesion classification and extracted features from whole images. Furthermore, the proposed method obtained 90.3% sensitivity, 95% confidence interval, and 89.9% specificity. The presented methodology would like to reduce overfitting to the maximum level in the future.

Vani, Kavitha, and Subitha (2021) proposed self-organizing map (SOM) and CNN architecture used to detect melanoma. The proposed approach utilized 500 images from the ISIC archive, in which 350 images for training and 150 for testing were used. The proposed methodology consisted of a preprocessing step used to enhance images. Furthermore, the active contour was used for segmentation purposes to differentiate between infected and healthy regions. The accuracy attained by the proposed approach was 90%.

Nawaz et al. (2021) proposed faster region-based convolutional neural networks (FRCNNs) and SVM were utilized for melanoma localization and classification. Additionally, the dataset utilized by the proposed approach was ISIC-2016. The proposed methodology consisted of preprocessing step to enhance the quality of images. The accuracy achieved by the proposed approach was 89.1%, 85.9% sensitivity, and 87.0% specificity. In the future, the proposed method will be deployed for the detection of other skin diseases as well.

Raza et al. (2021) proposed pretrained models for ensemble learning such as Xception, InceptionV3, InceptionResNet-V2, DenseNet-121, and DenseNet-201 for melanoma classification. The dataset utilized by the proposed method was the Figshare benchmark dataset. The main purpose of the proposal was to increase the model's generalization ability and testing ability. The accuracy attained by the proposed approach was 97.93%, 97.50 specificity, and 97.83% sensitivity. In the future, the author will try to work on multi-classification.

Al-Hammouri, Fora, and Ibbini (2021) proposed an extreme learning machine (ELM) used to classify melanoma. Moreover, the dataset utilized by the proposed approach was MED-NODE, in which 100 images for each class were categorized after the melanoma and normal augmentation process. The ELM approach consists of three main layers; input, hidden (multi layers), and output layer weights can be calculated very fast to avoid overfitting issues. The accuracy achieved by the proposed approach was 97% from 11 features and 91% using 5 features. In the future, the author will try to implement this method with a large dataset and multi-classification.

Bansal, Garg, and Soni (2022) proposed EfficientNetB0 for the classification of melanoma. Additionally, the two datasets utilized by the proposed approach were HAM10000, and PH2. The features from the dermoscopic images were extracted from the ResNet50V2 combined HC (Hand Crafted) feature extraction technique. The proposed methodology attained an accuracy of 94.9% on HAM10000 and 98% on the PH2 dataset. In the future, the author will combine different types of features from the images and improve the feature selection process.

Zhao et al. (2022) proposed U-Net++ for melanoma segmentation, and previous studies were based on only Fully Connected Networks (FCN) and U-Net. In addition, the proposed methodology was based on the ISIC-2018 dataset, which consisted of 2,594 training, 100 for validation, and 1000 images for the testing dataset. The proposed model consisted of solving the problem of vanishing gradient problem. The proposed method achieved a Jaccard Index 84.73% for task 1. In the future, the author will try to enhance the model with an attention mechanism.

Pereira et al. (2022) proposed multiple instance learning (MIL) and other learning approaches used for melanoma classification and segmentation using 3D features. In addition, the proposed approach utilized the datasets PH2, MED-NODE, and Atlas. The deep learning algorithms performed the classification process using RGB and MIL performed the 3D feature extraction process. The proposed ensemble learning model obtained 90.82% accuracy, 78.57% sensitivity, and 92.82% specificity. In the future, utilize large datasets and depth surfaces to enhance the classification process.

Alahmadi (2022) proposed a multiscale attention U-Net for melanoma skin cancer detection. In addition, the proposed approach's datasets were ISIC-2017, PH2, and ISIC-2018. To overcome the limitation of the traditional U-Net model, an attention process was inserted into the bottleneck of the hierarchical representation. The results achieved by the ISIC-2017 dataset were F1 score 90%, sensitivity 88%, accuracy 95%, and specificity 97%. Moreover, the results obtained by the ISIC-2018 dataset were 89% F1 score, 84% sensitivity, 95% accuracy, and 97% specificity. The performance of the PH2 dataset was 96% accuracy, 94% sensitivity, and 96% specificity (Table 7.1).

Table 7.1 A Comparative Study of Skin Cancer Analysis Using Deep Learning

References	Authors	Disease Detection	Classifiers	Datasets	Results
Garcia (2021)	Garcia.	Melanoma	ResNet50	27,531 images were used ISIC dataset	F1 score 53%, precision 32%
Thurnhofer-Hemsi and Domínguez (2020)	Thurnhofer et al.	Melanoma	DenseNet201	HAM1000	DenseNet201 achieved 96% accuracy
Zhang et al. (2020)	Zhang et al.	Melanoma and non-melanoma	Optimized CNN	22,000 images were used	Accuracy achieved by the proposed method was 80%
Pacheco and Krohling (2020)	Pacheco et al.	Melanoma and non-melanoma	CNN architecture	The dataset contained 1,612 images	95% accuracy is achieved
Mahbod et al. (2019)	Mahbod et al.	Melanoma and seborrheic keratosis	Alex Net, VGG16, and ResNet-18	ISIC-2017 dataset was used for experimentation	The accuracy achieved by melanoma was 83.83%, and seborrheic keratosis was 97.55 %
Vasconcelos and Vasconcelos (2020)	Vasconcelos et al.	Melanoma	DCNN	The dataset used by the proposed method was ISBI 2016	The accuracy achieved by the proposed method was 83%

(Continued)

Table 7.1 (Continued)

References	Authors	Disease Detection	Classifiers	Datasets	Results
Thurnhofer-Hemsi and Domínguez (2021)	Hemsi and Domínguez	Skin cancer with seven types of moles	DenseNet201	HAM10000 consists of 10,050 images	The accuracy achieved by the proposed method was 95%
Ali et al. (2021)	Ali et al.	Malignant moles	DCNN model	HAM10000	The accuracy achieved by the proposed method in training was 93.16%, and testing was 91.93%
Jiang et al. (2021)	Jiang and Jin	Malignant, benign, and inflammatory dermatoses	DRA Net	Histopathological images, which contained 1,167 images	Accuracy 86.8%
Pacheco and Krohling (2021)	Pacheco and Krohling	Melanoma and non-melanoma	Meta-Block algorithm	The dataset used by the proposed method was ISIC-2019 and PAD-UFES-20	The proposed method achieved 96% accuracy
Nida et al. (2022)	Nida et al.	Melanoma	Retina-Net, Conditional Random Field (CRF)	PH2, ISIC-2017, and ISIC-2018	Accuracy 94%, sensitivity 93%, and specificity 97%

(Continued)

Table 7.1 (Continued)

References	Authors	Disease Detection	Classifiers	Datasets	Results
Reis et al. (2022)	Reis et al.	Malignant	InSiNet	HAM10000, ISIC–2018	94.49% accuracy on ISIC–2018, 91.89%
Hurtado and Reales (2021)	Hurtado and Reales	Malignant	ANN, SVM, and KNN	Images captured through a digital camera (local dataset)	The most promising accuracy was given by ANN, which was 87.1%, and later improved from 84.3%
Toğaçar et al. (2021)	Toğaçar et al.	Malignant	MobileNetV2	1,497 malignant and 1,800 benign images	The accuracy achieved by the proposed approach was 95.27%
Zhang (2021)	Zhang	Melanoma	EfficientNet-B6	ISIC 2020	91.7 AUC–ROC score
Soenksen et al. (2021)	Soenksen et al.	Melanoma	DCNN	38,283 images	90.3% sensitivity, 95% confidence interval, and 89.9% specificity
Vani et al. (2021)	Vani et al.	Melanoma	CNN	500 images	90% accuracy
Nawaz et al. (2021)	Nawaz et al.	Melanoma	FRCNN	ISIC–2016	Accuracy 89.1 %, 85.9% sensitivity, and 87.0 % specificity

(Continued)

Table 7.1 (Continued)

References	Authors	Disease Detection	Classifiers	Datasets	Results
Raza et al. (2021)	Raza et al.	Melanoma	Xception, InceptionV3, InceptionResNet-V2, DenseNet-121, and DenseNet-201	Figshare benchmark dataset	Accuracy 97.93%, 97.50 specificity, and 97.83% sensitivity
Al-Hammouri et al. (2021)	Hammouri et al.	Melanoma	Extreme learning machine (ELM)	MED-NODE	97% accuracy
Bansal et al. (2022)	Bansal et al.	Melanoma	EfficientNetB0	HAM10000, and PH2	94.9% on HAM10000 and 98% on the PH2 dataset
Zhao et al. (2022)	Zhao et al.	Melanoma	U-Net++	ISIC-2018	The Jaccard Index for task 1 is 84.73%
Pereira et al. (2022)	Pereira et al.	Melanoma	Multiple instance learning (MIL)	PH2, MED-NODE, and Atlas	90.82 % accuracy, 78.57% sensitivity, and 92.82% specificity
Alahmadi (2022)	Alahmadi	Melanoma	Multiscale Attention U-Net	ISIC-2017	ISIC-2017 dataset with 90% F1 score, sensitivity 88%, accuracy 95%, and specificity 97%

7.2.1 Machine Learning

A branch of artificial intelligence (AI) known as machine learning uses prediction, historical, and past data to predict the outcome; for example, viruses and malware detection systems, weather forecasting systems, and fraud detection systems are based on machine learning (Hurtado & Reales, 2021). However, machine learning plays a significant role in life since a large bunch of data surrounds our lives and everybody wants to achieve remarkable victory in every competition; so, in difficult and complex situations, machine learning performs automated tasks and takes predicted decisions very quickly (Figures 7.4–7.6) (Mijwil, 2021).

Almansour and Jaffar (2016) proposed an SVM algorithm for melanoma skin cancer detection. Sixty-nine images were collected from the Denis database used in the suggested technique. Local binary pattern (LBP) and gray-level co-occurrence matrix (GLCM) were the primary methods used to extract features. Furthermore, GLCM was not as effective as LBP, but the proposed approach achieved 90.32% accuracy, 85.84% sensitivity, and 93.97% specificity.

Adjed et al. (2016) proposed detecting skin cancer disease using the SVM algorithm. For better detection of disease, they applied wavelets and curvelets. They used ROI's database for the proposed approach and provided 655 images. LBP was utilized to differentiate between melanoma and non-melanoma diseases by

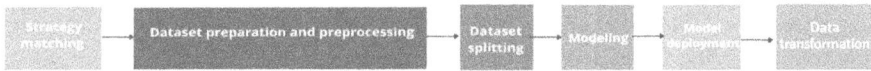

Figure 7.4   Machine learning architecture.

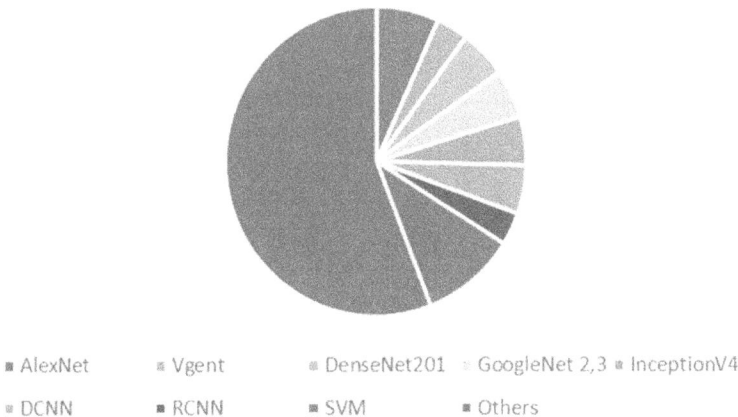

- AlexNet
- Vgent
- DenseNet201
- GoogleNet 2,3
- InceptionV4
- DCNN
- RCNN
- SVM
- Others

Figure 7.5   Classifiers used in literature review for skin cancer detection.

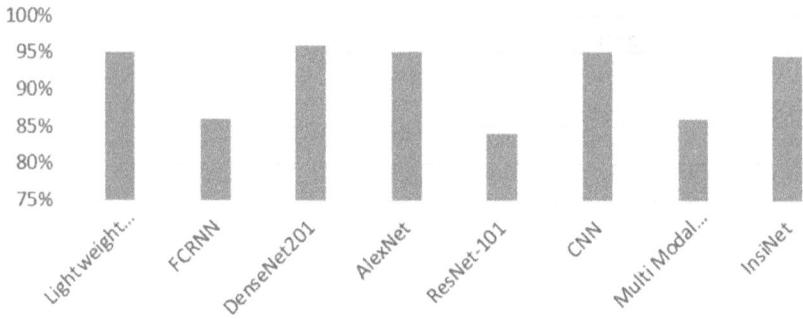

Figure 7.6   Comparison of classifiers with their accuracies.

extracting features from the images. The proposed approach achieved 76.1% accuracy, 75.6% sensitivity, and 76.6% specificity.

Hameed et al. (2020) proposed a multi-class multi-level (MCML) classifier to detect skin cancer disease. Mobile-enabled expert systems should be developed in areas where fewer medical facilities are available. The proposed method used 3,672 images, which were biopsy-proven and taken from the Dermis derma Quest database. In MCML, the noise was removed because of the preprocessing done by the traditional machine learning method. The accuracy achieved by the proposed method was 96.47%.

Hameed, Shabut, and Hossain (2018) proposed melanoma, eczema, benign psoriasis, and acne detection with the help of quadratic SVM and CAD systems. The proposed method involves preprocessing, segmentation, feature extraction, and classification. For accurate and reliable results, deep neural networks should be used. Furthermore, a total of 1,800 images were utilized in MATLAB 2018 for experimentation purposes. The proposed technique achieved 86% accuracy.

Mustafa, Dauda, and Dauda (2017) proposed an SVM classifier that was used for the detection of melanoma skin cancer. The computer can better visualize the patterns that humans are unable to identify. The proposed method used a total of 80 images that were taken from the Derma Quest database. The proposed method used light to enhance visual graphics for grab-cut segmentation. The proposed method achieved an accuracy of 80%, a precision of 86.21%, and a specificity of 55.36%.

Tan, Zhang, and Jiang (2016) proposed SVM and a genetic algorithm (GA) for the classification of skin cancer detection using dermoscopic images. For further improvement, GA would be combined with hybrid feature optimization. The system was developed to reduce noise from the images, fetch features from lesions, and select features for further classification. The proposed method used 1,300 dermoscopic images from the Dermfit database. The proposed method achieved an accuracy of 88%, a sensitivity of 83%, and a specificity of 89%.

Javaid, Sadiq, and Akram (2021) proposed that quadratic discriminant, SVM, and random forest were used for the classification of benign and malignant tumors, in addition to the OTSU algorithm used for segmentation. After the segmentation of gray-level features, histogram-oriented features were extracted from the segmented images. The dataset used by the proposed method was ISBI-2016, which already contained ground truth and labeled RGB images. The accuracy achieved by the random forest was 93.89%, the quadratic discriminant was 90.84%, and the SVM was 88.17%.

Luu, Le, and Phan (2021) proposed a random forest technique for the classification of squamous cell carcinoma (SCC), basal cell carcinoma (BCC), melanoma, and regular features of skin lesions. The dataset used for the proposed approach was 282 BCC, 231 SCC, 52 melanoma, and 42 normal images. The average precision achieved by the proposed technique was 93%. This study provided a cost-effective and accurate solution for skin cancer diagnosis.

7.3 Discussion

Skin is one of the most important parts of the human body since it protects us from the harmful effects of the environment. This chapter has studied and analyzed different research papers on diagnosing skin cancer lesions using deep learning and machine learning. Additionally, skin cancer is categorized into two types—the first is melanoma, and the second is non-melanoma. Moreover, melanoma is the worst among all skin cancers that have occurred in history. The ACS declares that the total number of cases reported in 2022 of melanoma in men and women is 99,780. Melanoma develops in cells known as melanocytes and spreads when melanocytes grow out of control. It appears when the skin is exposed to sunlight, such as arms, lips, nose, face, hands, etc. Melanoma can be treated if it is detected early; otherwise, patients will die. There are many types of melanomas, such as nodular melanoma and malignant melanoma. Mainly, most cases fall under the category of non-melanoma types such as BCC, SCC, and SGC. All three of these cells are found in the middle layer of the epidermis. Types of non-melanoma are easier to treat and diagnose compared to melanoma, which is a hard one. In addition, doctors use a biopsy to treat early skin cancer, which involves the removal of the record from suspected skin lesions.

Furthermore, medical detection is done to identify whether skin cancer is deadly or not and to discriminate the symptoms, whether it is melanoma or non-melanoma. Furthermore, deep learning algorithms solve the problem of skin cancer detection and perform the same function as the human brain. It has been used in various fields, including voice recognition, pattern matching, and bioinformatics. Traditionally, data is collected through the digital camera because it is used to arrange many images from various datasets. After collecting images, the data has been appropriately cleaned, such as for noise, hair removal, better contrast, and resizing the images. After improving the quality of the images, the processed data moves on to the segmentation process. After segmentation, the data is again tested and trained to predict whether it is melanoma or non-melanoma skin cancer. For the sake of diagnosis in deep learning, CNN and its various architectures have been analyzed with their results using deep learning algorithms like Res Net, U-Net, FCRCNN, enhanced CNN, Alex-Net, and many more. This chapter analyzed different datasets with their accuracies, sensitivity, specificity, and precision parameters. Among all the algorithms, CNN architectures achieved the highest accuracy, which is 98% in Table 7.2. In machine learning, SVM is used in most cases in diagnosing skin cancer lesions.

Moreover, only SVM and CNN showed great results when combined with Alex-Net and the GA. When deep learning is compared with machine learning, deep learning algorithms have shown excellent results. Machine learning is still present here but performs well when combined with different deep learning algorithms.

Table 7.2   A Comparative Study of Machine Learning Skin Cancer Analysis

References	Authors	Disease Detection and Classification	Classifiers	Datasets	Results
Almansour and Jaffar (2016)	AL Mansour et al.	Melanoma	SVM classifier	The proposed method used 69 images from the Dermis database	Accuracy 90.32%, sensitivity 84.84%, and specificity 93.97%
Adjed et al. (2016)	Added et al.	Melanoma and non-melanoma	SVM classifier	Proposed method used 655 images from the ROIs database	Accuracy 76.1%, sensitivity 75.6%, and specificity 76.6%
Hameed et al. (2020)	Hameed et al.	Melanoma and eczema	Multiclass multilevel (MCML)	The proposed method used 3,672 images which were biopsy-proven and taken from the Dermis derma Quest database	The accuracy achieved by the proposed method was 96.47%
Hameed et al. (2018)	Hameed et al.	Melanoma, acne, eczema, psoriasis, and benign	Quadratic SVM classifier with CAD	The proposed method used 1,800 images	Accuracy 86%

(Continued)

Table 7.2 (Continued)

References	Authors	Disease Detection and Classification	Classifiers	Datasets	Results
Mustafa et al. (2017)	Mustafa et al.	Melanoma	SVM classifier	The proposed method used a total of 80 images	Accuracy 80%, precision 86.21%, and specificity 55.36%
Tan et al. (2016)	Tan et al.	Benign and malignant	SVM and GA	The proposed method used 1,300 dermoscopic images	Accuracy 88%, sensitivity 83%, and specificity 89%
Javaid et al. (2021)	Javaid et al.	Benign and malignant	SVM, random forest, and quadratic discriminant	ISBI 2016	Accuracy random forest was 93.89% Quadratic discriminant was 90.84%, and the SVM was 88.17%
Luu et al. (2021)	Luu et al.	SCC, BCC, melanoma, and normal features of skin lesions	Random forest technique	The dataset contained 282 BCC, 231 SCC, 52 melanoma, and 42 normal images	The average precision achieved by the proposed technique was 93%

But let us look at deep learning algorithms. A single CNN achieved incredible accuracy compared to machine learning algorithms. Furthermore, various types of datasets and their explanations have been discussed. However, these datasets are HAM1000, PH2, ISIC, Derm IS, Dermnet NZ, and Dermnet.

7.4 Conclusion

Traditionally, dermatologists detect skin cancer through manually scanned images. However, this method was old, unreliable, and time-consuming because skin cancer patients died due to its late detection. Melanoma and non-melanoma both are dangerous types of skin cancer, but melanoma is the worst. Due to advancements in the field of AI, many automated and fast techniques were discovered by researchers due to health concerns. Different types of researchers have made their contributions to machine learning and deep learning areas of research. This chapter discusses various deep learning and machine learning techniques for a fast and reliable way to detect skin cancer. However, different datasets have been evaluated using dermoscopic images from publicly available dermatology databases. Moreover, current research cannot solve the problems, such as when the patient asks for skin cancer symptoms that appear on their body. Thus, in the future, for efficient skin cancer detection, researchers will solve problems regarding unbalanced datasets and low-resolution images and perform full-body photography to speed up skin lesion detection. The idea of auto-organization has emerged from the area of deep learning and will automate the whole process. Currently, the auto-organization model is still in the development phase and continues to evolve. Furthermore, it can drastically increase the efficiency of medical image processing, where minor features are essential for diagnosing the disease at critical times.

Acknowledgment

This work was supported by the Riphah Artificial Intelligence Research (RAIR) Lab, Riphah International University, Faisalabad Campus, Pakistan.

References

Adjed, F., Faye, I., Ababsa, F., Gardezi, S. J., & Dass, S. C. (2016). Classification of skin cancer images using local binary pattern and SVM classifier. In *AIP Conference Proceedings*, vol. 1787, no. 1, AIP Publishing.

Ahmad, M. F., Akbar, S., Hassan, S. A. E., Rehman, A., & Ayesha, N. (2021). Deep learning approach to diagnose Alzheimer's disease through magnetic resonance images. 2021 International Conference on Innovative Computing (ICIC).

Akbar, S., Akram, M. U., Sharif, M., Tariq, A., & Yasin, U. U. (2017). Decision support system for detection of papilledema through fundus retinal images. Journal of Medical Systems, 41, 1–16.

Alahmadi, M. D. (2022). Multiscale attention U-Net for skin lesion segmentation. IEEE Access, 10, 59145–59154.

Al-Hammouri, S., Fora, M., & Ibbini, M. (2021). Extreme learning machine for melanoma classification. 2021 IEEE Jordan International Joint Conference on Electrical Engineering and Information Technology (JEEIT).

Ali, M. S., Miah, M. S., Haque, J., Rahman, M. M., & Islam, M. K. (2021). An enhanced technique of skin cancer classification using deep convolutional neural network with transfer learning models. Machine Learning with Applications, 5, 100036.

Almansour, E., & Jaffar, M. A. (2016). Classification of dermoscopic skin cancer images using color and hybrid texture features. International Journal of Computer Science and Network Security, 16(4), 135–139.

Arif, R., Akbar, S., Farooq, A. B., Hassan, S. A., & Gull, S. (2022). Automatic detection of leukemia through convolutional neural network. 2022 International Conference on Frontiers of Information Technology (FIT).

Bansal, P., Garg, R., & Soni, P. (2022). Detection of melanoma in dermoscopic images by integrating features extracted using handcrafted and deep learning models. Computers & Industrial Engineering, 168, 108060.

Basurto-Lozada, P., Molina-Aguilar, C., Castaneda-Garcia, C., Vázquez-Cruz, M. E., Garcia-Salinas, O. I., Álvarez-Cano, A., …, Possik, P. A. (2021). Acral lentiginous melanoma: Basic facts, biological characteristics and research perspectives of an understudied disease. Pigment Cell & Melanoma Research, 34(1), 59–71.

Fahad, H., Ghani Khan, M. U., Saba, T., Rehman, A., & Iqbal, S. (2018). Microscopic abnormality classification of cardiac murmurs using ANFIS and HMM. Microscopy Research and Technique, 81(5), 449–457.

Farooq, A. B., Akbar, S., Arif, R., Hassan, S. A., & Gull, S. (2023). Melanoma classification through deep learning using dermoscopic images. 2023 International Conference on IT and Industrial Technologies (ICIT).

Garcia, S. I. (2021). Meta-learning for skin cancer detection using deep learning techniques. arXiv:2104.10775.

Gull, S., Akbar, S., & Naqi, S. M. (2023). A deep learning approach for multi-stage classification of brain tumor through magnetic resonance images. International Journal of Imaging Systems and Technology, 33(5), 1745–1766.

Gull, S., Akbar, S., & Shoukat, I. A. (2021). A deep transfer learning approach for automated detection of brain tumor through magnetic resonance imaging. 2021 International Conference on Innovative Computing (ICIC).

Hameed, N., Shabut, A. M., Ghosh, M. K., & Hossain, M. A. (2020). Multi-class multi-level classification algorithm for skin lesions classification using machine learning techniques. Expert Systems with Applications, 141, 112961.

Hameed, N., Shabut, A., & Hossain, M. A. (2018). A computer-aided diagnosis system for classifying prominent skin lesions using machine learning. 2018 10th Computer Science and Electronic Engineering (CEEC).

Hassan, S. A., Akbar, S., & Khan, H. U. (2024). Detection of central serous retinopathy using deep learning through retinal images. Multimedia Tools and Applications, 83(7), 21369–21396.

Hurtado, J., & Reales, F. (2021). A machine learning approach for the recognition of melanoma skin cancer on macroscopic images. TELKOMNIKA (Telecommunication Computing Electronics and Control), 19(4), 1357–1368.

Husham, A., Hazim Alkawaz, M., Saba, T., Rehman, A., & Saleh Alghamdi, J. (2016). Automated nuclei segmentation of malignant using level sets. Microscopy Research and Technique, 79(10), 993–997.

Iftikhar, S., Fatima, K., Rehman, A., Almazyad, A. S., & Saba, T. (2017). An evolution based hybrid approach for heart diseases classification and associated risk factors identification. Biomedical Research, 28(8), 3451–3455.

Ijaz, A., Akbar, S., AlGhofaily, B., Hassan, S. A., & Saba, T. (2023). Deep learning for pneumonia diagnosis using CXR images. 2023 Sixth International Conference of Women in Data Science at Prince Sultan University (WiDS PSU).

Jamal, A., Hazim Alkawaz, M., Rehman, A., & Saba, T. (2017). Retinal imaging analysis based on vessel detection. Microscopy Research and Technique, 80(7), 799–811.

Javaid, A., Sadiq, M., & Akram, F. (2021). Skin cancer classification using image processing and machine learning. 2021 International Bhurban Conference on Applied Sciences and Technologies (IBCAST).

Javed, R., Rahim, M. S. M., Saba, T., & Rehman, A. (2020). A comparative study of features selection for skin lesion detection from dermoscopic images. Network Modeling Analysis in Health Informatics and Bioinformatics, 9(1), 4.

Jiang, S., Li, H., & Jin, Z. (2021). A visually interpretable deep learning framework for histopathological image-based skin cancer diagnosis. IEEE Journal of Biomedical and Health Informatics, 25(5), 1483–1494.

Kassani, S. H., & Kassani, P. H. (2019). A comparative study of deep learning architectures on melanoma detection. Tissue and Cell, 58, 76–83.

Khan, A., Akbar, S., Alghanim, A., Hassan, S. A., & Ayesha, N. (2023). Automated hybrid model for detection and classification of brain tumor. 2023 Sixth International Conference of Women in Data Science at Prince Sultan University (WiDS PSU).

Luu, N. T., Le, T.-H., & Phan, Q.-H. (2021). Characterization of Mueller matrix elements for classifying human skin cancer utilizing random forest algorithm. Journal of Biomedical Optics, 26(7), 075001.

Mahbod, A., Schaefer, G., Wang, C., Ecker, R., & Ellinge, I. (2019). Skin lesion classification using hybrid deep neural networks. ICASSP 2019-2019 IEEE International Conference on Acoustics, Speech and Signal Processing (ICASSP).

Mijwil, M. M. (2021). Skin cancer disease images classification using deep learning solutions. Multimedia Tools and Applications, 80(17), 26255–26271.

Mustafa, S., Dauda, A. B., & Dauda, M. (2017). Image processing and SVM classification for melanoma detection. 2017 International Conference on Computing Networking and Informatics (ICCNI).

Naqi, S. A. E. A., Akbar, S., Iqbal, K., Hassan, S. A., & Gull, S. (2023). An automated hybrid glaucoma detection framework through retinal images. 2023 International Conference on IT and Industrial Technologies (ICIT).

Nawaz, M., Masood, M., Javed, A., Iqbal, J., Nazir, T., Mehmood, A., & Ashraf, R. (2021). Melanoma localization and classification through faster region-based convolutional neural network and SVM. Multimedia Tools and Applications, 80(19), 28953–28974.

Nida, N., Shah, S. A., Ahmad, W., Faizi, M. I., & Anwar, S. M. (2022). Automatic melanoma detection and segmentation in dermoscopy images using deep RetinaNet and conditional random fields. Multimedia Tools and Applications, 81, 1–21.

Pacheco, A. G., & Krohling, R. A. (2020). The impact of patient clinical information on automated skin cancer detection. Computers in Biology and Medicine, 116, 103545.

Pacheco, A. G., & Krohling, R. A. (2021). An attention-based mechanism to combine images and metadata in deep learning models applied to skin cancer classification. IEEE Journal of Biomedical and Health Informatics, 25(9), 3554–3563.

Pereira, P. M., Thomaz, L. A., Tavora, L. M., Assuncao, P. A., Fonseca-Pinto, R., Paiva, R. P., & Faria, S. M. (2022). Multiple instance learning using 3D features for melanoma detection. IEEE Access, 10, 76296–76309.

Raza, R., Zulfiqar, F., Tariq, S., Anwar, G. B., Sargano, A. B., & Habib, Z. (2021). Melanoma classification from dermoscopy images using ensemble of convolutional neural networks. Mathematics, 10(1), 26.

Reis, H. C., Turk, V., Khoshelham, K., & Kaya, S. (2022). InSiNet: A deep convolutional approach to skin cancer detection and segmentation. Medical & Biological Engineering & Computing, 60, 643–662.

Safdar, K., Akbar, S., & Shoukat, A. (2021). A majority voting based ensemble approach of deep learning classifiers for automated melanoma detection. 2021 International Conference on Innovative Computing (ICIC).

Schwartz, R. A., & Schwartz, R. A. (1988). Squamous cell carcinoma. Skin Cancer: Recognition and Management, pp. 36–47. Springer.

Shirazi, S. N., Akbar, S., Hassan, S. A., & Urooj, F. (2022). Computer-aided diagnosis of cataract disease through retinal images. 2022 International Conference on IT and Industrial Technologies (ICIT).

Shoukat, A., Akbar, S., Hassan, S. A., Iqbal, S., Mehmood, A., & Ilyas, Q. M. (2023). Automatic diagnosis of glaucoma from retinal images using deep learning approach. Diagnostics, 13(10), 1738.

Sikkandar, M. Y., Alrasheadi, B. A., Prakash, N., Hemalakshmi, G., Mohanarathinam, A., & Shankar, K. (2021). Deep learning based an automated skin lesion segmentation and intelligent classification model. Journal of Ambient Intelligence and Humanized Computing, 12(3), 3245–3255.

Soenksen, L. R., Kassis, T., Conover, S. T., Marti-Fuster, B., Birkenfeld, J. S., Tucker-Schwartz, J., …, Senna, M. M. (2021). Using deep learning for dermatologist-level detection of suspicious pigmented skin lesions from wide-field images. Science Translational Medicine, 13(581), eabb3652.

Tan, T. Y., Zhang, L., & Jiang, M. (2016). An intelligent decision support system for skin cancer detection from dermoscopic images. 2016 12th International Conference on Natural Computation, Fuzzy Systems and Knowledge Discovery (ICNC-FSKD).

Thurnhofer-Hemsi, K., & Domínguez, E. (2020). A convolutional neural network framework for accurate skin cancer detection. Neural Processing Letters, 1–21.

Thurnhofer-Hemsi, K., & Domínguez, E. (2021). A convolutional neural network framework for accurate skin cancer detection. Neural Processing Letters, 53(5), 3073–3093.

Toğaçar, M., Cömert, Z., & Ergen, B. (2021). Intelligent skin cancer detection applying autoencoder, MobileNetV2 and spiking neural networks. Chaos, Solitons & Fractals, 144, 110714.

Tschandl, P., Rosendahl, C., & Kittler, H. (2018). The HAM10000 dataset, a large collection of multi-source dermatoscopic images of common pigmented skin lesions. Scientific Data, 5(1), 1–9.

Urooj, F., Akbar, S., Hassan, S. A., & Gull, S. (2023). Computer-aided system for pneumothorax detection through chest X-ray images using convolutional neural network. 2023 International Conference on IT and Industrial Technologies (ICIT).

Vani, R., Kavitha, J., & Subitha, D. (2021). Novel approach for melanoma detection through iterative deep vector network. Journal of Ambient Intelligence and Humanized Computing, 1–10. doi: https://doi.org/10.1007/s12652-021-03242-5

Vasconcelos, C. N., & Vasconcelos, B. N. (2020). Experiments using deep learning for dermoscopy image analysis. Pattern Recognition Letters, 139, 95–103.

Vestergaard, M., Macaskill, P., Holt, P., & Menzies, S. (2008). Dermoscopy compared with naked eye examination for the diagnosis of primary melanoma: A meta-analysis of studies performed in a clinical setting. British Journal of Dermatology, 159(3), 669–676.

Waheed, Z., Waheed, A., Zafar, M., & Riaz, F. (2017). An efficient machine learning approach for the detection of melanoma using dermoscopic images. 2017 International Conference on Communication, Computing and Digital Systems (C-CODE).

Wang, G., Wang, Y., Li, H., Chen, X., Lu, H., Ma, Y., …, Tang, L. (2014). Morphological background detection and illumination normalization of text image with poor lighting. PLoS One, 9(11), e110991.

Wei, L., Ding, K., & Hu, H. (2020). Automatic skin cancer detection in dermoscopy images based on ensemble lightweight deep learning network. IEEE Access, 8, 99633–99647.

Wong, C., Strange, R., & Lear, J. (2003). Basal cell carcinoma. BMJ, 327(7418), 794–798.

World Health Organization (WHO). (2021). Available at: https://www.who.int/news-room/questions-and-answers/item/radiation-ultraviolet-(uv)-radiation-and-skin-cancer#:~:text=Currently%2C%20between%202%20and%203,skin%20cancer%20in%20their%20lifetime (accessed September 19, 2021).

Zhang, N., Cai, Y.-X., Wang, Y.-Y., Tian, Y.-T., Wang, X.-L., & Badami, B. (2020). Skin cancer diagnosis based on optimized convolutional neural network. Artificial Intelligence in Medicine, 102, 101756.

Zhang, R. (2021). Melanoma detection using convolutional neural network. 2021 IEEE International Conference on Consumer Electronics and Computer Engineering (ICCECE).

Zhao, C., Shuai, R., Ma, L., Liu, W., & Wu, M. (2022). Segmentation of skin lesions image based on U-Net++. Multimedia Tools and Applications, 81(6), 8691–8717.

Chapter 8

Enhancing Heart Disease Diagnosis with XAI-Infused Ensemble Classification

Naveed Abbas[1], Talha Tasleem[1], Abdul Hai[1],
Zieb Rabie Alqahtani[2], and Bandar Ali
Mohammed Alrami Alghamdi[3]

[1]*Department of Computer Science, Islamia College, Peshawar, Pakistan*
[2]*Vicube Lab, Faculty of Computing, University Technology, JB, Malaysia*
[3]*Faculty of Computer Studies, Arab Open University, Riyadh,*
  Kingdom of Saudi Arabia

8.1 Introduction

The heart, a vital and rapidly functioning organ, demands meticulous care. Given the prevalence of heart-related diseases, predictive analysis and comparative research become imperative. Late disease detection, often caused by inaccurate instruments, leads to unfortunate patient outcomes, underscoring the urgent need for enhanced predictive algorithms. Machine learning (ML) serves as an effective testing method, rooted in the principles of training and evaluation (Fahad et al., 2018). It is a subset of artificial intelligence (AI), a broad domain where machines emulate human capabilities. ML systems, specifically, are trained to analyze and harness data, sometimes referred to as machine intelligence when these technologies converge. In this study, we harness biological parameters like cholesterol levels, blood pressure, gender, age, and more as testing data. These parameters form the basis for comparing the accuracy of various algorithms (Husham et al., 2016). The proposed study explores four distinct

DOI: 10.1201/9781032626345-8

ML algorithms: DT, RF, KNN, and SVM. Through this comparison, we aim to identify the most effective method among them. ML falls under the umbrella of AI and is further enriched by deep learning models (Aghamohammadi et al., 2019). The predictive capabilities of an ML model are rooted in its exposure to training data. By leveraging past experiences, the model gains insights to guide predictions on new data instances. ML and AI represent rapidly advancing domains, particularly within the healthcare sector, offering tailored clinical support. In this realm, healthcare data encompasses both electronic health records (EHR) and data collected from Internet of Things (IoT) devices. Given the structured and unstructured data mix, humans face challenges in extracting actionable insights and informed decisions from these diverse data sources (Dhillon & Singh, 2019). Leveraging IoT and ML methodologies, healthcare services can readily extend to individuals in distant regions as well as those seeking initial medical guidance. The amalgamation of ML and AI has already demonstrated its efficacy in processing medical images for disease detection, identification, and prognosis (Hussain et al., 2020; Jabeen et al., 2018). The convergence of cloud-integrated solutions with IoT advancements facilitates the efficient delivery of healthcare services and the maintenance of patients' eMR (Srinivasu et al., 2021). Notably, mobile edge computing plays a pivotal role in providing timely computational services for the industrial (IIoT) (Ma et al., 2021). Felkey & Fox (2016) explored the practicality of mobile apps that consistently monitor patient medication adherence and caregiver engagement. This aids in the management of patients' eMR and facilitates efficient patient–physician communication. IBM Watson systems leverage AI-powered technologies within the medical field to extract insights about drug discovery, identify cancerous cells, and explore the intricacies of the immune system's response to cancer. Within the Internet of Medical Things framework, AI and ML leverage deep learning through convolutional neural networks (CNN) to predict heart diseases (Iftikhar et al., 2017; Pan et al., 2020; Saba & Rehman, 2013).

In this research, four distinct ML models are employed for the classification of heart diseases, alongside their associated explanations as an XAI. The evaluation of performance metrics is conducted both with and without explanations. The four specific models utilized in this context encompass the decision tree (DT), random forest (RF), support vector machine, and KNN (Adadi & Berrada, 2018). Notably, the primary emphasis of this study centers around the utilization of the SHAP method. Furthermore, based on the insights provided by the explanations, factors like feature contributions and feature weights are considered for feature selection. The features that are shortlisted through this process are then utilized as inputs for the RF model to perform subsequent classification, with a subsequent analysis of the resulting metrics.

The goals of the present research are outlined as follows in a bullet-point format:

■ Utilizing XAI ML methods to showcase model features and produce desired predictions, facilitates doctors in ascertaining prediction outcomes and diagnosing heart diseases effectively.

■ Among the four utilized ML models employed for classification, RF demonstrated the most favorable outcomes in terms of performance metrics.

■ The heart disease classification process is established, and predictions for patients with cardiovascular conditions are conducted using attributes such as "age," "sex," "cholesterol," "Max HR," and "chest pain." Additional details and features of the dataset can be found in Table 8.1.

■ Statistical measures for all factors related to heart diseases within a sample dataset are examined.

■ The most significant four features have been highlighted according to their contributions in the RF classifier. These top four features were selected based on their contributions as determined by the explainable techniques applied to the RF classifier.

■ The assessment of XAI-driven prediction of cardiovascular disease with ML classifiers entails an analysis of its performance through various statistical metrics.

There are six separate components in the current study, AI, XAI, and ML classifiers are highlighted in Section 8.1 as being crucial in the healthcare industry. This is followed by a thorough analysis of the body of research in Section 8.2. The definition of XAI is provided in Section 8.3. The approaches which include multiple ML algorithms and their experimental results are examined in Section 8.4. In Section 8.5, the outcomes of the trials are broken down, and in Section 8.6, the study's conclusion is distilled from the data and prospective future directions are outlined.

8.2 Related Work

Integrating into healthcare apps unquestionably plays a crucial function in the world of medicine (Chaudhry et al., 2017). However, the outcomes produced by ML models must be capable of elucidating the rationale behind the machine's choices and providing validation for the credibility of the forecasts (Larabi-Marie-Sainte et al., 2019; Tjoa & Guan, 2020). The potential of integrating AI with intelligent wearable devices holds significant promise in advancing healthcare. Embedding healthcare functionalities into smart wearables, like smartwatches, enables the gathering, forecasting, and analysis of health information. The incorporation of an explainable AI system is crucial for increasing confidence and reliability in the findings. As XAI's demand arises due to the challenges posed by opaque ML models, this has given rise to concerns regarding accountability, transparency, and trustworthiness in the generated outcomes. Consequently, it becomes crucial to develop methodologies utilizing explainable AI systems (Mughal, Sharif, Muhammad, & Saba, 2018b). This approach ensures that predictions rendered by AI systems are comprehensible, thus assisting medical practitioners in accurate patient diagnoses. This, in turn, nurtures a sense of confidence and reliability in the predictions derived from ML models (Janssen et al., 2022; Muhsin et al., 2014). AI certainly occupies a vital role in the healthcare domain, particularly in conjunction with healthcare applications. Nonetheless, the results produced by ML models must possess the ability to elucidate the machine's decisions, thereby reinforcing the credibility of the predictions (Tjoa & Guan, 2020). Guleria et al. (2022) have presented a sophisticated framework aimed at predicting heart disease by employing advanced deep learning methodologies. Researchers undertook ML experiments centered on coronary artery disease (CAD) within the Nigerian context. Among the evaluated models, the RF model proved to be the most precise in its predictive capabilities, closely trailed by the SVM, which showcased the most favorable sensitivity outcomes (Khan et al., 2022b; Saba et al., 2018; Samaras et al., 2023). Moreover, RF classifier demonstrated remarkable efficiency in predicting coronary artery stenosis among Taiwanese individuals with CAD, notably achieving a remarkable AUC value (Hsu et al., 2021; Naz et al., 2019). AI possesses the capability to categorize data and generate predictions through the aid of ML models. However, the lack of a comprehensive explanation for the relationships between input and output often results in predictive outcomes that lack accountability, transparency, and a clear grasp. The concept of XAI aims to enhance the interpretability of AI systems for human users, working to make their functions more intelligible and logically cohesive (Mughal et al., 2018a; Sharif et al., 2019). The terms transparency, interpretability, and explanation are often used interchangeably. Interpretability is associated with the degree to which a model can be understood (Gilpin et al., 2018), although it is also sometimes used in place of the term explain ability (Muhsin et al., 2014). Transparency can encompass a comprehensive lucidity that imparts collaborators with pertinent understandings of the model's functioning. This entails elucidations of training methodologies, scrutiny of training data distribution, code releases, and particulars at the level of specific traits (Javed et al., 2020). Alternatively, transparency can signify a distinct level of precision regarding the model's operation, divergent from opacity (Fellous et al., 2019). Fellous and coauthors (Calegari, Ciatto, Dellaluce, & Omicini, 2019), have investigated the implementation of XAI techniques in the field of neurosciences. In contrast, Dave and colleagues (Saba, Al-Zahrani, & Rehman, 2012) have explored the utilization of XAI methods using datasets associated with heart disease. Their objective is to enhance the trust of healthcare practitioners in AI systems, particularly by addressing outcomes stemming from opaque models in patient diagnosis (Khan et al., 2022a). The primary objective of XAI is to create AI systems that exhibit qualities such as comprehensibility, accountability, reliability, observability, interpretability, and explanatory capacity (Calegari, Ciatto, Dellaluce, & Omicini, 2019; Saba et al., 2012). The act of interpreting outcomes holds immense significance, particularly when they play a role in decision-making, particularly within the vital healthcare sector that directly impacts human lives. The core focus of the XAI domain is centered on elevating the efficacy of ML models by providing thorough explanations for the obtained results. Porto et al. (Porto, Molina, Berlanga, & Patricio, 2021; Rehman, 2023) have predicted cardiovascular disease using the heart dataset.

8.3 Development of a Cardiovascular Disease Prediction Using Explainable AI

AI methods contribute to resolving intricate tasks and achieving high levels of accuracy by mastering complex computational challenges (West, 2018). To enhance the efficacy of AI, XAI has been introduced, aiming to bolster the capabilities of ML models. XAI not only improves prediction accuracy in ML models but also offers insights into the functioning of ML models, especially in the context of deep learning and neural network models. Convolutional neural network (CNN)-based models have been employed for the detection of childhood pneumonia from chest X-ray images (Saba et al., 2018). DL models are employed for tasks like CT scan analysis, chest X-ray image assessment, heart disease prognosis (Yousaf et al., 2019), and reliable detection of lung ailments from medical images (Rehman, 2023). Additionally, these models have been leveraged to explore the predictive role of RhoB in rectal cancer patients (Sudheesh et al., 2023). The XAI framework entails that discussions or recommendations emerging from ML models are accompanied by comprehensive explanations (Ahmad et al., 2022). This practice instills confidence in accepting the generated outputs, as there exists a coherent rationale for the outcomes of ML models, particularly those categorized as black-box models. Black-box ML models employ various strategies to attain explainability, encompassing techniques such as (a) visualization approaches, (b) model explanation methods, (c) feature selection procedures, (d) assessment of feature relevance, (e) model simplification techniques, (f) provision of model explanations through examples, and (g) textual explanations, among others. The incorporation of XAI into the ML model framework addresses three fundamental inquiries: why, when, and how? These inquiries are primarily concerned with the predictions generated by the ML model, the confidence placed in its forecasts, and the mechanisms to rectify errors within the ML model. The integration of XAI and ML becomes especially crucial when the results derived from the ML model carry implications for human lives or society at large (Aggarwal et al., 2022). This is particularly pertinent in fields like healthcare, education, finance, weather forecasting, and medicine. For instance, in scenarios involving the prediction of a patient's disease using an ML model, the involvement of an XAI model becomes pivotal in deciding whether to rely on the ML model's predictions. XAI helps clarify the predictions generated by the ML model, the particular features selected for training the ML algorithms, and more. Figure 8.1a presents the implementation of ML methodology without XAI, while Figure 8.1b presents the implementation of ML methodology with XAI.

Figure 8.1b depicts the improved ML model, enhanced with XAI. The answers to the three essential questions – why, when, and how – are provided through the XAI module, which features an explanatory interface. The integration of XAI with black-box ML models becomes essential to expound upon the outcomes produced by ML and to elucidate the decision-making process. Through adequate explainability and transparency, healthcare professionals can place their trust in

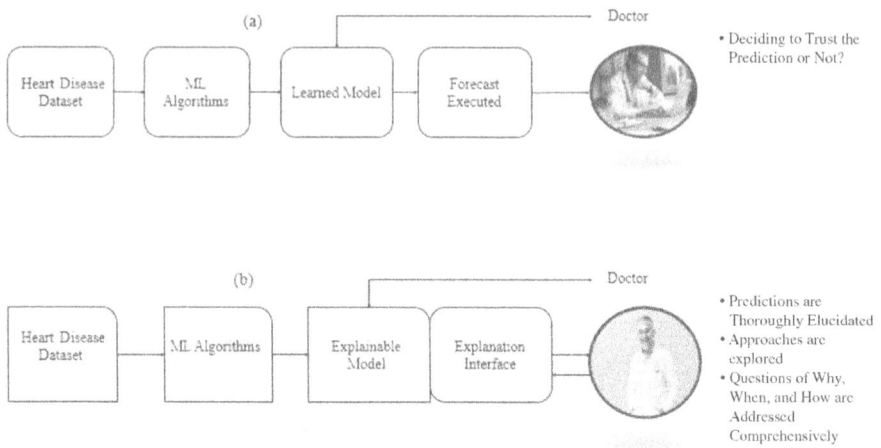

Figure 8.1 **(a) Implementation of ML methodology without the incorporation of explainable AI. (b) Enhanced ML approach integrated with explainable AI techniques.**

the predictions made by ML models. The conclusions drawn by ML models, particularly those utilizing deep neural networks, often possess intricate complexity and are challenging to grasp. As a result, medical practitioners and staff necessitate comprehensive explanations for predictive decisions, facilitating clinical assistance (Callahan & Shah, 2017).

8.4 Approach of Explainable AI across Different Classifiers

The proposed study employs an experimental approach that utilizes ML techniques to forecast cardiovascular risk. Within supervised ML, input data is matched with corresponding desired output labels, facilitating classification (Sadad et al., 2021). The model is then trained using ML algorithms while being guided by supervision, which subsequently enables predictions (Besse et al., 2019). Conversely, unsupervised learning involves unlabeled input data and focuses on clustering rather than classification (Guidotti et al., 2018). For this experiment, supervised ML algorithms are applied to the dataset presented in Table 8.1. Specifically, the experiment employs SVM, KNN, DT, and RF algorithms to predict heart disease. The predictive attributes include "age," "ST slope," and "cholesterol." These algorithms are compared based on accuracy and ROC curve values. The results furnish values generated by the ML model, indicating which patients are likely to have the disease and correctly identifying them as such (Aggarwal et al., 2022). Furthermore, the

Table 8.1   Heart Disease Dataset Variables and Their Description

S. No.	Attribute	Description
1	Age	Age of patients, in years
2	Sex	M = 1; F = 0
3	Chest pain type	1 is conventional angina, 2 is atypical angina, and 3 is non-angina chest discomfort, pain; 4 is asymptomatic
4	BP	Blood pressure at rest (in mmHg) at the time of hospital admission
5	Cholesterol	mg/dl of serum cholesterol
6	FBS over 120	Fasting blood sugar greater than 120 mg/dl (true or false)
7	EKG result	0 is normal; (1) having an irregular ST-T wave; (2) having left ventricular hypertrophy
8	MAX HR	Reached the highest possible heart rate
9	Exercise angina	Angina brought on by exercise (yes or no, 0)
10	ST depression	Exercise-induced ST depression compared to rest
11	Slope of ST	The peak workout ST segment's slope (1 is upsloping, 2 is flat, and 3 is down sloping).
12	Number of vessels	Number of main vessels (0–3) that are fluorescein-stained
13	Thallium	Defect categories include normal (3), fixed (6), and reversible (7)
14	Heart disease	Heart disease status (presence or absence)

outcomes spotlight cases where patients are misclassified as not having the disease when they do. The suggested model, coupled with the XAI framework for feature processing, is depicted in the block diagram in Figure 8.2.

In the domain of supervised learning, input variables are labeled and linked to their respective output variables. The ML classifier undergoes training using an existing dataset, during which model parameters can be selected. Feature extraction techniques can also be employed to optimize the model's effectiveness by selecting relevant features from the training dataset. Following training, the model becomes proficient at classifying input data and making the intended predictions.

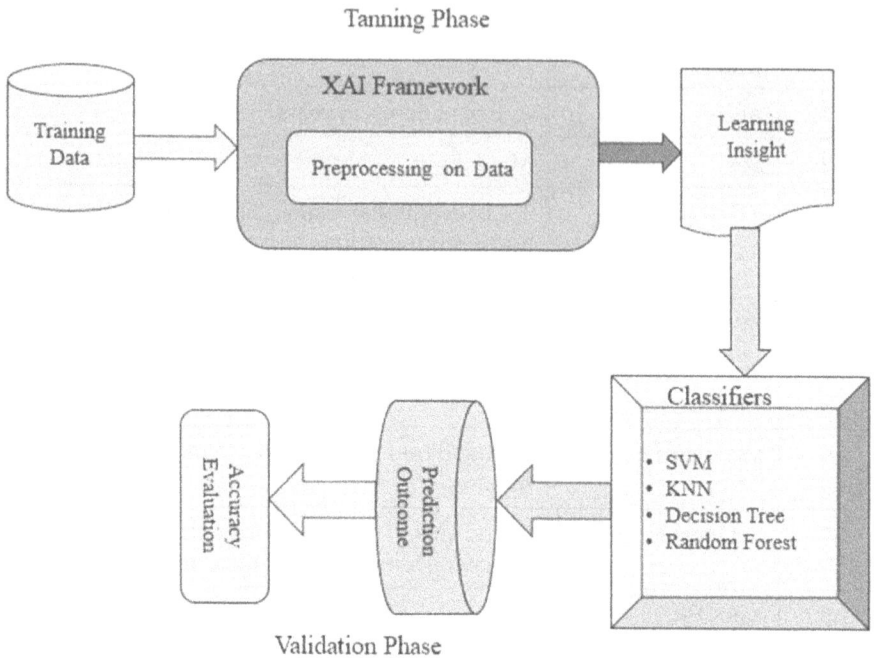

Figure 8.2 XAI framework employed in the feature processing to forecast heart disease.

8.4.1 Support Vector Machine (SVM)

This ML technique utilizes the concept of hyperplanes to classify data into distinct classes. The training dataset comprises (xi, yi) pairs, where $I = 1, 2, 3, ..., n$, with xi representing the ith vector and yi the target vector. The nature and number of hyperplanes determine the specific support vector (SV) method. For instance, if a straight line is employed as the hyperplane, it is referred to as linear SV. In the case of SVM, an accuracy rate of 84.1584% has been achieved. When utilizing all 13 attributes from the Cleveland dataset, an accuracy rate of 83.49% was attained (Pouriyeh et al., 2017). SVM constructs its model by establishing a hyperplane that effectively separates the provided data points. This separation is accomplished by maximizing the distance between the two clusters (Tahir et al., 2019; Xia, 2016). It identifies the nearest data vectors to the decision boundary within the training dataset, referred to as SVs, and then utilizes these SVs to classify specific test vectors (Son et al., 2010). The equation for determining the hyperplane is given by Equation (8.1):

$$F(i) = \beta + \omega_i T_i \qquad (8.1)$$

The hyperplane can be expressed as $|\beta + \omega_i T_i| = 1$, where β is the threshold value, ω_i is the weight vector, and T_i is the scalar offset. The instances in the training set closest to the hyperplane are called support vectors and denoted by i. For instance, a support vector machine method was used to predict how well patients with heart failure followed their medication (Guleria et al., 2022).

8.4.2 K-Nearest Neighbor (KNN)

The data are grouped based on how close they are to each other in terms of location. The groups of data that are near each other are called neighbors, and the user can decide how many neighbors to use for the analysis. The choice of the number of neighbors is crucial for the dataset. When $k = 3$, it implies there are three distinct data groups. Each group is represented in a two-dimensional space with coordinates (Xi, Yi), where Xi corresponds to the x-axis, Y to the y-axis, and $i = 1, 2, 3, …, n$. In a study conducted by Pouriyeh et al., an accuracy rate of 83.16% was obtained with a value of $K = 9$ (Sen, Hajra, & Ghosh, 2020; Abbas et al., 2015). In the KNN algorithm, the calculation involves determining the Euclidean distance. The distance between two points p and q, with Cartesian coordinates $(m1, n1)$ and $(m2, n2)$, is represented by Equation (8.2) (Haseeb et al., 2020; Abbas et al., 2018).

$$d\left(a, \beta\right) = \sqrt{\left(a_1 - \beta_1\right)^2 + \left(a_2 - \beta_2\right)^2} \tag{8.2}$$

8.4.3 DT

A DT functions as a classification algorithm well-suited for handling both categorical and numerical data. It is employed to construct tree-like structures that aid in decision-making. DTs are commonly utilized tools for handling medical datasets due to their simplicity and ease of analysis. The tree-shaped graph representation of data is straightforward to interpret and study. Three different types of nodes are used in the DT model:

Root Nodes: The pivotal node upon which all other nodes hinge.
Interior Nodes: Manage different characteristics or features.
Leaf Nodes: Represent the outcomes of individual tests.

Data are split within the tree based on attributes that offer the highest information gain or lowest entropy. The entropy of each attribute is calculated to gauge the extent to which it reduces uncertainty mentioned through Equations (8.3) and (8.4).

$$\text{entropy} = \sum_{i=1}^{e} - P_i \log_2 P_i \tag{8.3}$$

$$\text{Gain}(S, A) = \text{entrop}(s) - \sum_{\text{VE} = \text{values}(A)\frac{|SV|}{|S|}} \text{entropy (SV)} \qquad (8.4)$$

The entropy Equation (8.3) employs P_{ij} to denote the probability of each node, and the entropy of each node is determined based on this probability. The node with the highest entropy value is designated as the root node, and this process is reiterated for the remaining nodes until the entire tree is constructed or all nodes are accounted.

When the distribution of nodes is imbalanced, the creation of the tree can lead to overfitting issues, which negatively impacts calculations. This imbalance is one of the reasons why DTs tend to exhibit lower accuracy compared to SVM. Even though DT analysis presents data in a tree-like structure, resulting in higher accuracy compared to other algorithms, there is a possibility of overclassifying the data due to the examination of only one attribute at a time for decision-making. Chauhan et al.'s DT demonstrated an accuracy rate of 71.43% (Haseeb et al., 2020). In contrast, another study achieved a relatively lower accuracy of 42.8954% (Bouali & Akaichi, 2014).

8.5 Description of the Dataset and Implementation Environment

8.5.1 Data Collection

The dataset used in this analysis is sourced from the UCI repository, a reputable and extensively verified resource endorsed by numerous researchers and the UCI authority (Shahmiri, 2016). Specifically, we utilized the Cleveland Heart dataset from the UCI ML repository. This dataset comprises 14 variables and 303 observations. It includes 13 predictor variables and 1 categorical outcome variable, denoted as "Heart disease." The predictor variables encompass numerical attributes such as age, trtbps, chol, thalach, and old peak, as well as categorical attributes like sex, exercise angina, chest pain type, fbs, ekg, slope of ST, and thallium.

8.5.1.1 Attribute Selection

The attributes of the dataset encompass the distinct characteristics of the data employed within the system. In the context of heart prediction, certain attributes encompass factors like an individual's heart rate, gender, age, and additional factors, as indicated in Table 8.1.

Table 8.2 provides insight into the implementation environment and the framework utilized for simulation. This table outlines the resources employed during the simulation process to achieve optimal model performance. The statistical metrics for each of these attributes are outlined in Table 8.3.

Table 8.2 Specifics Regarding the Parameters of the Implementation Environment Utilized in the Present Study Are Provided

Experiment Configuration	Specification
Operating systems	Microsoft Windows 10
System type	x64-based type
Processor	Intel Corei5 2360H-1165 CPU @ 2.5 GHz
Architecture	64-bit
Processor graphics in use	Intel(R) Iris Xe Graphics
Installed Physical (RAM)	5 GB
Software used	Matlab R2021a, Weka 3.8.5

Table 8.3 Display Statistical Metrics and Information Related to the Feature Sets

Attribute	Min	Mean	Max	Std	Description
Age	29	54.4	77	9.10	Age of patients, in years
Sex	0	0.67	1	0.46	Male = 1; female = 0
Chest pain type	1.0	3.17	4	0.95	1 is conventional angina, 2 is atypical angina, and 3 is non-angina chest discomfort, pain; 4 is asymptomatic
BP	94	131	200	17.8	Blood pressure at rest (in mmHg) at the time of hospital admission
Cholesterol	126	249	564	51.6	mg/dl of serum cholesterol
FBS over 120	0	0.14	1	0.35	Fasting blood sugar greater than 120 mg/dl (true or false)
EKG result	0	1.02	2	0.99	0 is normal; (1) having an irregular ST-T wave; (2) having left ventricular hypertrophy
Max HR	71	149	202	23.1	Reached the highest possible heart rate
Exercise angina	0	0.32	1	0.47	Angina brought on by exercise (yes or no, 0)

(Continued)

Table 8.3   (Continued)

Attribute	Min	Mean	Max	Std	Description
ST depression	0	1.05	6	1.14	Exercise-induced ST depression compared to rest
Slope of ST	1	1.58	3	0.61	The peak workout ST segment's slope (1 is upsloping, 2 is flat, and 3 is down sloping)
Number of vessels	0	0.67	3	0.94	Number of main vessels (0–3) that are fluorescein-stained
Thallium	3	4.69	7	1.94	Defect categories include normal (3), fixed (6), and reversible (7)
Heart disease	0	0.54	1	0.49	Heart disease status (presence or absence)

8.6 Results and Conversations

The proposed approach involves utilizing explainable artificial intelligence (XAI) for applying ML classifiers to predict cardiovascular disease. Several performance indicators, including area under the curve (AUC), accuracy, true positive rate (TPR), recall, and precision are measured to assess the method (Chen, Liu, & Peng, 2019). The decision-making process becomes more trustworthy because of the application of XAI approaches, which improve the properties of the model's interpretability. To ensure the model's effectiveness, values from the confusion matrix are employed (Jamal et al., 2017). True positives are instances of irregularities that have been accurately identified, while true negatives represent correctly identifying negative cases of normalcy. False positives occur when normal cases are mistakenly identified as positive, and false negatives arise when cases that should be identified as positive are classified as negative. The comparison of results from the dataset involves four machine-learning models: DT, RF, KNN, and SVM. The RF algorithm achieves the highest accuracy of 99.1% after being trained on the dataset, outperforming the other algorithms. This indicates RF's effectiveness in accurately predicting instances of cardiovascular disease based on the provided data.

The SVM took 8.223 seconds for training, utilizing a linear kernel function employing the one-versus-one multiclass approach. KNN achieved an accuracy of 79.5% in a training time of 6.706 seconds. The DT required 5.678 seconds for training and achieved an accuracy of 95.4%. Moving on to the RF model, it yielded the lowest accuracy at 99.5%. However, its training time was shorter than the other two models, specifically 5.678 seconds.

Table 8.4 Performance Metrics of Different Classifiers

Model	Accuracy (%)	TNR/ Specifics (%)	TPR/ Recall (%)	F Score (%)	Precision (%)	Training Time (s)
KNN	71.1	69.7	81.1	78.6	76.2	6.706
SVM	95.5	71.7	92.5	85.7	79.8	8.223
DT	95.4	72.6	91.4	84.8	80.1	6.833
RF	99.1	70.5	93.1	86.9	79.9	6.678

RF achieves higher classification accuracy than the DT. As a result, we will omit the DT and instead, in the forthcoming section focused on utilizing XAI techniques for explanation, we will opt for RF as the fundamental algorithm (Saba et al., 2018a).

A post-justification of the model's forecasted results is given at the post-modeling stage's last step. Here, the results lack inherent self-explanation and remain obscure to the model's initial design. Given that black-box models inherently lack transparency, to make these models more accessible by removing internal logic or output patterns, techniques including leveraging model features, local logic, and global logic are used. Consequently, in this segment of the XAI process, a comparison ensues between the results generated by both types of models. The performance metrics is presented in Table 8.4.

Using test findings, the ROC curve is used in training to categorize a patient's illness state as positive or negative. It identifies the optimal threshold value that offers the most effective symptomatic performance (Narkhede, 2018; Abbas et al., 2019b). The present model incorrectly classified 7% of the data as positive, according to the RF model, which has a false positive rate (FPR) of 0.7. A TPR of 0.91 clear shows that the model accurate classification rate is 91%. The ROC curve is renowned as the probability curve, where the TPR is plotted on the vertical axis and the FPR on the horizontal axis. The trade-off between the TPR and the FPR across diverse probability thresholds is succinctly described. This trade-off is observed in a predictive software model for heart disease, which employs varying probability thresholds (Rehman et al., 2023). The interpretation of model performance is facilitated through ROC curves, which are depicted for the KNN, SVM, DT, and RF trained models. The ROC curve graphically represents the TPR and FPR values of the trained ML models.

Table 8.5 presents that classifier outcomes are comparatively lower than those of the other models. These methods include identifying outliers, determining a maximum margin solution, and reducing the dangers of both underfitting and overfitting. Overfitting, which signifies a significant disparity between training and testing bias, can lead to misleading or even detrimental clinical decision-making (Kernbach & Staartjes, 2022).

Table 8.5   Evaluating and Contrasting the Area under the Curve (AUC) Values among Different ML Classifiers

Reference	Disease	Dataset	Classification Techniques	AUC (Best Classifier)
Megna et al. (2021)	Heart disease	Federicoll University	ADA,AdaBoost,LR, NB,RF,Rpart,SVM, XGBoot	LR archived 75%
Sharma et al. (2022)	Heart disease	Dataset from UK Biobank pertaining to cardiovascular conditions	Artificial neural network (ANN), naive Bayes, RF, Lasso, ridge regression (RR), SVM, LR	RF archived 79.9%
Mujeeb et al. (2019)	Heart disease	Kazakh ethnic group residing in Xinjiang	Naive Bayes, RF, SVM, XGB DT, kNN, LR	LR archived 87.2%
Patro, Padhy, and Chiranjevi, (2021)	Heart disease	Cleveland dataset by UCI, Statlog heart disease dataset	LR, multiple linear regression, RR, DT, SVM, kNN, naive Bayes	Naive Bayes archived 83%
Yuvalı, Yaman, and Tosun (2022)	Coronary artery disease (CAD)	Dataset from NEU Hospital used for heart disease analysis	KNN, SVM, RF, ANN, naive Bayes, LR	LR archived 81.3%
XAI proposed classifiers	Heart disease	The UCI repository's Cleveland dataset is tailored for heart disease analysis	kNN, SVM, DT, RF	RF archived 99.1%

The effectiveness of the proposed ML classifiers driven by XAI surpasses that of traditional classification models. Additionally, the XAI framework provides greater interpretability and instills confidence in the decisions made. While evaluating real-world scenarios, the performance of the proposed model diverges significantly from the dataset employed in the evaluation. This divergence represents a potential challenge for the model. Analyzing real-time case studies involves multiple underlying factors, as training samples should ideally originate from the same demographic population. People residing in the same demographic region often share similar lifestyles and health standards. However, obtaining sufficient training and testing data is a complex endeavor, intertwined with technical and economic considerations. In future research, addressing the aforementioned issue in obtaining real-time data and assessing the ensemble model within the XAI framework could be a focal point.

8.7 Conclusion

In the healthcare industry, AI is playing a crucial role together with ML and IoT, emerging as a powerful tool for developing and implementing intelligent systems (Keleş et al., 2011). Applications powered by AI not only help patients save time and money, but they also provide initial clinical support. The combination of ML models and AI applications improves diagnostics, prognostics, procedures, and interpretations, and patient investigations with heightened precision. These technologies assist medical professionals, including physicians and radiologists, in reaching more definitive outcomes. In certain illnesses, accurate interpretation is a challenge, but the synergy of AI, ML, and IoT technologies is proving to be a blessing for patients situated in remote regions (Abbas et al., 2019a). This synergy provides initial aid, cost-savings, and relief from discomfort. This study delves into the contributions of AI and ML in healthcare, describing their benefits and difficulties in the sector. The study investigates a ML-based experimental strategy for cardiac disease prediction. Of note, the RF algorithm stands out in terms of performance, achieving an accuracy rate of 99.1% among all classifiers employed in heart disease classification.

The proposed study explores the ML algorithms SVM, KNN, DT, and RF. The research examines XAI methods in-depth, aiming to enhance the clarity and analysis of data from a dataset that is specifically focused on cardiac disease. An acknowledged limitation of existing models lies in the dataset's constrained attribute scope and sample size. Nevertheless, the study comprehensively elucidates classification models and delves into the outcomes when coupled with XAI techniques. The application of different ML classification and clustering algorithms on various healthcare datasets is one potential future attempt. This exploration aims to harness the capabilities of AI, ML, and IoT-rich intelligent systems within the healthcare sector. Expanding the research into the realms of deep learning and neural networks using larger cardiovascular disease datasets is also envisioned. Furthermore, integrating trained ML models into well-defined explainable AI interface systems is crucial. Such integration ensures that predictive outcomes from these models are both understandable and reliable for medical professionals and clinical support staff. In the present study, an XAI-driven approach for classifiers predicting heart disease is evaluated using a singular dataset, the Cleveland dataset. The model may be statistically analyzed using a variety of datasets, such as the UK Biobank dataset, the University Federico II dataset, the Statlog heart disease dataset, and the NEU Hospital dataset for heart disease, among others.

Acknowledgment

The authors acknowledge the Faculty of Computer Studies, Arab Open University, Riyadh, KSA, for their unconditional support.

References

Abbas, N., Mohamad, D., Abdullah, A. H., Saba, T., Al-Rodhaan, M., & Al-Dhelaan, A. (2015). Nuclei segmentation of leukocytes in blood smear digital images. Pakistan Journal of Pharmaceutical Sciences, 28(5), 1801–1806.

Abbas, N., Saba, T., Mohamad, D., Rehman, A., Almazyad, A. S., & Al-Ghamdi, J. S. (2018). Machine aided malaria parasitemia detection in Giemsa-stained thin blood smears. Neural Computing and Applications, 29, 803–818.

Abbas, N., Saba, T., Rehman, A., Mehmood, Z., Javaid, N., Tahir, M., ..., Shah, R. (2019a). Plasmodium species aware based quantification of malaria parasitemia in light microscopy thin blood smear. Microscopy Research and Technique, 82(7), 1198–1214.

Abbas, N., Saba, T., Rehman, A., Mehmood, Z., Kolivand, H., Uddin, M., & Anjum, A. (2019b). Plasmodium life cycle stage classification based quantification of malaria parasitaemia in thin blood smears. Microscopy Research and Technique, 82(3), 283–295.

Adadi, A., & Berrada, M. (2018). Peeking inside the black-box: A survey on explainable artificial intelligence (XAI). IEEE Access, 6, 52138–52160.

Aggarwal, R., Podder, P., & Khamparia, A. (2022). ECG classification and analysis for heart disease prediction using XAI-driven machine learning algorithms. In Biomedical Data Analysis and Processing Using Explainable (XAI) and Responsive Artificial Intelligence (RAI) (pp. 91–103). Springer.

Aghamohammadi, M., Madan, M., Hong, J. K., & Watson, T. (2019). Predicting heart attack through explainable artificial intelligence. Computational Science–ICCS 2019: 19th International Conference, Faro, Portugal, June 12–14, 2019, Proceedings, Part II 19. Springer.

Ahmad, G. N., Fatima, H., Ullah, S., & Saidi, A. S. (2022). Efficient medical diagnosis of human heart diseases using machine learning techniques with and without GridSearchCV. IEEE Access, 10, 80151–80173.

Besse, P., Castets-Renard, C., Garivier, A., & Loubes, J. M. (2019). Can everyday AI be ethical? Machine learning algorithm fairness. Statistiques et Société, 6(3), 105–112.

Bouali, H., & Akaichi, J. (2014). Comparative study of different classification techniques: Heart disease use case. 2014 13th International Conference on Machine Learning and Applications. IEEE.

Calegari, R., Ciatto, G., Dellaluce, J., & Omicini, A. (2019). Interpretable narrative explanation for ML predictors with LP: A case study for XAI. CEUR Workshop Proceedings (Vol. 2404, pp. 105–112). Sun SITE Central Europe, RWTH Aachen University.

Callahan, A., & Shah, N. (2017). Machine Learning in Healthcare: Key Advances in Clinical Informatics. Elsevier: Amsterdam, The Netherlands.

Chaudhry, J., Saleem, K., Islam, R., Selamat, A., Ahmad, M., & Valli, C. (2017, October). AZSPM: Autonomic zero-knowledge security provisioning model for medical control systems in fog computing environments. 2017 IEEE 42nd Conference on Local Computer Networks Workshops (LCN Workshops) (pp. 121–127). IEEE.

Chen, P.-H.C., Liu, Y., & Peng, L. (2019). How to develop machine learning models for healthcare. Nature Materials, 18(5), 410–414.

Dhillon, A., & Singh, A. (2019). Machine learning in healthcare data analysis: A survey. Journal of Biology and Today's World, 8(6), 1–10.

Fahad, H. M., Ghani Khan, M. U., Saba, T., Rehman, A., & Iqbal, S. (2018). Microscopic abnormality classification of cardiac murmurs using ANFIS and HMM. Microscopy Research and Technique, 81(5), 449–457.

Felkey, B.G., & Fox, B.I. (2016). Is this the first adherence-focused multidisciplinary care team app? Hospital Pharmacy, 51(1), 94–95.

Fellous, J. M., Sapiro, G., Rossi, A., Mayberg, H., & Ferrante, M. (2019). Explainable artificial intelligence for neuroscience: Behavioral neurostimulation. Frontiers in Neuroscience, 13, 1346.

Gilpin, L. H., Bau, D., Yuan, B. Z., Bajwa, A., Specter, M., & Kagal, L. (2018). Explaining explanations: An overview of interpretability of machine learning. 2018 IEEE 5th International Conference on Data Science and Advanced Analytics (DSAA). IEEE.

Guidotti, R., Monreale, A., Ruggieri, S., Turini, F., Giannotti, F., & Pedreschi, D. (2018). A survey of methods for explaining black box models. ACM Computing Surveys (CSUR), 51(5), 1–42.

Guleria, P., Naga Srinivasu, P., Ahmed, S., Almusallam, N., & Alarfaj, F. K. (2022). XAI framework for cardiovascular disease prediction using classification techniques. Electronics, 11(24), 4086.

Haseeb, K., Islam, N., Saba, T., Rehman, A., & Mehmood, Z. (2020). LSDAR: A lightweight structure based data aggregation routing protocol with secure Internet of Things integrated next-generation sensor networks. Sustainable Cities and Society, 54, 101995.

Hsu, Y. C., Tsai, I. J., Hsu, H., Hsu, P. W., Cheng, M. H., Huang, Y. L., …, Lin, C. Y. (2021). Using anti-malondialdehyde modified peptide autoantibodies to import machine learning for predicting coronary artery stenosis in Taiwanese patients with coronary artery disease. Diagnostics, 11(6), 961.

Husham, A., Hazim Alkawaz, M., Saba, T., Rehman, A., & Saleh Alghamdi, J. (2016). Automated nuclei segmentation of malignant using level sets. Microscopy Research and Technique, 79(10), 993–997.

Hussain, N., Khan, M. A., Sharif, M., Khan, S. A., Albesher, A. A., Saba, T., & Armaghan, A. (2020). A deep neural network and classical features based scheme for objects recognition: An application for machine inspection. Multimedia Tools and Applications, 5, 1–23.

Iftikhar, S., Fatima, K., Rehman, A., Almazyad, A. S., & Saba, T. (2017). An evolution based hybrid approach for heart diseases classification and associated risk factors identification. Biomedical Research, 28(8), 3451–3455.

Jabeen, S., Mehmood, Z., Mahmood, T., Saba, T., Rehman, A., & Mahmood, M. T. (2018). An effective content-based image retrieval technique for image visuals representation based on the bag-of-visual-words model. PLoS One, 13(4), e0194526.

Jamal, A., Hazim Alkawaz, M., Rehman, A., & Saba, T. (2017). Retinal imaging analysis based on vessel detection. Microscopy Research and Technique, 80(7), 799–811.

Janssen, F. M., Aben, K. K., Heesterman, B. L., Voorham, Q. J., Seegers, P. A., & Moncada-Torres, A. (2022). Using explainable machine learning to explore the impact of synoptic reporting on prostate cancer. Algorithms, 15(2), 49.

Javed, R., Rahim, M. S. M., Saba, T., & Rehman, A. (2020). A comparative study of features selection for skin lesion detection from dermoscopic images. Network Modeling Analysis in Health Informatics and Bioinformatics, 9, 1–13.

Keleş, A., Keleş, A., & Yavuz, U. (2011). Expert system based on neuro-fuzzy rules for diagnosis breast cancer. Expert Systems with Applications, 38(5), 5719–5726.

Kernbach, J.M., & Staartjes, V.E. (2022). Foundations of machine learning-based clinical prediction modeling: Part II—generalization and overfitting. Machine Learning in Clinical Neuroscience: Foundations and Applications, 15–21. Springer

Khan, M. A., Akram, T., Sharif, M., Javed, K., Raza, M., & Saba, T. (2020). An automated system for cucumber leaf diseased spot detection and classification using improved saliency method and deep features selection. Multimedia Tools and Applications, 79, 18627–18656.

Khan, M. A., Sharif, M. I., Raza, M., Anjum, A., Saba, T., & Shad, S. A. (2022a). Skin lesion segmentation and classification: A unified framework of deep neural network features fusion and selection. Expert Systems, 39(7), e12497.

Khan, M. A., Sharif, M. I., Raza, M., Anjum, A., Saba, T., & Shad, S. A. (2022b). Skin lesion segmentation and classification: A unified framework of deep neural network features fusion and selection. Expert Systems, 39(7), e1249718.

Larabi-Marie-Sainte, S., Aburahmah, L., Almohaini, R., & Saba, T. (2019). Current techniques for diabetes prediction: Review and case study. Applied Sciences, 9(21), 4604.

Ma, L., Wang, X., Wang, X., Wang, L., Shi, Y., & Huang, M. (2021). TCDA: Truthful combinatorial double auctions for mobile edge computing in Industrial Internet of Things. IEEE Transactions on Mobile Computing, 21(11), 4125–4138.

Megna, R., Petretta, M., Assante, R., Zampella, E., Nappi, C., Gaudieri, V., …, Cuocolo, A. (2021). A comparison among different machine learning pretest approaches to predict stress-induced ischemia at PET/CT myocardial perfusion imaging. Computational and Mathematical Methods in Medicine, 2021, 3551756.

Mughal, B., Muhammad, N., Sharif, M., Rehman, A., & Saba, T. (2018a). Removal of pectoral muscle based on topographic map and shape-shifting silhouette. BMC Cancer, 18(1), 1–14.

Mughal, B., Sharif, M., Muhammad, N., & Saba, T. (2018b). A novel classification scheme to decline the mortality rate among women due to breast tumor. Microscopy Research and Technique, 81(2), 171–180.

Muhsin, Z. F., Rehman, A., Altameem, A., Saba, T., & Uddin, M. (2014). Improved quadtree image segmentation approach to region information. The Imaging Science Journal, 62(1), 56–62.

Mujeeb, S., Alghamdi, T. A., Ullah, S., Fatima, A., Javaid, N., & Saba, T. (2019). Exploiting deep learning for wind power forecasting based on big data analytics. Applied Sciences, 9(20), 4417.

Narkhede, S. (2018). Understanding AUC–ROC curve. Towards Data Science, 26(1), 220–227.

Naz, A., Javed, M. U., Javaid, N., Saba, T., Alhussein, M., & Aurangzeb, K. (2019). Short-term electric load and price forecasting using enhanced extreme learning machine optimization in smart grids. Energies, 12(5), 866.

Pan, Y., Fu, M., Cheng, B., Tao, X., & Guo, J. (2020). Enhanced deep learning assisted convolutional neural network for heart disease prediction on the Internet of Medical Things platform. IEEE Access, 8, 189503–189512.

Patro, S. P., Padhy, N., & Chiranjevi, D. (2021). Ambient assisted living predictive model for cardiovascular disease prediction using supervised learning. Evolutionary Intelligence, 14(2), 941–969.

Porto, R., Molina, J. M., Berlanga, A., & Patricio, M. A. (2021). Minimum relevant features to obtain explainable systems for predicting cardiovascular disease using the stat log data set. Applied Sciences, 11(3), 1285.

Pouriyeh, S., Vahid, S., Sannino, G., De Pietro, G., Arabnia, H., & Gutierrez, J. (2017, July). A comprehensive investigation and comparison of machine learning techniques in the domain of heart disease. 2017 IEEE Symposium on Computers and Communications (ISCC) (pp. 204–207). IEEE.

Rehman, A. (2023). Brain stroke prediction through deep learning techniques with ADASYN strategy. 2023 16th International Conference on Developments in eSystems Engineering (DeSE), Istanbul, Turkiye, pp. 679–684.

Rehman, A., Saba, T., Mujahid, M., Alamri, F.S., & ElHakim, N. (2023). Parkinson's disease detection using a hybrid LSTM-GRU deep learning model. Electronics, 12(13), 2856.

Saba, T., Al-Zahrani, S., & Rehman, A. (2012). Expert system for offline clinical guidelines and treatment. Life Science Journal, 9(4), 2639–2658.

Saba, T., Bokhari, S. T. F., Sharif, M., Yasmin, M., & Raza, M. (2018). Fundus image classification methods for the detection of glaucoma: A review. Microscopy Research and Technique, 81(10), 1105–1121.

Saba, T., & Rehman, A. (2013). Effects of artificially intelligent tools on pattern recognition. International Journal of Machine Learning and Cybernetics, 4, 155–162.

Saba, T., Rehman, A., Mehmood, Z., Kolivand, H., & Sharif, M. (2018a). Image enhancement and segmentation techniques for detection of knee joint diseases: A survey. Current Medical Imaging, 14(5), 704–715.

Sadad, T., Rehman, A., Munir, A., Saba, T., Tariq, U., Ayesha, N., & Abbasi, R. (2021). Brain tumor detection and multi-classification using advanced deep learning techniques. Microscopy Research and Technique, 84(6), 1296–1308.

Samaras, A. D., Moustakidis, S., Apostolopoulos, I. D., Papageorgiou, E., & Papandrianos, N. (2023). Uncovering the black box of coronary artery disease diagnosis: The significance of explainability in predictive models. Applied Sciences, 13(14), 8120.

Sen, P.C., Hajra, M., & Ghosh, M. (2020). Supervised classification algorithms in machine learning: A survey and review. Emerging Technology in Modelling and Graphics: Proceedings of IEM Graph 2018. Springer.

Shahmiri, S. (2016). Wearing your data on your sleeve: Wearables, the FTC, and the privacy implications of this new technology. Texas Review of Entertainment & Sports Law, 18, 25.

Sharif, U., Mehmood, Z., Mahmood, T., Javid, M. A., Rehman, A., & Saba, T. (2019). Scene analysis and search using local features and support vector machine for effective content-based image retrieval. Artificial Intelligence Review, 52, 901–925.

Sharma, D., Gotlieb, N., Farkouh, M. E., Patel, K., Xu, W., & Bhat, M. (2022). Machine learning approach to classify cardiovascular disease in patients with nonalcoholic fatty liver disease in the UK Biobank Cohort. Journal of the American Heart Association, 11(1), e022576.

Son, Y. J., Kim, H. G., Kim, E. H., Choi, S., & Lee, S. K. (2010). Application of support vector machine for prediction of medication adherence in heart failure patients. Healthcare Informatics Research, 16(4), 253–259.

Srinivasu, P. N., Bhoi, A. K., Nayak, S. R., Bhutta, M. R., & Woźniak, M. (2021). Blockchain technology for secured healthcare data communication among the non-terminal nodes in IoT architecture in 5G network. Electronics, 10(12), 1437.

Sudheesh, R., Mujahid, M., Rustam, F., Mallampati, B., Chunduri, V., de la Torre Díez, I., & Ashraf, I. (2023). Bidirectional encoder representations from transformers and deep learning model for analyzing smartphone-related tweets. PeerJ Computer Science, 9, e1432.

Tahir, B., Iqbal, S., Usman Ghani Khan, M., Saba, T., Mehmood, Z., Anjum, A., & Mahmood, T. (2019). Feature enhancement framework for brain tumor segmentation and classification. Microscopy Research and Technique, 82(6), 803–811.

Tjoa, E., & Guan, C. (2020). A survey on explainable artificial intelligence (XAI): Toward medical XAI. IEEE Transactions on Neural Networks and Learning Systems, 32(11), 4793–4813.

West, D.M. (2018). The Future of Work: Robots, AI, and Automation. Brookings Institution Press.

Xia, T. (2016). Support vector machine based educational resources classification. International Journal of Information and Education Technology, 6(11), 880.

Yousaf, K., Mehmood, Z., Saba, T., Rehman, A., Munshi, A. M., Alharbey, R., & Rashid, M. (2019). Mobile-health applications for the efficient delivery of health care facility to people with dementia (PwD) and support to their carers: A survey. BioMed Research International, 2019, no. 1, p. 7151475.

Yuvalı, M., Yaman, B., & Tosun, Ö. (2022). Classification comparison of machine learning algorithms using two independent CAD datasets. Mathematics, 10, 311. https://doi.org/10.3390/math10030311.

Chapter 9

Transparency in HealthTech: Unveiling the Power of Explainable AI

Shiza Maham[1], Abdullah Tariq[1], Muhammad Usman Ghani Khan[2], and Amjad R. Khan[3]

[1]*University of Engineering and Technology, Lahore, Pakistan*

[2]*National Centre of Artificial Intelligence, KICS UET, Lahore, Pakistan*

[3]*Information Systems Department, CCIS Prince Sultan University, Riyadh, Kingdom of Saudi Arabia*

9.1 Introduction

In the era of rapid technological advancements, the global landscape is witnessing significant disruptions caused by various artificial intelligence (AI) technologies. While holding immense potential, these innovations have given rise to growing concerns regarding their far-reaching implications on both societal and individual levels (Malhi et al., 2019). As AI continues to influence diverse aspects of our lives, the need for a framework that ensures its ethical, transparent, and accountable use becomes increasingly apparent. Enter Responsible AI, a concept developed to address these concerns and guide the deployment of AI technologies in a manner that aligns with ethical standards and societal values (Mujeeb et al., 2019; Saba et al., 2022).

In the vast realm of healthcare, where precision and understanding can be a matter of life and death, the integration of technology has proclaimed a transformative era. Explainable artificial intelligence (XAI) stands at the forefront of technological advancements, particularly in the healthcare sector. Unlike traditional

DOI: 10.1201/9781032626345-9

black-box AI models, XAI prioritizes not only accuracy in predictions and decision-making but also the provision of comprehensible explanations for its outputs (Iftikhar et al., 2017; Jamal, Hazim Alkawaz, Rehman, & Saba, 2017) This paradigm shift is especially critical in healthcare, where transparency and interpretability are paramount in gaining trust and fostering collaboration between AI systems and healthcare professionals. In recent years, the emergence of XAI has been a game changer in the healthcare landscape. Traditionally, the inner workings of AI algorithms were like a mystical process, generating outcomes without offering a clear window into the decision-making process (Rehman & Saba, 2014; Sharif et al., 2019). The real-world implications of the lack of interpretability in AI models have become evident in several healthcare sectors (Fahad et al., 2018; Rehman et al., 2022). One such example is in the field of medical imaging, where deep learning (DL) models are increasingly used for tasks like radiology image analysis. If a model identifies a tumor or an anomaly in an image, the ability to explain why it made that specific diagnosis becomes crucial for the radiologist or treating physician. Consider a scenario where an AI model detects a potential pathology in a medical image, but the explanation behind this detection is unclear. Without a transparent rationale, the healthcare professional may be left questioning the reliability of the AI system (Gunraj et al., 2022). This lack of trust can lead to the rejection of AI-generated insights or, at the very least, create an environment of uncertainty in which the human expert feels compelled to reevaluate the AI recommendations independently. Moreover, the inability to understand the reasoning behind AI-driven suggestions can have significant consequences in critical decision-making processes such as treatment planning (Meethongjan et al., 2013). By overturning the system's choice, it also enables the system to optimize the algorithm to lessen bias. As a result, it gives healthcare models safety and equity and encourages people to trust in the process of making decisions (Jabeen et al., 2018; Jamal et al., 2017). XAI is applicable to a wide range of ML methods, including random forests, logistic regression, etc. The explanatory domain within the framework of the XAI model is divided into local and global methodologies. The global technique requires an explanation of the entire model, whereas the local technique requires a reason that is limited to specific predictions (Hussain et al., 2020; Mohseni, Zarei, & Ragan, 2021).

Figure 9.1 illustrates the global XAI forecast spanning from 2020 to 2030, revealing a compound annual growth rate of 21.5% (2023).

9.1.1 XAI Insights

XAI represents a groundbreaking frontier within the field of ML, explicitly focusing on unraveling the responses of AI systems to decisions made within opaque structures. The application of XAI extends beyond theoretical realms, offering the potential to construct recommendation systems tailored for healthcare sectors

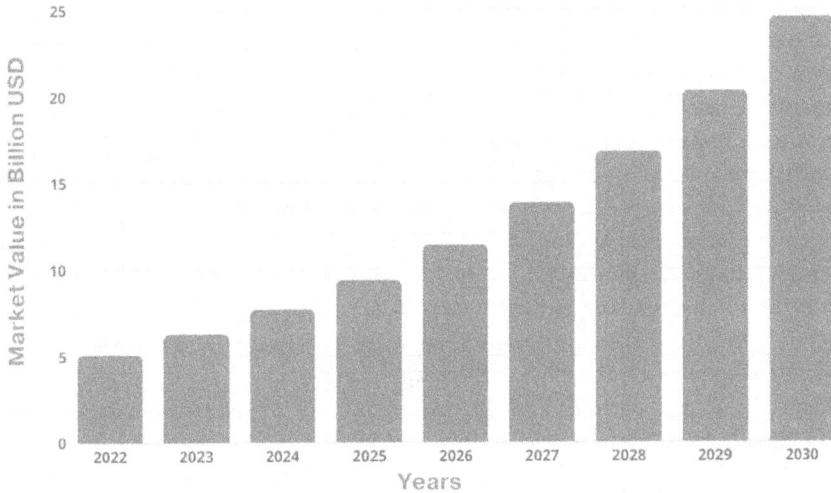

Figure 9.1   Global market for XAI from 2022 to 2030.

(Fan et al., 2022). Traditional ML algorithms often need help to provide clear explanations for the decisions they make, leaving users in the dark about the rationale behind specific choices. This opacity is particularly evident in widely adopted deep neural network techniques, which, despite delivering impressive performance, lack transparency in revealing the details of decision-making processes (Graziani et al., 2020). The challenge lies in balancing the undeniable benefits of enhanced performance with the need for comprehensibility and trust in AI technologies. In the context of healthcare, where precise decision-making is paramount, the XAI paradigm becomes increasingly indispensable (Haseeb et al., 2020). While capable of achieving remarkable outcomes, black-box models risk hindering their integration into clinical practice due to a need for more transparency and interpretability. As technological capabilities advance and vast amounts of data become more accessible, AI has made significant strides in augmenting intelligence, enriching data analysis, and automating various functions (Lundberg, & Lee, 2017). This progress extends beyond medical contexts, encompassing a broad spectrum of computer and signal processing-related studies. However, the realization of AI's full potential relies on overcoming the challenges posed by the explainability and transparency of existing systems, especially in critical domains like healthcare (Lopes et al., 2022).

9.1.1.1 Emergence of DL

DL stands as a revolutionary set of methodologies that has significantly transformed the landscape of ML in recent years (Naz et al., 2019). Unlike traditional ML approaches, DL is not confined to a single algorithm but encompasses a diverse set of methods that give rise to neural networks with deep layers. DL networks are known for being complex, featuring multiple layers that enable them to extract hierarchical representations from data. This depth allows DL models to capture intricate patterns and relationships within complex datasets, leading to superior performance in various domains (Larabi-Marie-Sainte, Aburahmah, Almohaini, & Saba, 2019). However, the power of DL comes at a cost, demanding exceptionally high computational capabilities and the deployment of node clusters to handle the computational load efficiently. One of the remarkable strengths of DL algorithms lies in their consistent outperformance of other methods, particularly evident in tasks such as image detection, natural language processing, and speech synthesis (Triantafyllopoulos et al., 2023). These applications showcase the ability of DL to identify complex patterns and nuances, making it a preferred choice for tasks requiring advanced pattern recognition. The accuracy of DL models is intimately tied to the size of the training data. Larger datasets provide more prosperous and more diverse information for the model to learn from, enhancing its ability to generalize to new, unseen data (Husham et al., 2016). Consequently, the scalability of DL models heavily depends on the availability of diverse datasets. Even with its strengths, DL is not without its drawbacks. Training DL models can be expensive regarding computational resources and time (Javed et al., 2020). The complexity of these models necessitates sophisticated hardware requirements, often requiring specialized GPUs or TPUs to handle the intense computations involved in the training process. Another limitation is the black-box nature of DL algorithms (Khan et al., 2020). Understanding how these algorithms converge and make decisions can be elusive, rendering them less interpretable compared to simpler models. This lack of transparency may raise concerns in applications where interpretability and explainability are crucial, such as medical diagnoses (Khan et al., 2022).

9.1.2 Objectives of XAI

The primary goal of XAI is to address the "why and how" questions associated with a given answer. For instance, XAI aims to explain why a specific answer was generated and how it was derived. This process enhances user empowerment, trust, transparency, compliance, and accountability in AI systems (refer to Figure 9.2).

A. Transparency

XAI seeks to improve the transparency and human understandability of AI models' decision-making processes (Simonyan & Zisserman, 2014). This is vital, particularly in domains like healthcare, banking, and autonomous cars, where

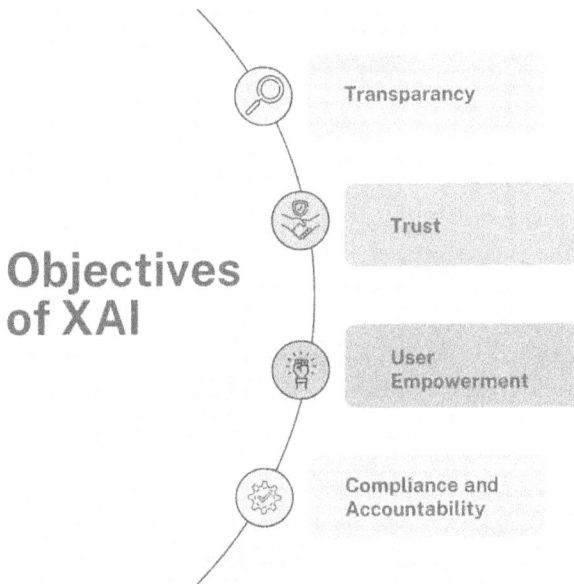

Figure 9.2   XAI objectives.

choices significantly impact. In order to make it easier for users—including non-experts—to understand the logic behind AI suggestions or forecasts, it also aims to shed light on how AI models reach particular conclusions.

B. Trust

XAI aims to enhance trust in AI systems by making their behavior more transparent and accountable. Users are more likely to trust AI models if they can comprehend the rationale behind their decisions. It can help identify and address biases in AI models, reducing the risk of unintended consequences. This is essential for ensuring fairness and avoiding discrimination in decision-making.

C. User Empowerment

XAI encourages user involvement in the decision-making process. By providing understandable explanations, users can have more informed interactions with AI systems and actively participate in refining or challenging the decisions made by the model (Saba et al., 2018a, 2018b). It can also facilitate collaboration between AI systems and human experts. When AI systems provide clear explanations, experts from various domains can work together more effectively, leveraging the strengths of both human and machine intelligence.

D. Compliance and Accountability

XAI is crucial for meeting regulatory requirements that mandate transparency and accountability in AI systems. Regulations such as the general data protection regulation (GDPR) in Europe emphasize the need for explainability in automated decision-making. XAI helps in identifying errors or flaws in AI models, enabling developers to correct and improve the system. This accountability is essential for minimizing the impact of AI mistakes.

9.1.3 Market Dynamics and Statistical Analysis

XAI is swiftly establishing itself as a critical player in pivotal industries, encompassing healthcare, environmental sciences, retail, transportation, media and entertainment, automotive, supply chain management, marketing, finance, telecommunication, etc. This state-of-the-art technology is reshaping the market dynamics by delivering a spectrum of advantages, such as enhanced client retention, streamlined inventory supervision, advanced design interpretability, resilient performance, scalability, and accurate cost estimation. Figure 9.3 depicts that in the past few years, there has been a notable surge in research findings related to XAI in healthcare (Ibrahim et al., 2019). The graph visually highlights the expanding body of knowledge in this area, demonstrating the heightened attention given to exploring how AI can be effectively explained and interpreted in the medical field (Husham et al., 2016).

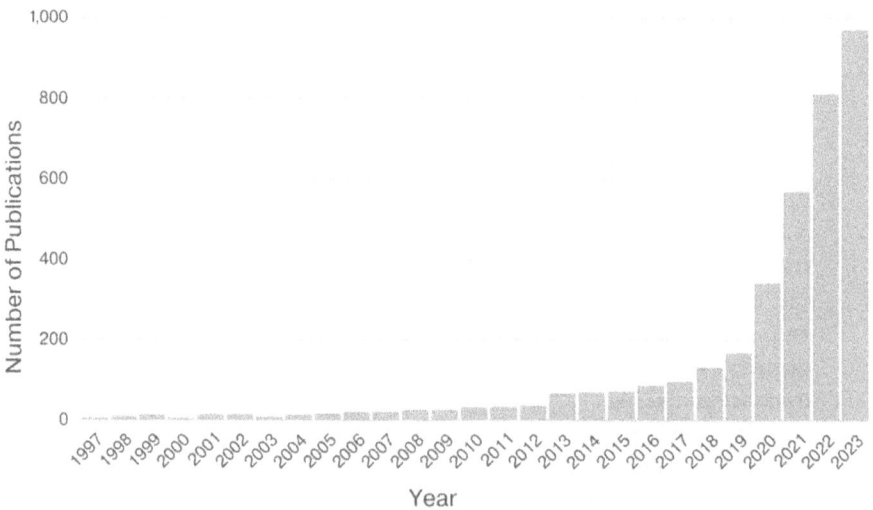

Figure 9.3 The graph illustrates the progressive growth in the volume of publications on XAI from 1997 to 2023. The horizontal axis represents the respective publication years, while the vertical axis quantifies the cumulative publications count for each corresponding year. This comprehensive analysis focuses on the number of scholarly works cataloged on PubMed as of the latest update on December 6, 2023 (accessible at https://pubmed.ncbi.nlm.nih.gov). The search queries employed for this survey included variations such as "explainable AI," "explainable artificial intelligence," and the acronym "XAI." Furthermore, the search criteria encompassed the intersection of these XAI-related terms with subjects pertaining to medical and healthcare contexts.

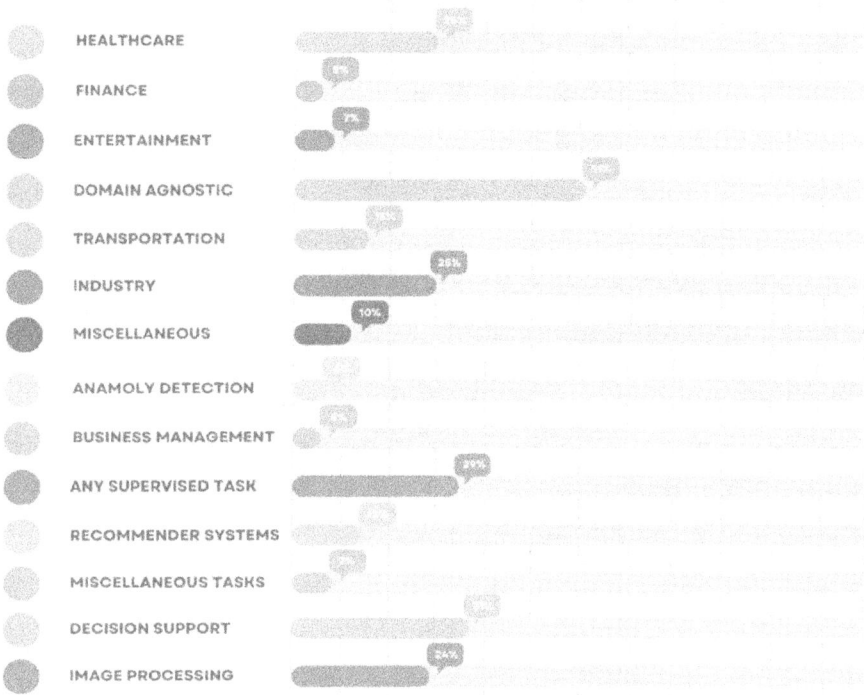

Figure 9.4   Research statistics for XAI across various applications encompassing domain-specific (a) and task-oriented (b) perspectives.

Figure 9.4 depicts the distribution of research articles across various application domains and tasks. Specifically, Figure 9.4a illustrates a domain-agnostic distribution where the healthcare sector emerges prominently, emphasizing the crucial role of XAI in delivering comprehensive explanations within this domain. Figure 9.4b delves into the significance of XAI in task-driven AI and ML applications. These applications are pivotal in supporting decision-making processes across diverse sectors, including recommendation models, prediction models, image processing, and business administration. The sub-figures collectively underscore the growing influence of XAI in both domain-agnostic and task-driven contexts (Islam, Ahmed, Barua, & Begum, 2022).

Several cutting-edge projects at the intersection of XAI and healthcare are making significant strides. The projects mentioned in Table 9.1 collectively exemplify the evolution of XAI in healthcare toward transparency, precision, and improved patient outcomes.

Table 9.1 EXAI's Practical Implementations in the Healthcare Sector through Real-World Industry Projects

Project Name	Objective	Start Date	End Date	Organization	Deliverables
DeepMind Health (Scaling Streams with Google, **2023**)	To utilize AI for various healthcare applications, including patient monitoring and predictive analytics	2016	Ongoing	DeepMind (a subsidiary of Alphabet)	Improved patient outcomes and early detection of deteriorating health
IBM Watson for Oncology (IBM, 2023) Park et al. (2023)	To assist oncologists in treatment decisions by analyzing and interpreting medical literature.	2014	Ongoing	IBM Watson Health	Enhanced treatment plans and increased access to medical knowledge.
Explainable AI in NHS (NHSX, 2023) Lip et al. (2024)	To implement XAI in the National Health Service (NHS) to enhance transparency in decision-making.	2019	Ongoing	National Health Service (NHS)	Improved trust in AI systems and better collaboration with clinicians.
PathAI (PathAI, 2023)	To develop interpretable AI solutions for pathology and diagnostic purposes	2016	Ongoing	PathAI	Enhanced accuracy in pathology diagnosis and improved patient care
Microsoft InnerEye (Microsoft, 2023) **Rakib et al. (2018)**	To utilize AI to assist in the analysis of medical imaging data, particularly in cancer treatment	2018	Ongoing	Microsoft	Improved radiology diagnostics and personalized treatment plans

9.2 Methods

The challenge in ML models lies in the increasing complexity, making it challenging to evaluate them. The deep neural networks stand out as the most intricate and accurate models, exhibiting exceptional performance (Liu et al., 2021). However, a significant drawback is the lack of understanding regarding how these results are generated. XAI addresses this complexity by branching out into simple algorithms requiring minimal to no explanation and more complicated methods. XAI methods are divided into two main categories—transparent and post hoc approaches. Delving deeper, some explanations pertain to individual instances. The comprehensive hierarchy of XAI approaches is shown in Figure 9.5.

9.2.1 Post Hoc Approaches

In XAI, post hoc procedures are strategies and tactics that offer justifications for model predictions subsequent to the model's decision-making process (Saba & Rehman, 2013). These methods are employed to interpret the output of a trained ML model, especially when the model itself is complex and lacks inherent interpretability. Post hoc explanations are valuable in understanding why a model made a particular prediction, which is crucial for building trust in AI systems and ensuring their ethical use (Murdoch et al., 2019). The post hoc method of explanation is further categorized into two parts—model-specific and model-agnostic.

9.2.1.1 Model-specific Techniques

Model-specific techniques are designed for use with specific types of models and are not universally applicable. They are employed based on particular requirements,

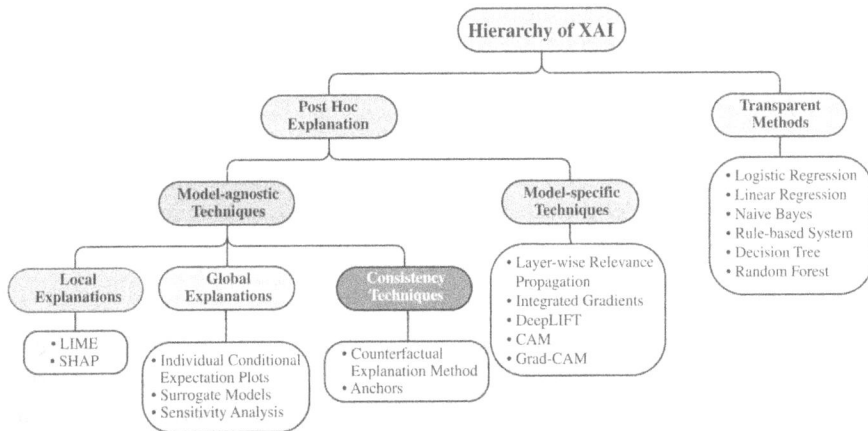

Figure 9.5　A thorough structure of XAI approaches.

with dependencies that restrict their compatibility with all models. One example is CAM. CAM generates an activation map for a specific class, indicating the distinct image regions utilized by CNN to recognize that particular category (Yousaf et al., 2019). This method is tailored to work with CNN or models featuring similar convolutional layers. Another technique, GRAD-CAM (Selvaraju et al., 2016), leverages gradients of the class projected onto the feature map from the last convolutional layer of the neural network. This provides insights into the features extracted by CNN for result generation (Hu et al., 2022). The output is represented in red and green colors, where red denotes the model's predicted attention area and green surrounds it, indicating a low probability for the presence of the discussed object. While GRAD-CAM is an improved version of CAM, it shares the limitation of exclusively working with CNNs. On the other hand, deep label-special feature map (Deep LIFT) (Li et al., 2021) distinguishes itself from prior approaches by decomposing global feature sets into label-specific features. It utilizes the graph convolutional network to enhance its functionality by capturing relationships between labels (Muhsin et al., 2014).

9.2.1.2 Model-agnostic Techniques

Model-agnostic refers to a characteristic of techniques which are not dependent on the internal structure or details of a specific ML model (Tahir et al., 2019). In other words, a model-agnostic approach is designed to be broadly applicable across different models, regardless of their underlying architecture, complexity, or algorithms (Le et al., 2021). Model-agnostic XAI techniques aim to provide interpretability and explanations for the predictions or decisions made by ML models without requiring specific knowledge about how those models are internally constructed (Mundher et al., 2014). These methods are often applied externally to a trained model, allowing users to gain insights into the model's decision-making process without being constrained by the intricacies of the model itself. The critical advantage of model-agnostic approaches is their versatility, as they can be used across various ML models, including both simple and complex ones, making them particularly useful in scenarios where different models may be employed for other tasks or in different contexts. Furthermore, it is divided into two categories based on the scope of explanations, i.e., local and global explanations. Moreover, the consistency technique also falls under the category of model agnostic techniques.

A. Local Explanations

Local explanations refer to descriptions of conclusions that are tied to specific instances. An example of this is LIME (Dieber & Kirrane, 2020). The methodology involves selecting a set of instances in the surrounding area of a specific prediction. These neighboring occurrences are then used to train a model that is simple and easily interpretable. This often involves a linear model that estimates the performance and outcomes of the model in the local region.

Another example is SHAP. SHAP values can be employed to elucidate any model's output in the ML domain. These values originate from the concept of cooperative game theory and represent the calculation of each player's contribution to a game's winning. In the context of AI and ML, we can interpret these values as the contribution of each feature in determining the final result (Rehman, 2023). The higher the SHAP value a feature has, the more significant its contribution to the outcome (Mughal et al., 2018a, 2018b).

B. Global Explanations

Another facet of model-agnostic techniques involves providing global explanations. Certain researchers have endeavored to adapt active local XAI concepts to derive explanations, thereby extracting answers in a manner that facilitates achieving global results for the model. A research study (Ribeiro, Singh, & Guestrin, 2016) introduced SP-LIME as a global approach. SP-LIME operates by offering global explanations, extracting crucial features from each local instance presented to the model (Saba et al., 2012). SP-LIME stands out as the preferred choice when considering a more reliable approach. It utilizes an explanation matrix to aggregate global results from the localized values provided by LIME. This approach is nonredundant and builds upon the foundation laid by LIME. Another study (Lundberg et al., 2019) introduced an approach employing the SHAP method for globally scoped result detection. Within this framework, a Tree Explainer was employed. The underlying mechanism of this framework involves determining local values, akin to SHAP values, and configuring them to discern global results (Yang, & Yu, 2021). The new iteration of SHAP, utilizing this framework, offers an explanation that is both local and global without compromising stability and accuracy. Global interpretations encompass dependence plots, summaries, feature importance, and other relevant factors. In 2019, a method known as "Global Attribution Analysis" (GAA) was introduced (Ibrahim et al., 2019). GAA generates global attribution for a single element and subsequently explains it. Each global attribution elucidates a specific aspect of the model, contributing to an overall understanding of the model's functioning. Additionally, surrogate models are employed to extract global explanations of the primary model. A surrogate model can take the form of any transparent model, and their interpretations can be utilized to evaluate our model comprehensively after obtaining the full results (Sadad et al., 2021).

C. Consistency Techniques

The third model-agnostic technique is the consistency technique, a method ensuring that explanations provided by XAI remain consistent with the behavior of the AI models they explain. This is important because if an explanation is inconsistent with the model, it can be misleading or harmful. Anchoring is part of the consistency approach (van der Velden et al., 2020). This technique involves utilizing examples or reference points to clarify the predictions made by an AI model. For instance, if an AI model predicts the likelihood of a patient developing a heart condition, the explanation might compare the patient's risk factors to those of other patients who have experienced the condition. Moreover, the counterfactual explanation method is another consistency approach that explains the predictions of an AI model by highlighting subtle changes that could lead the model to make different decisions or predictions (Vayá et al., 2020). This method is based on the concept that the most effective way to comprehend why a model made a specific prediction is to observe the results if the given input was slightly altered (Wang et al., 2021).

9.2.2 Transparent Approaches

Methods that have easily interpreted and illustrated internal workings and decision-making processes are those used in transparent approaches. These strategies are beneficial when there is a manageable amount of complexity or linearity in the interactions between internal features. The transparent models are easy to interpret, and the scalability of such methods used on large datasets can be obtained. Naive Bayes, decision trees, linear regression, and logistic regression are a few types of transparent models. Linear regression represents a fundamental ML algorithm and serves as the foundation for many contemporary modeling tools (Su et al., 2012). The results from linear regression can be easily interpreted through graphical representation, providing users with a clear understanding of why specific outcomes were derived from the model. Naive Bayes, another straightforward model, relies on the naive Bayes theorem. Similar to linear regression, its outcomes are interpretable and can be articulated effectively. The naive Bayes model enables users to comprehend the rationale behind its predictions.

On the other hand, the decision tree algorithm organizes results in a tree-like structure. Visualizing decision trees graphically facilitates a clear understanding of the decision sequence and the impact of different features on the final prediction. It is worth noting that none of these models involve hidden layers, as seen in neural networks.

9.3 Conclusion and Future Directions

XAI stands as an emerging discipline focused on bolstering user confidence through active user involvement and addressing issues related to transparency. Given the intricate nature of decision-making in critical domains like medicine, the growing significance of XAI is undeniable. This study presents a comprehensive examination of XAI models applied within the scope of healthcare 5.0, specifically focusing on tasks related to medical imaging. The scope of medical imaging tasks explored in this study encompasses classification, detection, segmentation, and the generation of clinical reports. Our analysis of current trends reveals a rising prevalence of comprehensive methodologies, where diverse forms of explanation are integrated. Instances of these more holistic approaches encompass the fusion of textual and visual explanations. The diverse landscape of medical imaging modalities, including but not limited to X-rays, CT scans, Fundus images, and MRIs, serves as pivotal input data for these models, facilitating the recognition of medical imaging patterns through a spectrum of sophisticated algorithms. The organization of information in this study follows a systematic approach, structuring imaging techniques based on the XAI framework. The majority of existing XAI methods are post hoc in nature. This preference is likely due to the convenience they offer to end users like clinicians and researchers, who find it easier to apply techniques such as Grad-CAM and LIME. Nevertheless, it is recommended to create an explainability model specifically for critical medical scenarios. In future, large vision models (LVM) will be very useful and overcome all traditional methods of visual explanations. By aligning information according to the XAI framework and categorizing it based on anatomical considerations and datasets, this study not only facilitates a clearer understanding of the subject matter but also lays a foundation for researchers to make informed strides in advancing medical research and applications but we cannot ensure comprehensive coverage of all aspects within the field. Despite the possibility that some aspects of the work in the domain may not have been included, we have carefully outlined our search strategy to ensure openness in the selection of papers.

References

Dieber, J., & Kirrane, S., 2020. Why model why? Assessing the strengths and limitations of LIME. arXiv:2012.00093.

Dutta, J., Puthal, D., & Yeun, C.Y. Next generation healthcare with explainable AI: IoMT-edge-cloud based advanced eHealth. doi: 10.1109/GLOBECOM54140.2023.10436967

Fahad, H. M., Ghani Khan, M. U., Saba, T., Rehman, A., & Iqbal, S. (2018). Microscopic abnormality classification of cardiac murmurs using ANFIS and HMM. Microscopy Research and Technique, 81(5), 449–457.

Fan, Z., Gong, P., Tang, S., Lee, C. U., Zhang, X., Song, P., Chen, S., & Li, H. (2022). Joint localization and classification of breast tumors on ultrasound images using a novel auxiliary attention-based framework. arXiv:2210.05762.

Graziani, M., Andrearczyk, V., Marchand-Maillet, S., & Müller, H. (2020). Concept attribution: Explaining CNN decisions to physicians. Computers in Biology and Medicine, 123, 103865.

Gunraj, H., Sabri, A., Koff, D., & Wong, A. (2022). COVID-Net CT-2: Enhanced deep neural networks for detection of COVID-19 from chest CT images through bigger, more diverse learning. Frontiers in Medicine, 8, 729287.

Haseeb, K., Islam, N., Saba, T., Rehman, A., & Mehmood, Z. (2020). LSDAR: A lightweight structure based data aggregation routing protocol with secure Internet of Things integrated next-generation sensor networks. Sustainable Cities and Society, 54, 101995.

Hu, B., Vasu, B., & Hoogs, A. (2022). X-MIR: EXplainable medical image retrieval. In Proceedings of the IEEE/CVF Winter Conference on Applications of Computer Vision (pp. 440–450).

Husham, A., Hazim Alkawaz, M., Saba, T., Rehman, A., & Saleh Alghamdi, J. (2016). Automated nuclei segmentation of malignant using level sets. Microscopy Research and Technique, 79(10), 993–997.

Hussain, N., Khan, M. A., Sharif, M., Khan, S. A., Albesher, A. A., Saba, T., & Armaghan, A. (2020). A deep neural network and classical features based scheme for objects recognition: An application for machine inspection. Multimedia Tools and Applications, 83(5), 1–23.

IBM Products. Available at: https://www.ibm.com/watson-health/oncology (accessed November 23, 2023).

Ibrahim, M., Louie, M., Modarres, C., & Paisley, J. (2019, January). Global explanations of neural networks: Mapping the landscape of predictions. In Proceedings of the 2019 AAAI/ACM Conference on AI, Ethics, and Society (pp. 279–287).

Iftikhar, S., Fatima, K., Rehman, A., Almazyad, A. S., & Saba, T. (2017). An evolution based hybrid approach for heart diseases classification and associated risk factors identification. Biomedical Research, 28(8), 3451–3455.

Islam, M. R., Ahmed, M. U., Barua, S., & Begum, S. (2022). A systematic review of explainable artificial intelligence in terms of different application domains and tasks. Applied Sciences, 12(3), 1353.

Jabeen, S., Mehmood, Z., Mahmood, T., Saba, T., Rehman, A., & Mahmood, M. T. (2018). An effective content-based image retrieval technique for image visuals representation based on the bag-of-visual-words model. PLoS One, 13(4), e0194526.

Jamal, A., Hazim Alkawaz, M., Rehman, A., & Saba, T. (2017). Retinal imaging analysis based on vessel detection. Microscopy Research and Technique, 80(7), 799–811.

Javed, R., Rahim, M. S. M., Saba, T., & Rehman, A. (2020). A comparative study of features selection for skin lesion detection from dermoscopic images. Network Modeling Analysis in Health Informatics and Bioinformatics, 9, 1–13.

Khan, M. A., Akram, T., Sharif, M., Javed, K., Raza, M., & Saba, T. (2020). An automated system for cucumber leaf diseased spot detection and classification using improved saliency method and deep features selection. Multimedia Tools and Applications, 79, 18627–18656.

Khan, M. A., Sharif, M. I., Raza, M., Anjum, A., Saba, T., & Shad, S. A. (2022). Skin lesion segmentation and classification: A unified framework of deep neural network features fusion and selection. Expert Systems, 39(7), e12497.

Larabi-Marie-Sainte, S., Aburahmah, L., Almohaini, R., & Saba, T. (2019). Current techniques for diabetes prediction: Review and case study. Applied Sciences, 9(21), 4604.

Le, N. Q. K., Kha, Q. H., Nguyen, V. H., Chen, Y. C., Cheng, S. J., & Chen, C. Y. (2021). Machine learning-based radiomics signatures for EGFR and KRAS mutations prediction in non-small-cell lung cancer. International Journal of Molecular Sciences, 22(17), 9254.

Li, J., Yang, Z., & Yu, Y. (2021, September). A medical AI diagnosis platform based on vision transformer for coronavirus. 2021 IEEE International Conference on Computer Science, Electronic Information Engineering and Intelligent Control Technology (CEI) (pp. 246–252). IEEE.

Li, J., Zhang, C., Zhou, J. T., Fu, H., Xia, S., & Hu, Q. (2021). Deep-LIFT: Deep label-specific feature learning for image annotation. IEEE Transactions on Cybernetics, 52(8), 7732–7741.

Lip, Gerald, Alex Novak, Mathias Goyen, Katherine Boylan, & Amrita Kumar (2024). Adoption, orchestration, and deployment of artificial intelligence within the National

Health Service—facilitators and barriers: an expert roundtable discussion. BJR| Artificial Intelligence 1(1), ubae009.

Lopes, P., Silva, E., Braga, C., Oliveira, T., & Rosado, L. (2022). XAI systems evaluation: A review of human and computer-centred methods. Applied Sciences, 12(19), 9423.

Lundberg, S. M., Erion, G., Chen, H., DeGrave, A., Prutkin, J. M., Nair, B., Katz, R., Himmelfarb, J., Bansal, N., & Lee, S. I. (2019). Explainable AI for trees: From local explanations to global understanding. arXiv:1905.04610.

Lundberg, S. M., & Lee, S. I. (2017). A unified approach to interpreting model predictions. Advances in Neural Information Processing Systems (p. 30). NIPS.

Malhi, A., Kampik, T., Pannu, H., Madhikermi, M., & Främling, K. (2019, December). Explaining machine learning-based classifications of in-vivo gastral images. In 2019 Digital Image Computing: Techniques and Applications (DICTA) (pp. 1–7). IEEE.

Meethongjan, K., Dzulkifli, M., Rehman, A., Altameem, A., & Saba, T. (2013). An intelligent fused approach for face recognition. Journal of Intelligent Systems, 22(2), 197–212.

Microsoft (2023). Project InnerEye : Democratizing medical imaging AI. Microsoft Research. Available at: https://www.microsoft.com/en-us/research/project/medical-image-analysis/ (accessed November 23, 2023).

Mohseni, S., Zarei, N., & Ragan, E. D. (2021). A multidisciplinary survey and framework for design and evaluation of explainable AI systems. ACM Transactions on Interactive Intelligent Systems (TIIS), 11(3–4), 1–45.

Mughal, B., Muhammad, N., Sharif, M., Rehman, A., & Saba, T. (2018a). Removal of pectoral muscle based on topographic map and shape-shifting silhouette. BMC Cancer, 18(1), 1–14.

Mughal, B., Sharif, M., Muhammad, N., & Saba, T. (2018b). A novel classification scheme to decline the mortality rate among women due to breast tumor. Microscopy Research and Technique, 81(2), 171–180.

Muhsin, Z. F., Rehman, A., Altameem, A., Saba, T., & Uddin, M. (2014). Improved quadtree image segmentation approach to region information. The Imaging Science Journal, 62(1), 56–62.

Mujeeb, S., Alghamdi, T. A., Ullah, S., Fatima, A., Javaid, N., & Saba, T. (2019). Exploiting deep learning for wind power forecasting based on big data analytics. Applied Sciences, 9(20), 4417.

Mundher, M., Muhamad, D., Rehman, A., Saba, T., & Kausar, F. (2014). Digital watermarking for images security using discrete Slantlet transform. Applied Mathematics & Information Sciences, 8(6), 2823.

Murdoch, W. J., Singh, C., Kumbier, K., Abbasi-Asl, R., & Yu, B. (2019). Interpretable machine learning: Definitions, methods, and applications. arXiv:1901.04592.

Naz, A., Javed, M. U., Javaid, N., Saba, T., Alhussein, M., & Aurangzeb, K. (2019). Short-term electric load and price forecasting using enhanced extreme learning machine optimization in smart grids. Energies, 12(5), 866.

NHSX. (2023). The NHS AI Lab. Available at: https://www.nhsx.nhs.uk/ai-lab/ (accessed November 23, 2023).

Park, Taeyoung, Philip Gu, Chang-Hee Kim, Kwang Taek Kim, Kyung Jin Chung, Tea Beom Kim, Han Jung, Sang Jin Yoon, & Jin Kyu Oh (2023). Artificial intelligence in urologic oncology: the actual clinical practice results of IBM Watson for Oncology in South Korea. Prostate International, 11(4), 218–221.

PathAI. (2023). Available at: https://www.pathai.com/ (accessed November 23, 2023).

Rakib, Gazi Abdur, Rudaiba Adnin, Shekh Ahammed Adnan Bashir, Chashi Mahiul Islam, Abir Mohammad Turza, Saad Manzur, Monowar Anjum Rashik et al. (2022). InnerEye: A tale on images filtered using Instagram filters-how do we interact with them and how can we automatically identify the extent of filtering? In International Conference on Mobile and Ubiquitous Systems: Computing, Networking, and Services (pp. 494–514). Cham: Springer Nature Switzerland.

Rehman, A. (2023). Brain stroke prediction through deep learning techniques with ADASYN strategy. 2023 16th International Conference on Developments in eSystems Engineering (DeSE) (pp. 679–684). Istanbul, Türkiye.

Rehman, A., & Saba, T. (2014). Features extraction for soccer video semantic analysis: Current achievements and remaining issues. Artificial Intelligence Review, 41, 451–461.

Rehman, A., Saba, T., Kashif, M., Fati, S. M., Bahaj, S. A., & Chaudhry, H. (2022). A revisit of Internet of Things technologies for monitoring and control strategies in smart agriculture. Agronomy, 12(1), 127.

Ribeiro, M. T., Singh, S., & Guestrin, C. (2016). "Why should I trust you?": Explaining the predictions of any classifier. KDD (pp. 1135–1144). ACM.

Saba, T., Al-Zahrani, S., & Rehman, A. (2012). Expert system for offline clinical guidelines and treatment. Life Science Journal, 9(4), 2639–2658.

Saba, T., Bokhari, S. T. F., Sharif, M., Yasmin, M., & Raza, M. (2018b). Fundus image classification methods for the detection of glaucoma: A review. Microscopy Research and Technique, 81(10), 1105–1121.

Saba, T., & Rehman, A. (2013). Effects of artificially intelligent tools on pattern recognition. International Journal of Machine Learning and Cybernetics, 4, 155–162.

Saba, T., Rehman, A., Mehmood, Z., Kolivand, H., & Sharif, M. (2018a). Image enhancement and segmentation techniques for detection of knee joint diseases: A survey. Current Medical Imaging, 14(5), 704–715.

Saba, T., Rehman, A., Sadad, T., Kolivand, H., & Bahaj, S. A. (2022). Anomaly-based intrusion detection system for IoT networks through deep learning model. Computers and Electrical Engineering, 99, 107810.

Sadad, T., Rehman, A., Munir, A., Saba, T., Tariq, U., Ayesha, N., & Abbasi, R. (2021). Brain tumor detection and multi-classification using advanced deep learning techniques. Microscopy Research and Technique, 84(6), 1296–1308.

Selvaraju, R. R., Das, A., Vedantam, R., Cogswell, M., Parikh, D., & Batra, D. (2016). Grad-CAM: Why did you say that? arXiv:1611.07450.

Sharif, U., Mehmood, Z., Mahmood, T., Javid, M. A., Rehman, A., & Saba, T. (2019). Scene analysis and search using local features and support vector machine for effective content-based image retrieval. Artificial Intelligence Review, 52, 901–925.

Simonyan, K., & Zisserman, A. (2014). Very deep convolutional networks for large-scale image recognition. arXiv:1409.1556.

Tahir, B., Iqbal, S., Usman Ghani Khan, M., Saba, T., Mehmood, Z., Anjum, A., & Mahmood, T. (2019). Feature enhancement framework for brain tumor segmentation and classification. Microscopy Research and Technique, 82(6), 803–811.

Triantafyllopoulos, A., Schuller, B.W., İymen, G., Sezgin, M., He, X., Yang, Z., Tzirakis, P., Liu, S., Mertes, S., André, E., & Fu, R. (2023). An overview of affective speech synthesis and conversion in the deep learning era. Proceedings of the IEEE, 111(10), 1355–1381.

van der Velden, B. H., Janse, M. H., Ragusi, M. A., Loo, C. E., & Gilhuijs, K. G. (2020). Volumetric breast density estimation on MRI using explainable deep learning regression. Scientific Reports, 10(1), 18095.

Vayá, M. D. L. I., Saborit, J. M., Montell, J. A., Pertusa, A., Bustos, A., Cazorla, M., Galant, J., Barber, X., Orozco-Beltrán, D., García-García, F., & Caparrós, M. (2020). BIMCV COVID-19+: A large annotated dataset of RX and CT images from COVID-19 patients. arXiv:2006.01174.

Wang, H., Wang, S., Qin, Z., Zhang, Y., Li, R., & Xia, Y. (2021). Triple attention learning for classification of 14 thoracic diseases using chest radiography. Medical Image Analysis, 67, 101846.

Yousaf, K., Mehmood, Z., Saba, T., Rehman, A., Munshi, A. M., Alharbey, R., & Rashid, M. (2019). Mobile-health applications for the efficient delivery of health care facility to people with dementia (PwD) and support to their carers: A survey. BioMed Research International, 2019, 7151475.

Chapter 10

Therapeutic Virtual Reality Exposure Therapies for Nyctophobia and Claustrophobia with Active Heart Rate Monitoring

Zubaira Naz[2], Ayesha Azam[1,2], Muhammad Usman Ghani Khan[1,2], and Noor Ayesha[3]

[1]Department of Computer Science, University of Engineering and Technology, Lahore, Pakistan

[2]Al-Khwarizmi Institute of Computer Science, University of Engineering and Technology, Lahore, Pakistan

[3]Center of Excellence in Cyber Security (CYBEX), Prince Sultan University Riyadh, Kingdom of Saudi Arabia

10.1 Introduction

A phobia is a persistent and incapacitating fear, significantly impairing an individual's ability to carry out daily tasks. One type of impairment is avoiding what they fear (Schowalter 1994). People who had suffered a brain injury are more prospective to get some kind of phobia. Phobias are typically categorizing into anxiety disorders: social anxiety disorder, specific anxiety disorder, panic and generalized disorders that further divided into environmental, situation, or injury types

DOI: 10.1201/9781032626345-10

(Muris et al. 2017). In the United States, it is estimated by the interview data from National Comorbidity Survey Replication (NCS-R) that more than 12.5% of adults have had a specific phobia some time in their life, and women are the most likely to get phobias than men; nevertheless, anyone can get phobia. Exposure therapies had been considered to be effective to treat the phobias (Hofmann & Smits 2008; Norton & Price 2007). Traditional therapies have also been facilitated and optimized through the development of disruptive technologies, such as virtual reality (VR) (Maples-Keller et al. 2017) (Jabeen et al., 2018). VR is a visual computerized simulation that generates realistic experiential sensations. VR allows users to immerse themselves in the virtual world through interactive equipment, such as Oculus or other head-mounted displays (Concannon, Esmail, and Roduta Roberts 2019; Harrington et al. 2018). Additionally, VR provides interaction between humans and machines, which is not possible with 3D or 360 videos (Fox, Arena, and Bailenson 2009). It has been demonstrated that the VR treatment methods benefit phobic individuals both mentally and physically. As after taking VR therapy sessions, patients with panic disorder and agoraphobia (PDA) exhibited increment in their courage (Peñate, Pitti, & Bethencourt 2008). By progressively adapting patients to their phobias, VR can help patients feel comfortable and conduct their daily activities without avoiding what they fear. A few of the common phobias are claustrophobia and nyctophobia.

The rest of the chapter is organized as follows: Section 10.2 presents the previous work proposed by researchers for phobia treatments. Section 10.3 is our proposed methodology of developing VR game, integrating with heart monitoring device and evaluation method. Section 10.4 presents the results of our proposed methodology, which is the VR game and evaluated by adults. Finally, Section 10.5 presents the conclusion from our research work.

10.2 Literature Review

In recent years, numerous studies have examined how effective VR is at treating various phobias. A study was conducted by E. Shanthini et al. (Shanthini et al. 2022) in 2022, in which they developed 3D virtual environments for the treatment of nyctophobia, acrophobia, entomophobia, and aquaphobia (Bagha & Shaw, 2011). They also monitored the patient's heart rate using gravity heart rate monitor sensor during exposure therapy in order to assess the impact of these therapies on user's phobia. The designed environments exposed users to high building, insects, waters, darkness etc. However, neither the authors conducted a study to analyze the stress levels and impact of their prototype, nor they add gazed based interactivity in the environments. In another article (Muris et al. 2017). Helle et al. (2022) presented a VR-based exposure therapy, stimulating an elevator, designed for claustrophobic patients. The major focus of the chapter was on evaluating the usability and usefulness of VR exposure therapy by clinicians

(Rehman, 2023). Seven clinicians, including psychiatric nurse, environmental therapist, and psychologists, used the application and data was collected through SUS survey, interviews, and observations made by experts. The results of their study stated that VR-based exposure therapies are useful and able to manage different anxiety attacks (Mughal et al. 2018a,b).

A study was published by R.S. Sree et al. (Sharmikha Sree, Meera, Deepika, et al. 2022) in 2022, in which they developed narrowed, dark, messy living room, bedroom, and kitchen 3D environments as an exposure therapy for claustrophobic patients (Saba et al. 2012). Their developed application has multiple levels, and next level is more confined place than the previous one. User can move from one place to another in environments by teleportation using eye gaze–based interactions. As a result of using Google Cardboard to view and use the application, they concluded that this exposure therapy using VR is cheap and overcomes the disadvantages of medication and other traditional therapies. Sree et al. (Sharmikha Sree, Meera, Priyadharshini, et al. 2022) integrated different 3D virtual environments for the treatment of claustrophobia as exposure therapies. Claustrophobic house, trial rooms, tunnels, public restroom have been researched and designed in 3D for different levels. They deployed their application on android and can be used using Google cardboard. They achieved teleportation to a place where user is looking at by eye gaze interaction techniques (Muhsin et al. 2014).

Cognitive behavioral therapy is something that can change the beliefs and habits of patients about their fears (Javed et al., 2020). Paulus et al. (2019) present an alternative tool to it, which is the porotype of virtual exposure therapy for nyctophobia, named Night Forest. This game has one player (boy scout), whose task is to look for logs in the dark forest (Husham et al. 2016). The researchers made the user experience realistic and amazing by adding natural sound of birds and footsteps (Bagha & Shaw 2011). They also conducted an experimental study to evaluate their protype and findings suggested that fear level of female users did not go down as compared to male users (Saba et al. 2018a,b). Nevertheless, they did not have features of teleportation or heart monitoring in their application. In another study, VR-based exposure therapy for nyctophobia was presented by Nimnual and Yossatorn (2019) in 2019. They developed the virtual environments in Unity 3D and deployed the application on the immersive VR headset. Further, they evaluated the satisfaction and usefulness of designed prototype by VR and medical experts and 20 nyctophobic patients. The patients were highly satisfied with the prototype and rated it 4.6 (mean) on a Liker scale. Francová, Jablonská, and Fajnerová (2023) conducted a feasibility study on phobic and control group to design and validate virtual environments for claustrophobic exposure therapy. The results from the study indicated VR exposure therapies have the potential to induce claustrophobia, and that virtual environments evoked a sense of presence. Table 10.1 presents these papers comparison with our contribution in tabular form.

Table 10.1 clearly demonstrates that none of the research work covers all the features in one framework. Some frameworks monitor heart rate but their protype

Table 10.1 Literature Comparison of Different VR Exposure Therapies for Phobia Treatment

Authors	Year	Phobias	Game/Environments	Gaze-based Interactivity	Evaluated	Heart Rate Monitoring	Real-time Heart Rate Display	Deploy to
Paulus et al. (2019)	2019	Nyctophobia	Game	No	Yes	No	No	Mobile VR
Nimnual and Yossatorn (2019)	2019	Nyctophobia	Environment	No	No	No	No	Head-mounted display
Jashwanth et al. (2020)	2020	Acrophobia, nyctophobia, agoraphobia, kenophobia, claustrophobia, tachophobia	Environment	No	Yes	Yes	No	VR headset
Shanthini et al. (2022)	2022	Nyctophobia, acrophobia, entomophobia, and aquaphobia	Environment	No	No	Yes	No	Oculus
Helle et al. (2022)	2022	Claustrophobia	Environment	No	Yes	No	No	HTC VIVE

(Continued)

Table 10.1 (Continued)

Authors	Year	Phobias	Game/ Environments	Gaze-based Interactivity	Evaluated	Heart Rate Monitoring	Real-time Heart Rate Display	Deploy to
Sharmikha Sree, Meera, Deepika, et al. (2022)	2022	Claustrophobia	Environment	Yes	No	No	No	Google cardboard
Sharmikha Sree, Meera, Priyadharshini, et al. (2022)	2022	Claustrophobia	Environment	Yes	No	No	No	Google cardboard
Francová, Jablonská, and Fajnerová (2023)	2023	Claustrophobia	Environment	No	Yes	No	No	–
Proposed work	2024	Nyctophobia, claustrophobia	Games with dark and confined environment	Yes	Yes	Yes	Yes	VR headsets HTC VIVE

consists of only environment and no interaction for user, while others provide interactions but no stress level monitoring. Therefore, in this chapter, we aim to develop a framework for nyctophobic and claustrophobic patients as these are common phobias among children and adults and despite being common, very few studies use VR-based exposure therapies for these phobias' treatments. The main contribution of our work is proposed below:

- Developing immersive 3D games with dark and confined environment for nyctophobia and claustrophobia, and users will be given a task to collect as many crystals as they can to keep them engaged in the environment
- Heart rate monitoring while they are exposed to therapy to measure their stress levels to ensure that therapy is not demanding and they can gradually increase their tolerance to the feared circumstances. Real-time graphical feedback on the user's stress levels to improve the user's awareness of their physiological reaction to fear and anxiety. Users can also track their development as they conquer their phobias.
- Evaluation of application through STAI-Y1 (State Trait Anxiety Inventory)

As a whole, VR-based exposure therapies with heart rate monitoring and interactive features are effective for treating phobias. Eye gaze interaction has been incorporated for teleportation in virtual environments to enhanced user's sense of control in immersive environments. To evaluate the effectiveness and degree of improvement in participants phobia, STAI-Y1 was employed.

10.3 Methodology

The proposed work methodology breaks down into four stages, each of which focuses on creating an efficient VR exposure therapy for claustrophobia and nyctophobia patients (Jamal et al. 2017). The first section focuses on creating realistic 3D simulations of environments that make patients anxious and fearful, i.e., triggering their fears. Moreover, a crystal collection game has also been created to increase the framework's interaction and engagement (Hussain et al. 2020). The implementation of eye-gaze-based teleportation technique in Unity 3D is covered in the second section, to eliminate the need for patients to physically move around the 3D environment by allowing them to navigate around utilizing their eye gaze for locomotion in environment (Tahir et al. 2019). In the third section, the Oculus Quest 2 VR headset and heart rate monitoring sensors are integrated to track the stress levels throughout exposure therapy by viewing real-time heart rate data from the sensors on the VR headset (Iftikhar et al. 2017; Naz et al. 2019). Finally, a pilot study was conducted to evaluate the framework. For patients with claustrophobia and nyctophobia, a successful VR exposure therapy experience is delivered using this framework, Figure 10.1 depicting the methodology steps for it.

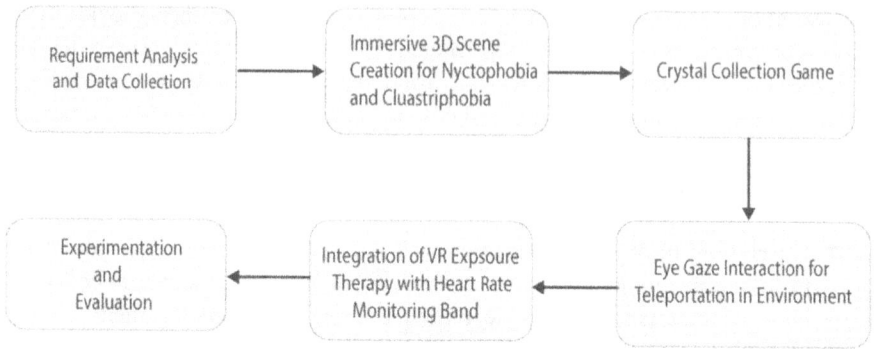

Figure 10.1 Methodology steps for the development of VR exposure therapy to treat phobias.

Figure 10.2 illustrates the flow diagram of propose VR exposure therapy framework to treat nyctophobia and claustrophobia. Subjects will wear the VR headset, and heart rate monitoring sensor on their fingertip. Controllers will be used to move around and interact with objects in the environment. Users can teleport to explore the environments, while collecting crystals. Monitored heart rate will be displayed graphically to user in the environment.

10.3.1 VR Exposure Therapies Framework

To design and develop 3D environments, unity 3D was first installed. Using Unity 3D for low-end devices like mobile phones is a great way to create complex objects. In addition, it provides a good experience for smaller teams, and it has a significantly larger asset storage than other game engines. Software and hardware requirements other than unity 3D for generating 3D virtual worlds and interactive

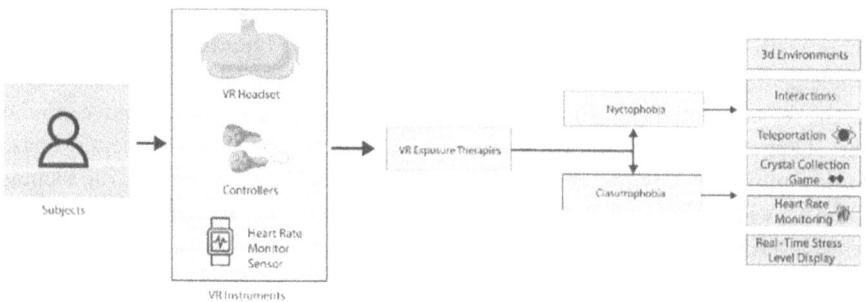

Figure 10.2 Flow diagram of VR exposure therapy to treat nyctophobia and claustrophobia.

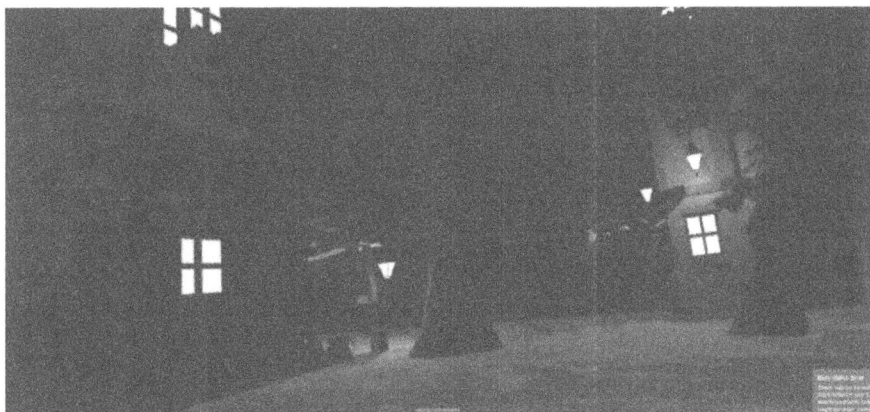

Figure 10.3   Dark, gloomy 3D environment for nyctophobia.

features are Visual Studio 2022, C# language, VR Headset (Oculus Quest 2), heart rate monitoring band sensor (MAX30102).

It was a complex process requiring careful planning and attention to detail to implement 3D environments for treating nyctophobia and claustrophobia. First, the specific triggers were researched for each condition before sourcing high-quality 3D assets from the Unity Asset Store. A dark, gloomy, and shady 3D environment is then created for nyctophobia (Figure 10.3), using Unity Asset Store assets. The environment is visually engaging and realistic to simulate scenarios that trigger fear and anxiety in patients. For claustrophobia treatment, the environment has multiple buildings and compact, narrowed, and small streets that the user has to navigate through (Figure 10.4). Details were carefully considered when designing these environments, ensuring every aspect was optimized for VR. Moreover, a crystal collection game was incorporated to provide further engagement and interactivity. As part of this game, players collect crystals within a 3D environment while facing their fears, distracting them from anxiety-provoking stimuli shown in Figure 10.5.

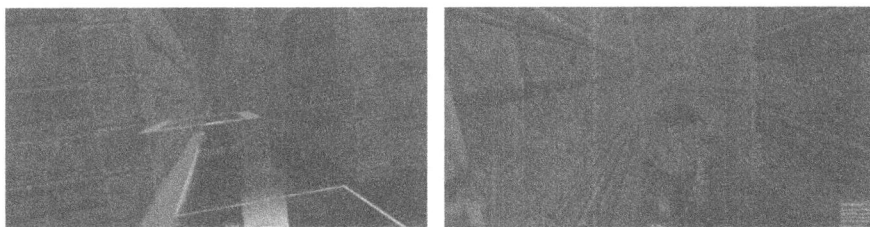

Figure 10.4   Three-dimensional confined places for claustrophobic patients.

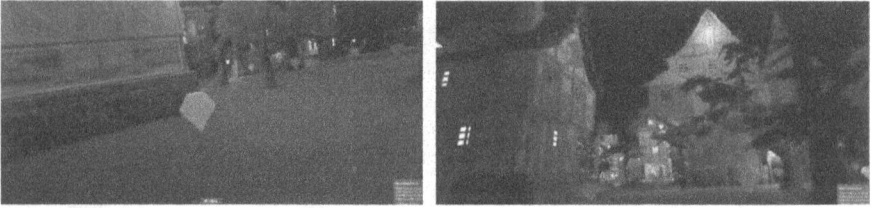

Figure 10.5 Crystal collection game.

10.3.2 Eye Gaze–based Teleportation

A popular locomotion method for VR, teleportation allows users to travel beyond the available tracking space without experiencing VR sickness (Khan et al. 2022; Saba & Rehman 2013). Eye gaze–based teleportation relies on the help of eye-tracking technology in head-mounted displays (Prithul et al. 2022). It is well understood that humans use gaze as a natural and intuitive means of interaction. Therefore, this interaction was employed in our framework to enhance VR immersive experience. Figure 10.6a shows the eye gaze feature in the nyctophobia environment and Figure 10.6b shows the eye gaze interactivity in claustrophobia. A gaze teleportation locomotion method in VR allows the user to teleport to the point they are looking at by pressing a button. It helps us to design intuitive locomotion interfaces to allow users to scale virtual worlds larger than their play space. Linn (2017) conducted a study involving 12 participants. He compared gaze teleportation to a conventional hand-tracking controller. Participants played Valve's The Lab with an HTC Vive and a Tobii Eyetracker. The VR System program with eye gaze–based interaction can be seen in Figure 10.7, and the interaction process involves (1) mapping the user's eye focus on the screen coordinates, (2) generating a primary ray (raycasting using the sphere) from the user's eye focus direction, (3) intersection analysis with scene objects, (4) identifying the object pointed by the sight, (5) handling the event associated with the object, and rendering a stereo pair for HMD (Piotrowski & Nowosielski 2020).

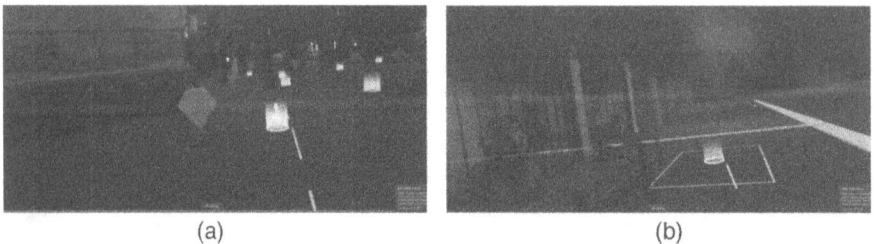

(a)   (b)

Figure 10.6 (a) Eye gaze interactivity in nyctophobia environment. (b) Eye gaze interactivity in claustrophobia environment.

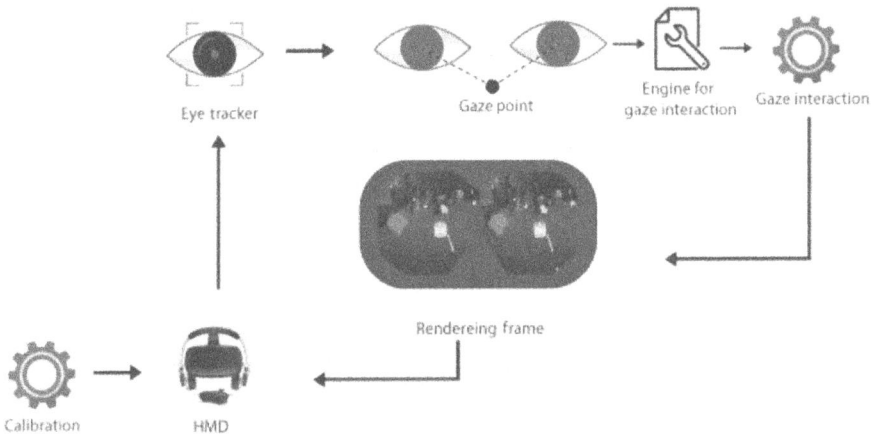

Figure 10.7   Program of VR system with eye gaze–based interaction.

Half of the participants utilized gaze teleportation to complete the tasks, while the other half used hand-tracking. They scored their experiences in terms of satisfaction, annoyance, effort, distance, occlusion, immersion, and motion sickness using Likert questions (Larabi-Marie-Sainte et al. 2019). Conclusively, findings state that gaze teleportation is an excellent fit for applications where users are expected to move in their concentration direction without being distracted. In Unity 3D, raycast is used to implement this interaction. However, eyes tend to wander around and follow contours; therefore, some ray casts miss targets by a hair's breadth. To overcome this problem, Algorithm 1 for gaze-based teleportation has been presented.

Algorithm 10.1: For selecting areas and point at which to teleport to

---

Input: Ray cast from camera in gaze direction
Output: Selected the target area or point at which to teleport to
Start:
  1. if ray cast hits point or area:
  2.   select it
  3. else:
  4.   find the lowest angle between the gaze vector and every point
  5.   if that angle is < 5°:
  6.   select it
  7. only mark selections if there was at least 200 ms since the last selection
  8. unselect the point if not reselected in 200 ms
End:

Linn (2017) devised the Algorithm 10.1 for gaze-based teleportation. The above-described problem can be handled by calculating the shortest angle between the eyes and all teleportation points. The angle comparison also overcomes the problem of objects in the distance that is too small to choose. Raycast is useful for finding nearby items and pinpointing the gaze point on bigger surfaces. They included a delay in order to adjust the selection to minimize flickering when the eye is at the edge of two closely situated locations. Two hundred millisecond was found to be an appropriate delay period without making the selections sluggish and while yet making the edge cases feel assured.

10.3.3 Integration of Heart Rate Monitoring Band with Framework

In order to measure the heart rate of users, VR application was integrated with a MAX30102 pulse sensor. This sensor works on the principle of photoplethysmography (PPG) using red and IR wavelengths (Naz et al. 2019). The sensor transfers an analog pulse signal to microcontroller through I2C bus. The sensor can be used on the fingertips, wrist, and earlobe, as represented in Figure 10.8. In our case, participants wear it on their fingertips. In order to measure heart rate, the raw pulse signal has to be processed (Yousaf et al. 2019). In the push to lessen the instrument size to make it wearable or versatile, it is presented to more noise. Inborn noise and movement antiques can be taken out by various techniques. PPG-based instruments like pulse oximeters work surprisingly well when the subject is in resting position. Nonetheless, in reality, the subject may not be required to act along these lines. The signal gets contorted on development of subjects, which could be automatic, for instance, when shuddering.

Different combinations of low-pass, band-pass, peak isolators and fast Fourier transform (FFT) were tested for best results with earlobe PPG signal. Experimental results show that very low-level motion artifacts can be efficiently removed with combination of a simple low pass and a peak isolation filter, but the method fails for greater motion artifacts. On the other hand, FFT keeps the results consistent with varying levels of noise. Frequency analysis is commonly carried out using FFT. Analyzing a signal in the frequency domain is achieved by performing the FFT. When there are more than two samples in the signal, FFT is the faster version of the discrete Fourier transform (DFT) (Joo & Oppenheim 1988). The N-point DFT can be computed using Equation (10.1) (Mohd Sani et al. 2015).

$$x_n = \frac{1}{N} \sum_{k=0}^{N-1} X_k \cdot e^{i2\pi kn/N}, \ n \in \mathbb{Z} \tag{10.1}$$

where x_n is the discrete-time signal with a period of N. In order to determine the frequency of the PPG signal, FFT was computed and analyzed. Once the frequency

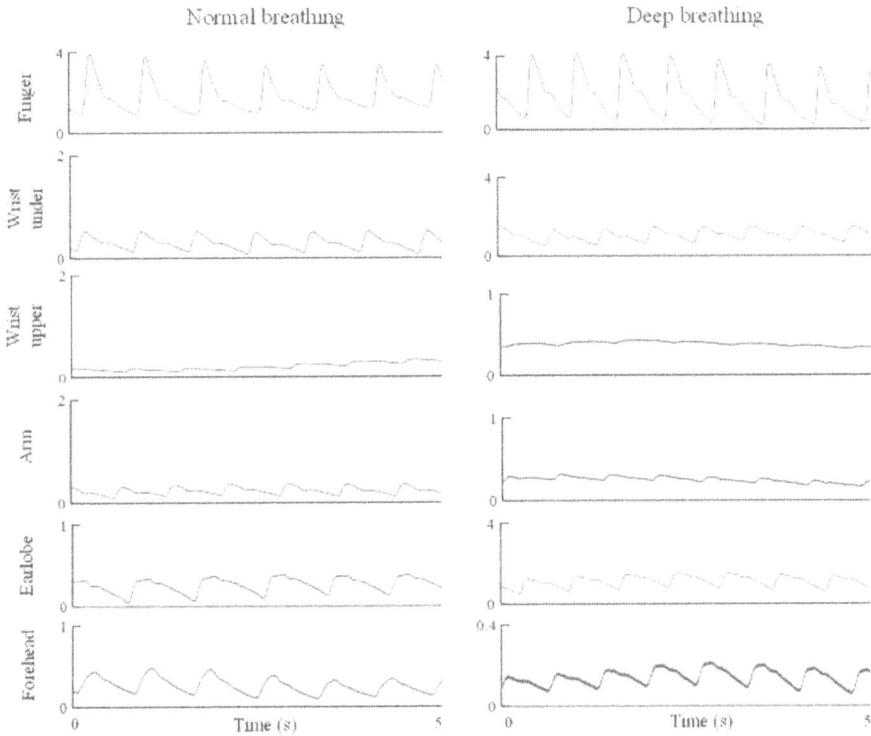

Figure 10.8   PPG signal from different body location.

of the signal was obtained from the spectrum, the heart rate was measured from Equation (10.2) (Joo & Oppenheim 1988).

$$\text{Heart rate} = \text{frequency} \times 60 \tag{10.2}$$

Different FFT windowing functions also have different effects on the results. Figure 10.9 shows the heart rate values generated after using different noise removal methods. It is clear from the chart that a low-pass filter with an FFT with a Nuttall window generates the closest average to actual HR value and has little standard deviation in comparison with other functions. The Nuttall window coefficients are given by Equation (10.3) ("Nuttall Window | RecordingBlogs" n.d.):

$$a(k) = 0.355768 - 0.487396\cos\left(\frac{2\pi k}{N-1}\right) + 0.144232\cos\left(\frac{4\pi k}{N-1}\right) \\ - 0.012604\cos\left(\frac{6\pi k}{N-1}\right) \tag{10.3}$$

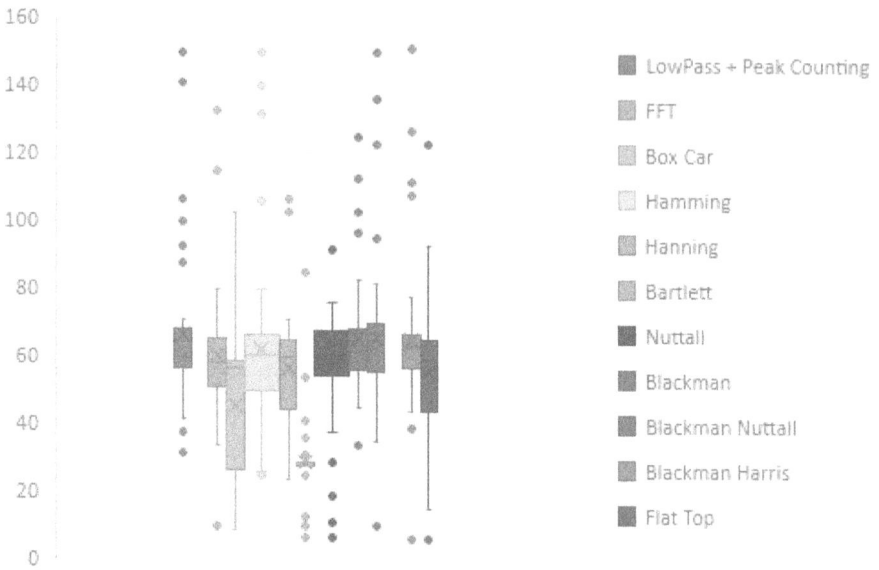

Figure 10.9   Heart rate values with different filters.

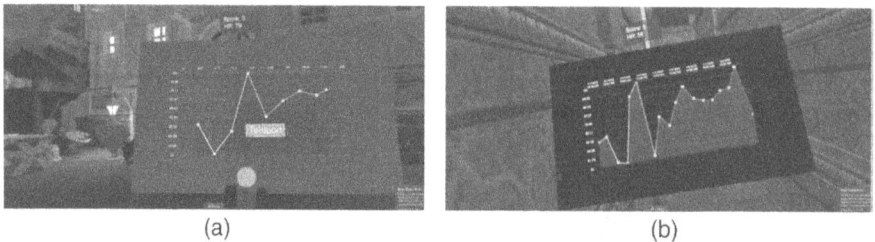

Figure 10.10   (a) Real-time heart rate monitoring graph in nyctophobia environment. (b) Real-time heart rate monitoring graph in claustrophobia environment.

where N is the length of the filter and $k = 0, 1, 2, ..., N − 1$. Finally, framework was deployed on the HTC VIVE and real-time monitored data of user was being graphically represented during the exposure therapy, as shown in Figure 10.10. This feature presents a visual representation of the individual's stress level, which is helpful to track the efficacy of the VR therapy.

10.4 Experiments and Results

This section presents the experiment conducted to assess the efficiency and usability of VR phobia treatment framework and analysis of the findings from the experiment. STAI was chosen as an evaluation method for our developed framework for phobia treatment. It is a widely used measure of trait and state anxiety developed in 1983 by Spielberger, Gorsuch, Lushene, Vagg, and Jacobs. It can be utilized in therapeutic settings to differentiate anxiety from depressive illnesses. During the test, a total of 20 traits and 20 states of anxiety are assessed. Items like "I feel rested; I have a lack of self-confidence" and "I feel frightened; I feel calm." "I worry too much about something that really doesn't matter," and "I am relaxed; I am content," are examples of trait and state anxiety items (Beckler 2010). Based on a 4-point scale, all objects are rated from "Almost Never" to "Almost Always." A higher score indicates a higher level of anxiety. In this study, only STAI-Y1 form was used which is for state anxiety inventory (Sadad et al. 2021). The state anxiety form consists of 20 statements, score ranges from 20 to 80 (higher score higher anxiety levels) (Julian 2011), and 4-point Likert scale for its rating is as follows:

- 1: Not at All
- 2: Somewhat
- 3: Moderately so
- 4: Very much so

Also, the heart rate changes were recorded in users over time after each session. In total, users use these VR phobia treatment frameworks twice, with a gap of a day. Each session consisted of 40–60 minutes, followed by questionnaire of STAI-Y1. They rated these question/statements of STAI-Y1 on the scale of 1–4 (Almost Never to Almost Always). Twenty participants were recruited, of which 8 suffered from claustrophobia and others from claustrophobia. Six were females (30%) and 14 (70%) were males. The average age of participants is Table 10.2 demonstrate the STAI-Y1 score against each participant after each session. STAI-Y1-1 states after session 1 and STAI-Y1-2 states after session 2 rating by users.

Depending on the severity of the anxiety, STAI scores are commonly subdivided into "no or low anxiety" if score range is 20–37, "moderate anxiety" if score range is 38–44, and "high anxiety" if score range is 45–80. In general, adult males have a heart rate of 70–72 beats per minute, while adult females have a heart rate of 78–82 beats per minute and this difference is due to the heart size in males and females (Prabhavathi et al. 2014). Table 10.2 presents STAI-Y1 score after first and second use of the phobia treatment framework. Also, the average heart (beats per minute) of patients during first and second use is also presented in Table 10.2. The average STAI-Y1 after first use is 57 which comes in the range of 45–80 and marked as "high anxiety." However, after second use, the mean score value of STAI reduces to 41 (comes under the range of 38–44), which was marked by researchers as "moderate anxiety." This decrease in anxiety after one use demonstrated the effectiveness of phobia treatment framework. These monitored heart rates also presented graphically in Figure 10.11, and clearly shows a decrease in heart rate in second use than the first use of phobia treatment framework.

Table 10.2   STAI-Y1 Scores, and Average Heart Rate after Each Use by Each Participant

Participant	STAI-Y1- 1	STAI-Y1-2	Heart Rate (After First Use) (bpm)	Heart Rate (After Second Use) (bpm)
P1	40	26	93	82
P2	37	21	89	88
P3	67	42	150	130
P4	55	35	105	105
P5	64	38	130	123
P6	46	30	167	165
P7	39	23	102	98
P8	69	43	165	120
P9	73	56	187	140
P10	56	33	142	124
P11	68	38	155	123
P12	45	31	103	78
P13	75	61	192	165
P14	56	42	120	96
P15	53	40	139	101
P16	71	59	182	155
P17	49	50	111	103
P18	58	52	102	76
P19	58	55	112	85
P20	73	63	206	172
Mean	**57**	**41**	**134**	**112**

Table 10.3 descripts the comparative analysis with exiting studies.

Other fear-inducing environments can be designed and added to the framework, such as car washes, tube trains, elevators, revolving doors, etc., for claustrophobic and basements, garages, cells, and other dark scenes for nyctophobia. VR can be used to treat other phobias as well, i.e., aerophobia, agoraphobia, acrophobia, etc.

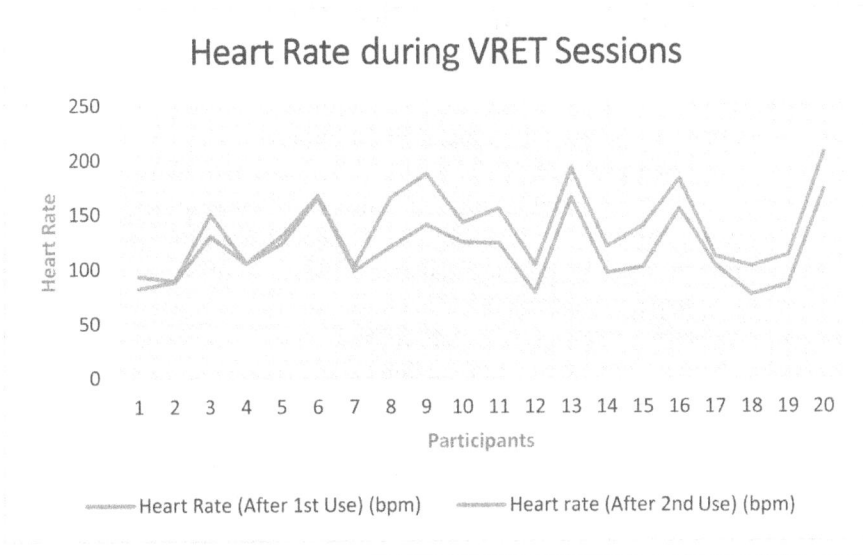

Figure 10.11   Heart rate graph of two sessions of VR environments.

Future research can use a variety of methods with a large number of participants to evaluate the effectiveness of this and other such frameworks (Meethongjan et al. 2013). It is also possible to administer a survey questionnaire following the therapy, asking questions as follows: Did they improve their fear control in subsequent therapy sessions as a result of the therapy? Were the participants able to complete all therapy stages in the first session? Is it possible for them to overcome their fears? Which environment causes the most anxiety? Such surveys will be useful in understanding which elements contribute to the widespread fear of phobias, as well as for future research (Sharmikha Sree, Meera, Priyadharshini, et al. 2022).

Table 10.3   A Definite Comparative Analysis with Existing Studies

Study	Phobia	Participants	HRM
Francová, Jablonská, and Fajnerová (2023)	Claustrophobia	18	No
Rizhan et al. (2021)	Claustrophobia	–	No
Helle et al. (2022)	Claustrophobia	7	No
Dawis and Setiawan (2022)	Nyctophobia	5	Yes
Proposed system	Claustrophobia and nyctophobia	20	Yes

10.5 Conclusion and Future Directions

VRET applications have become a powerful elective that can rise to the consequences of conventional medicines for phobias from an adequacy perspective. Nonetheless, they are likewise instruments fit for improving the mental treatment field. In the coming years, there will be a critical increment in the standard utilization of these VRET applications, as these are valuable for the treatment of phobias. So as to advance in this field, new exploration lines should locate the best methodologies to improve introduction treatment, decrease the repeat of fear, and increment the adequacy of presentation-based medicines. Our developed framework provides exposure therapies for claustrophobia (affects 5–10% of human population) and nyctophobia, both are very common occurring phobias among adults and children. The heart rate monitoring through sensors help in assessing the effectiveness of the exposure therapies over time. The findings expressed clearly that our therapeutic strategy help in decreasing the high rates in two sessions only. Further, participants were administered to STAI survey, and findings from this survey also demonstrated the decrease of anxiety and fear in second use than the first use. As a result, our therapy sessions were found to be beneficial in the treatment of claustrophobia and nyctophobia, allowing people to overcome their fears.

The future work of VR exposure therapies would include designing and developing immersive VR environments for different phobias, namely, arachnophobia (the fear of spiders), acrophobia (fear of heights), agoraphobia (the fear of open or crowded places), etc., other than claustrophobia and nyctophobia. The future work could possibly include using other methods for measuring the degree of improvement in phobic patients after VRET to evaluate its effectiveness other than STAI. Moreover, future studies should perform the experimentation on larger sample group to generalize results. Adding games, challenges, and other interaction mechanism could be another possible future work in this respect.

References

Bagha, S., & Shaw, L. (2011). A real time analysis of PPG signal for measurement of SpO_2 and pulse rate. International Journal of Computer Applications, 36(11), 45–50.

Concannon, B. J., Shaniff, E., & Mary, R.R. (2019). Head-mounted display virtual reality in post-secondary education and skill training. Frontiers in Education, 4, 80. https://doi.org/10.3389/FEDUC.2019.00080

Dawis, A. M., & Setiawan, I. (2022). Utilization of virtual reality technology in knowing the symptoms of acrophobia and nyctophobia. Journal of Applied Science and Technology, 2(2), 36–42. https://doi.org/10.30659/JAST.2.02.36-42

Fahad, H. M., Ghani Khan, M. U., Saba, T., Rehman, A., & Iqbal, S. (2018). Microscopic abnormality classification of cardiac murmurs using ANFIS and HMM. Microscopy Research and Technique, 81(5), 449–457.

Fox, Jesse, Arena, Dylan, & Bailenson, Jeremy N. (2009). Virtual reality: A survival guide for the social scientist. Journal of Media Psychology, 21(3), 95–113. https://doi.org/10.1027/1864-1105.21.3.95

Francová, Anna, Jablonská, Markéta, & Fajnerová, Iveta. (2023). Design and evaluation of virtual reality environments for claustrophobia. PRESENCE: Virtual and Augmented Reality, 32, 23–34. https://doi.org/10.1162/PRES_A_00385

Harrington, C. M., Dara, O. K., Quinlan, J. F., Ryan, D., et al. (2018). Development and evaluation of a trauma decision-making simulator in oculus virtual reality. The American Journal of Surgery, 215(1), 42–47. https://doi.org/10.1016/J.AMJSURG.2017.02.011

Helle, J., Heldal, I., Soleim, H., Geitung, A., & Larsen, T. F. (2022). Virtual reality exposure therapy for claustrophobia: Evaluating usability and usefulness by clinicians. In 2022 1st IEEE International Conference on Cognitive Aspects of Virtual Reality, CVR 2022, pp. 65–72. https://doi.org/10.1109/CVR55417.2022.9967569

Hofmann, S. G., & Smits, Jasper A. J. (2008). Cognitive-behavioral therapy for adult anxiety disorders: A meta-analysis of randomized placebo-controlled trials. The Journal of Clinical Psychiatry, 69(4), 621–632. https://doi.org/10.4088/JCP.V69N0415

Husham, A., Hazim Alkawaz, M., Saba, T., Rehman, A., & Saleh Alghamdi, J. (2016). Automated nuclei segmentation of malignant using level sets. Microscopy Research and Technique, 79(10), 993–997.

Hussain, N., Khan, M. A., Sharif, M., Khan, S. A., Albesher, A. A., Saba, T., & Armaghan, A. (2020). A deep neural network and classical features based scheme for objects recognition: An application for machine inspection. Multimedia Tools and Applications, 83, 14935–14957.

Iftikhar, S., Fatima, K., Rehman, A., Almazyad, A. S., & Saba, T. (2017). An evolution based hybrid approach for heart diseases classification and associated risk factors identification. Biomedical Research, 28(8), 3451–3455.

Jabeen, S., Mehmood, Z., Mahmood, T., Saba, T., Rehman, A., & Mahmood, M. T. (2018). An effective content-based image retrieval technique for image visuals representation based on the bag-of-visual-words model. PLoS One, 13(4), e0194526.

Jamal, A., Hazim Alkawaz, M., Rehman, A., & Saba, T. (2017). Retinal imaging analysis based on vessel detection. Microscopy Research and Technique, 80(7), 799–811.

Jashwanth, K., Shetty, S. R., Yashwanth, A. N., & Ravish, R. (2020). Phobia therapy using virtual reality. In 2020 IEEE International Conference for Innovation in Technology, INOCON 2020, pp. 1–6. https://doi.org/10.1109/INOCON50539.2020.9298227

Javed, R., Rahim, M. S. M., Saba, T., & Rehman, A. (2020). A comparative study of features selection for skin lesion detection from dermoscopic images. Network Modeling Analysis in Health Informatics and Bioinformatics, 9, 1–13.

Joo, Tae H., & Oppenheim, Alan V. (1988). Effects of FFT coefficient quantization on sinusoidal signal detection. In IEEE International Conference on Acoustics, Speech and Signal Processing: Proceedings, 1818–1821. https://doi.org/10.1109/ICASSP.1988.196975

Julian, Laura J. (2011). Measures of anxiety. Arthritis Care & Research, 63(11), S467–S472. https://doi.org/10.1002/ACR.20561

Khan, M. A., Sharif, M. I., Raza, M., Anjum, A., Saba, T., & Shad, S. A. (2022). Skin lesion segmentation and classification: A unified framework of deep neural network features fusion and selection. Expert Systems, 39(7), e12497.

Larabi-Marie-Sainte, S., Aburahmah, L., Almohaini, R., & Saba, T. (2019). Current techniques for diabetes prediction: Review and case study. Applied Sciences, 9(21), 4604.

Linn, Andreas. (2017). Gaze Teleportation in Virtual Reality. http://urn.kb.se/resolve?urn=urn:nbn:se:kth:diva-216585

Maples-Keller, Jessica L., Bunnell, Brian E., Kim, Sae Jin, & Rothbaum, Barbara O. (2017). The use of virtual reality technology in the treatment of anxiety and other psychiatric disorders. Harvard Review of Psychiatry, 25(3), 103. https://doi.org/10.1097/HRP.0000000000000138

Meethongjan, K., Dzulkifli, M., Rehman, A., Altameem, A., & Saba, T. (2013). An intelligent fused approach for face recognition. Journal of Intelligent Systems, 22(2), 197–212.

Mohd Sani, N. H., Mansor, W., Lee, Khuan Y., Zainudin, N. Ahmad, & Mahrim, S. A. (2015). Determination of heart rate from photoplethysmogram using fast Fourier transform. In 2015 International Conference on BioSignal Analysis, Processing and Systems (ICBAPS 2015), October, 168–170. https://doi.org/10.1109/ICBAPS.2015.7292239

Mughal, B., Muhammad, N., Sharif, M., Rehman, A., & Saba, T. (2018a). Removal of pectoral muscle based on topographic map and shape-shifting silhouette. BMC Cancer, 18(1), 1–14.

Mughal, B., Sharif, M., Muhammad, N., & Saba, T. (2018b). A novel classification scheme to decline the mortality rate among women due to breast tumor. Microscopy Research and Technique, 81(2), 171–180.

Muhsin, Z. F., Rehman, A., Altameem, A., Saba, T., & Uddin, M. (2014). Improved quadtree image segmentation approach to region information. The Imaging Science Journal, 62(1), 56–62.

Muris, P., Simon, E., Lijphart, H., Bos, A., Hale, W., Schmeitz, K., & Albano, A. M., et al. (2017). The youth anxiety measure for DSM-5 (YAM-5): Development and first psychometric evidence of a new scale for assessing anxiety disorders symptoms of children and adolescents. Child Psychiatry and Human Development, 48(1), 1–17. https://doi.org/10.1007/S10578-016-0648-1

Naz, A., Javed, M. U., Javaid, N., Saba, T., Alhussein, M., & Aurangzeb, K. (2019). Short-term electric load and price forecasting using enhanced extreme learning machine optimization in smart grids. Energies, 12(5), 866.

Nimnual, R., & Yossatorn, Y. (2019). Therapeutic virtual reality for nyctophobic disorder. In ACM International Conference Proceeding Series, February, 11–15. https://doi.org/10.1145/3332305.3332310

Norton, P. J., & Price, E. C. (2007). A meta-analytic review of adult cognitive-behavioral treatment outcome across the anxiety disorders. The Journal of Nervous and Mental Disease, 195(6), 521–531. https://doi.org/10.1097/01.NMD.0000253843.70149.9A

Paulus, E., Yusuf, F. P., Suryani, M., & Suryana, I. (2019). Development and evaluation on night forest virtual reality as innovative nyctophobia treatment. Journal of Physics: Conference Series, 1235(1), 012003. https://doi.org/10.1088/1742-6596/1235/1/012003

Peñate, W., Pitti, C. T., & Bethencourt, J. M. (2008). The effects of a treatment based on the use of virtual reality exposure and cognitive-behavioral therapy applied to patients with agoraphobia 1. International Journal of Clinical and Health Psychology, 8(1), 5–22.

Piotrowski, P., & Nowosielski, A. (2020). Gaze-based interaction for VR environments. Advances in Intelligent Systems and Computing, 1062, 41–48. https://doi.org/10.1007/978-3-030-31254-1_6

Prabhavathi, K., Selvi, K. T., Poornima, K. N., & Sarvanan, A. (2014). Role of biological sex in normal cardiac function and in its disease outcome: A review. Journal of Clinical and Diagnostic Research, 8(8), BE01. https://doi.org/10.7860/JCDR/2014/9635.4771

Prithul, A., Bhandari, J., Spurgeon, W., & Folmer, E. (2022). Evaluation of hands-free teleportation in VR. In Proceedings: SUI 2022: ACM Conference on Spatial User Interaction, December 2022. https://doi.org/10.1145/3565970.3567683

Rehman, A. (2023). Brain stroke prediction through deep learning techniques with ADASYN strategy. In 2023 16th International Conference on Developments in eSystems Engineering (DeSE), Istanbul, Turkiye, 679–684.

Rizhan, Wan, Shapri, Saadah Mohd Nur, Amin, Mat Atar Mat, & Muhamad, Mahathir. (2021). Mobile-based virtual reality application for experiencing and detecting claustrophobia. International Journal of Engineering Trends and Technology 69, 53–58. https://doi.org/10.14445/22315381/IJETT-V69I2P208

Saba, T., Al-Zahrani, S., & Rehman, A. (2012). Expert system for offline clinical guidelines and treatment. Life Science Journal, 9(4), 2639–2658.

Saba, T., Bokhari, S. T. F., Sharif, M., Yasmin, M., & Raza, M. (2018b). Fundus image classification methods for the detection of glaucoma: A review. Microscopy Research and Technique, 81(10), 1105–1121.

Saba, T., & Rehman, A. (2013). Effects of artificially intelligent tools on pattern recognition. International Journal of Machine Learning and Cybernetics, 4, 155–162.

Saba, T., Rehman, A., Mehmood, Z., Kolivand, H., & Sharif, M. (2018a). Image enhancement and segmentation techniques for detection of knee joint diseases: A survey. Current Medical Imaging, 14(5), 704–715.

Sadad, T., Rehman, A., Munir, A., Saba, T., Tariq, U., Ayesha, N., & Abbasi, R. (2021). Brain tumor detection and multi-classification using advanced deep learning techniques. Microscopy Research and Technique, 84(6), 1296–1308.

Schowalter, J. E. (1994). Fears and phobias. Pediatrics in Review, 15(10), 384–388. https://doi.org/10.1542/PIR.15-10-384

Set, Sampler (2010). State-trait anxiety inventory for adults. Garden, 1–75.

Shanthini, E., Sangeetha, V., Selvapriya, P., Shivani, B., Shanmuga Priya, M., & Anindita, K. (2022). Virtual therapy for phobias: A human computer interaction. Proceedings: 2022 IEEE World Conference on Applied Intelligence and Computing, AIC 2022, 349–353. https://doi.org/10.1109/AIC55036.2022.9848950.

Sharmikha Sree, R., Meera, S., Deepika, R., Kalpana, R. A., Ramya, N., & Ganga, A. (2022). Dealing with claustrophobia using virtual reality. AIP Conference Proceedings, 2464(1), 060007. https://doi.org/10.1063/5.0082647

Sharmikha Sree, R., Meera, S., Priyadharshini, S., & Gayathri, R. (2022). An integration of various virtual environments to overcome claustrophobia using virtual reality. Proceedings: International Conference on Applied Artificial Intelligence and Computing (ICAAIC 2022), 1621–27. https://doi.org/10.1109/ICAAIC53929.2022.9792837

Tahir, B., Iqbal, S., Usman Ghani Khan, M., Saba, T., Mehmood, Z., Anjum, A., & Mahmood, T. (2019). Feature enhancement framework for brain tumor segmentation and classification. Microscopy Research and Technique, 82(6), 803–811.

Yousaf, K., Mehmood, Z., Saba, T., Rehman, A., Munshi, A. M., Alharbey, R., & Rashid, M. (2019). Mobile-health applications for the efficient delivery of health care facility to people with dementia (PwD) and support to their carers: A survey. BioMed Research International, 2019, 7151475.

Chapter 11

Explainable Artificial Intelligence-Based Machine Analytics and Deep Learning in Medical Science

Morteza Soltani[1], Mehdi Davari[2], Mina Bahadori[1],
Ahmad Kokhahi[1], Mahsa Bahadori[3], and
Masoumeh Soleimani[1]

[1]*Department of Industrial Engineering, Clemson University,
Clemson, South Carolina, USA*
[2]*Department of Management, Isfahan Branch, Islamic Azad University,
Isfahan, Iran*
[3]*Department of Industrial Engineering, Islamic Azad University,
Mashhad, Iran*

11.1 Introduction

Artificial intelligence (AI) is a broad term encompassing the utilization of computers to simulate intelligent behavior with minimal human involvement. The inception of robots is widely acknowledged as the starting point of AI (Hamet and Tremblay, 2017). Since the development of the initial AI model designed to assist physicians, medicine has emerged as a primary domain for the application

DOI: 10.1201/9781032626345-11

205

of AI (Burton et al., 2019). Additional studies have further expanded the scope of AI applications, such as work on face detection in close-up shot video events using video mining (Khan et al., 2023), and a directional review by author on health monitoring methods in heart diseases based on a data mining approach (Harouni et al., 2022). These contributions illustrate the diverse applications of AI, ranging from video analysis to health monitoring, in different domains. The earliest work of medical AI can be traced back to the early 1970s, a period when the AI field was approximately 15 years old (Wikipedia, 2023). For example, in the early stages of AI development, there was significant interest in specific tasks, including the interpretation of electrocardiogram (ECG) signals (Kundu et al., 2000), disease diagnosis (De Dombal et al., 1972), selecting appropriate treatments (De Dombal et al., 1972), and analyzing clinical reasoning (Barnett et al., 1987). In the early stages of artificial intelligence in medical (AIM) research, scholars identified the suitability of AI techniques in the life sciences. This was prominently demonstrated in the Dendral experiments during the late 1960s and early 1970s. These experiments involved the collaboration of computer scientists such as Edward Feigenbaum, chemists such as Carl Djerassi, geneticists such as Joshua Lederberg, and philosophers of science such as Bruce Buchanan. Their collective efforts showcased the capability to represent and leverage expert knowledge in symbolic form. The 1970s witnessed a surge of interest in applying AI to biomedical contexts, fueled in part by the establishment of the SUMEX-AIM Computing Resource (Nordlinger et al., 2020) at Stanford University and a parallel facility at Rutgers University. These initiatives leveraged the emerging apparent to provide computing resources to a broad community of researchers, nationally and eventually internationally. This community utilized AI methods to address challenges in biology and medicine. Notably, several early AIM systems, including Internist-1 (Miller et al., 1985), CASNET (Weiss et al., 1978), and MYCIN (Shortliffe, 2012), were crafted using these shared national resources, with support from the Division of Research Resources at the National Institutes of Health. Currently, AI integration in healthcare has broadened to encompass tasks like patient data administration, healthcare services management, and predictive medicine. The heightened demand for these AI applications in the healthcare sector is driven by the persistent mental and physical strain experienced by healthcare practitioners, especially during the recent COVID-19 pandemic (Loh et al., 2021; Mollica and Fricchione, 2021). Consequently, extensive AI research aims to alleviate the workload burden on healthcare professionals and its role exhibited in Figure 11.1.

Additionally, the performance of DL is directly linked to the input size, making it particularly advantageous in medical scenarios where extensive datasets are commonplace (Maier et al., 2019). The utilization of the DL approach enhances the effectiveness of previous efforts based on ML models, particularly in the realms of biomedical image classification (Zhang et al., 2019) and segmentation

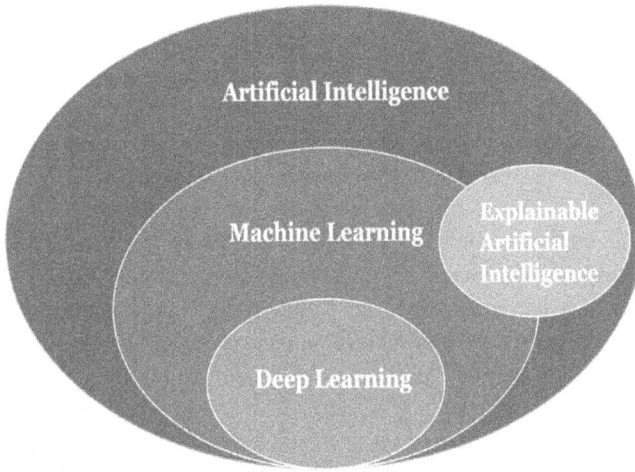

Figure 11.1 **The relationship between artificial intelligence, machine learning, deep learning, and explainable artificial intelligence (Zhang et al., 2022).**

(Haque and Neubert, 2020; Hesamian et al., 2019; Tajbakhsh et al., 2020). The issues surrounding the ability of ML to interpret and explain algorithms have become increasingly prominent. Numerous articles propose various measures and frameworks aimed at capturing interpretability, leading to the emergence of the topic of XAI as a focal point in the ML research community (Bahadori et al., 2024). To address this need for transparency, popular DL libraries have incorporated their own XAI libraries, such as PyTorch, Captum, and TensorFlow (Tjoa and Guan, 2020).

Figure 11.2 illustrates how XAI serves as a link connecting human–computer interaction (HCI) and artificial intelligence. XAI primarily aims to elucidate the interaction for end users, fostering the establishment of a reliable and trustworthy environment (Nazar et al., 2021).

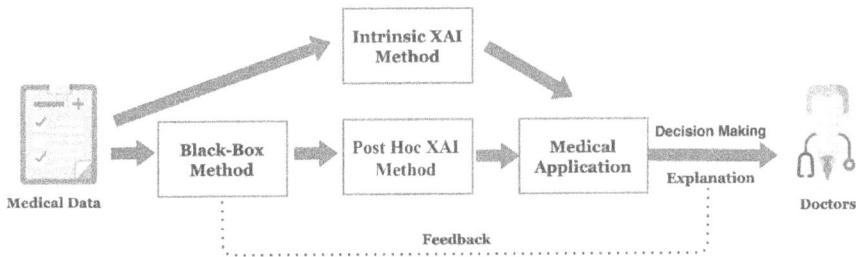

Figure 11.2 **General process of medical XAI application (Zhang et al., 2022).**

11.2 XAI Techniques

In medical science, the application of XAI is crucial for building trust and facilitating the adoption of AI-driven solutions. Interpretability is particularly essential in healthcare, where decisions can have significant consequences on patient outcomes (Alorf 2021). XAI techniques such as rule-based systems, decision trees, and model-agnostic methods like LIME (Local Interpretable Model-agnostic Explanations) and SHAP (SHapley Additive exPlanations) can help elucidate the factors influencing AI predictions. For instance, in diagnostic applications, an XAI approach can provide insights into the features or patterns in medical data that contribute to a specific diagnosis, aiding healthcare professionals in making informed decisions and enhancing overall patient care. The transparency offered by XAI not only improves accountability but also fosters collaboration between AI systems and human experts in the medical field. The taxonomy of XAI methods that is shown in Figure 11.3 refers to the systematic classification or categorization of various approaches and techniques that aim to enhance the interpretability and transparency of AI models.

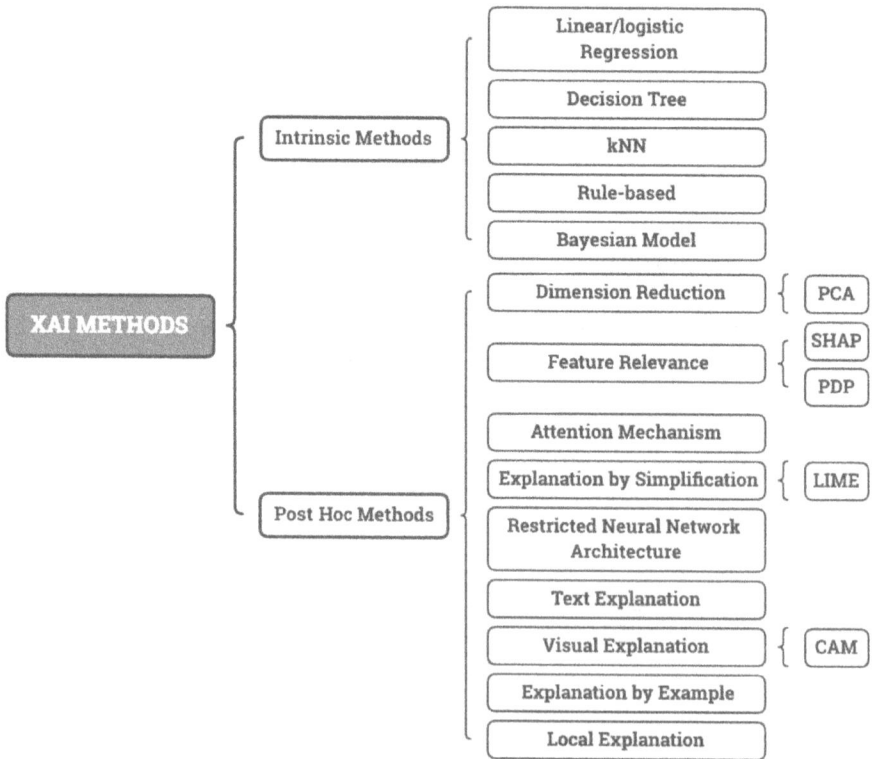

Figure 11.3 Classification of XAI techniques (Band et al., 2023).

In this section, we discuss different XAI techniques used in healthcare. We look at approaches like rule-based systems, fuzzy classifier, and model-agnostic methods such as LIME and SHAP. The focus is on showing how these techniques clarify the workings of AI in medical science, providing insights into why certain predictions are made.

11.2.1 SHapley Additive exPlanations (SHAP)

One of the techniques used in XAI is the Shapley additive explanations (SHAP). This technique tries to interpret the outputs of machine learning algorithms by using the obtained Shapley values of the game theory. Some of the papers using SHAP technique are summarized here.

The research developed accurate and interpretable machine learning models to predict first-time acute exacerbation of chronic obstructive pulmonary disease (COPD) at an individual level. Employing SHapley Additive exPlanations (SHAP) and a local explanation method, the gradient boosting machine (GBM) and support vector machine (SVM) models demonstrated superior discrimination ability, with the GBM model exhibiting a higher net benefit in identifying high-risk patients (Antoniadi et al. 2021). The integration of SHAP and the local explanation method not only enhanced model interpretability but also provided visual explanations of individualized risk predictions, aiding clinicians in understanding key features and the decision-making process (Kor et al., 2022). Shi et al. (2022) developed a machine learning algorithm to predict the malnutrition in children suffering from congenital heart disease (CHD). They implement five machine learning algorithms and measure the area under the receiver operating characteristic (ROC) curve to access their performances. They also implement SHAP to evaluate the feature that the models have chosen. Chen et al. (2021) try to predict the negative effect of surgeries by focusing on physiological signals. They propose an algorithm named PHASE (physiological signal embeddings) to achieve this purpose. In order to interpret the results gained from the model, they use Shapely values. Duckworth et al. (2021) try to determine the patients who need immediate help and hospital admission. They use supervised machine learning algorithms for making future predictions. They use COVID-19 as an example for evaluating the accuracy of proposed algorithm. They use SHAP to observe the amount of difference in feature's SHAP value in comparison with the total value. Zeng et al. (2021) focus on the congenital heart surgery. They train a machine learning algorithms for prediction of possible problems that the patients can face with after surgery. They use SHAP technique for interpretation of obtained results.

Lee et al. (2021) describe the development of cancer prediction models using data from the Korean National Insurance System Database. It focuses on predicting the incidence of cancers using machine learning algorithms like logistic regression, random forest, light gradient boosting machine (LGBM), and others. The SHAP method was utilized to interpret the LGBM model, revealing the most influential factors for cancer prediction, such as age and gender. The study demonstrates the potential of using national health data and machine learning to develop accurate and practical cancer prediction models. Beebe-Wang et al. (2021) focus on predicting imminent dementia in the aging population using machine learning. The study develops a model to predict dementia. SHAP was used to interpret the XGBoost model to identify the most influential features for dementia prediction. This approach emphasizes the importance of recent cognitive assessments.

Dissanayake et al. (2020) explore the development of a deep learning classifier for detecting heart anomalies without the need for heart sound segmentation. The study employs machine learning algorithms, particularly focusing on Mel-Frequency Cepstral Coefficients (MFCCs), to analyze heart sounds and classify them as normal or abnormal (Rawal et al., 2023). SHAP was used to interpret the classifier, highlighting the model's reliance on specific features like the S1 and S2 heart sound locations in the phonocardiogram (PCG) wave. The findings suggest that segmentation is not a necessary step for this classification task, as the model learns to focus on significant sound locations for accurate predictions. Jiang et al. (2021) investigate the risk factors for in-hospital mortality among sepsis survivors readmitted to the ICU. The study applies machine learning algorithms to analyze clinical data and predict mortality risks. The SHAP method is employed to interpret the GBM model to identify key factors contributing to mortality risk in sepsis survivors. This approach enhances the understanding of risk factors for in-hospital mortality in sepsis survivors exhibited in Figure 11.4.

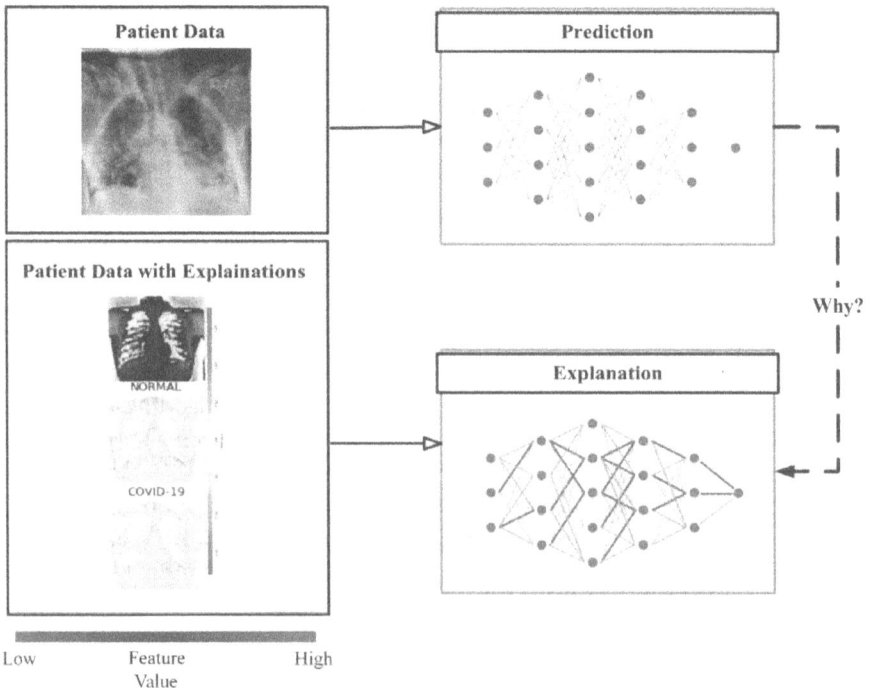

Figure 11.4   SHAP Explainer (Band et al., 2023).

11.2.2 Gradient-weighted Class Activation Mapping (GradCAM)

The other technique that is significantly explored in XAI for the purpose of visualizing and interpreting the decisions made by a deep neural network, specifically in facing of convolutional neural network (CNN), is Gradient-weighted Class Activation Mapping (GradCAM). In the following paragraph, we summarize some of the papers that implemented this technique in their research.

Figueroa et al. (2022) build a CNN algorithm for the classification of different cancer types. However, the explanation and interpretability of the model is under question since it can intensify the importance of factors which are less important. To rectify this problem, they propose a GradCAM model. Xu et al. (2021) propose an XAI system based on GradCAM for diagnosing fungal keratitis with the help of in vivo confocal microscopy images. Chetoui et al. (2021) construct a deep learning model for COVID-19 detection. They propose a novel scaling CNN algorithm, named Efficient Net. This algorithm takes a distinct approach compared to existing methods that adjust network parameters like width, depth, and resolution independently. Instead, Efficient Net uniformly scales each dimension by applying a specified set of scaling factors. Liu et al. (2021) discuss that clinical observers have a limited ability to accurately predict the presence of microvascular invasion (MVI) in preoperative assessments of hepatocellular carcinoma (HCC). They argue that this problem arises due to the fact that majority of this technique in this field rely on the computed tomography (CT) images. However, these approaches heavily connected to the human expertise and necessitate manual tumor contouring (Antony et al., 2021).

In proposed work, we have introduced a deep learning framework for preoperative MVI prediction that utilizes CT images from the arterial phase (AP). They use GradCAM technique for visualizing the output of the algorithm. Figure 11.5 displays

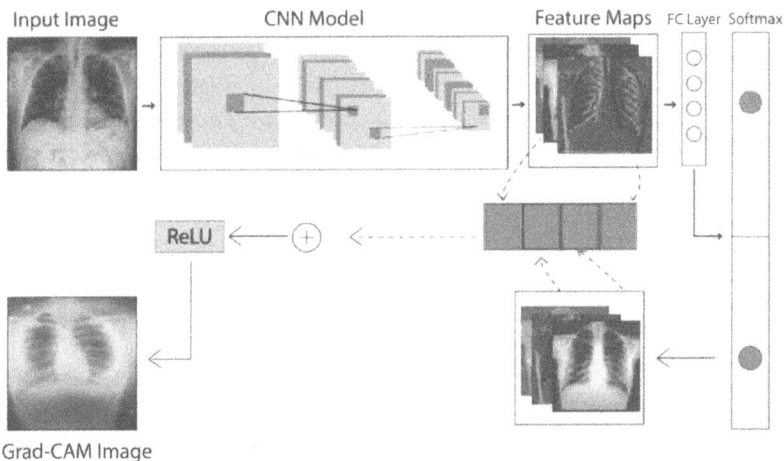

Figure 11.5   GradCAM explainer (Band et al., 2023).

patient data alongside localization maps, providing explanations for each. The process involves utilizing the Grad-CAM technique to generate a heat map from a chest X-ray image.

11.2.3 Local Interpretable Model-agnostic Explanations (LIME)

Local interpretable model-agnostic explanations (LIME) is a technique used in the field of machine learning to explain the predictions of any machine learning model so that people can easily interpret them. This technique is model-agnostic, meaning it can work for all the machine learning algorithms. Also, it is applicable on each individual data rather than the whole dataset. some papers regarding this technique are mentioned in this section.

Magesh et al. (2020) present a machine learning model that classifies DaTSCAN images for early Parkinson's disease detection, achieving high accuracy. The model uses a convolutional neural network (CNN) architecture enhanced by transfer learning, which significantly improves diagnosis accuracy. It employs LIME to provide visual explanations for its predictions, making the diagnostic process transparent and understandable. This approach ensures that the model's decisions are not only accurate but also interpretable. Palatnik de Sousa et al. (2019) focus on the use of LIME to enhance the interpretability of CNN models in classifying histopathology images for lymph node metastases. It compares different segmentation algorithms for generating super pixels, essential for LIME's visual explanations, and introduces a simpler square grid method. The results demonstrate that LIME can effectively reveal the CNN's focus areas in the images. This approach not only improves model transparency but also bridges the gap between AI and expert knowledge in medical diagnostics (Marani et al., 2023).

Figure 11.6 displays the gene ranking determined by prediction probabilities derived from feature extraction techniques. The LIME interpreter was employed for gene ranking, and the plot segregates AD and non-AD genes. The findings highlight the pivotal role of genes in Alzheimer's disease (AD) development, investigating the support vector classification (SVC) process to pinpoint key genes in AD, namely, OR8B8 and ATP6V1G. Furthermore, the analysis identifies the most crucial genes for non-AD, specifically HTR1F and OR6B2 (Kamal et al., 2021).

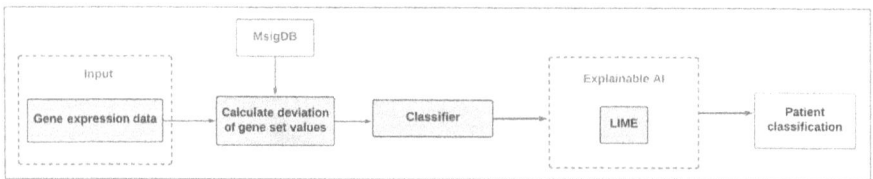

Figure 11.6   LIME explainer (Band et al., 2023).

11.2.4 Partial Dependence Plots (PDPs)

PDPs represent a methodological cornerstone in XAI, tracing their lineage to classical statistical literature's relentless pursuit of understanding variable relationships. The conceptualization of partial dependence found its genesis in the exploration of partial derivatives within early statistical works, laying a robust theoretical foundation that continues to influence subsequent advancements in interpretability (Wang et al., 2021).

11.2.5 Counterfactual Explanations

The counterfactual explanations technique within XAI plays a pivotal role in addressing the imperatives of fairness and interpretability within automated decision-making systems (Wachter et al., 2017). By offering alternative scenarios that, if implemented, would yield different model predictions, this method stands as a critical tool in enhancing the transparency and accountability of machine learning models. This becomes particularly crucial in sensitive applications governed by stringent regulations such as the General Data Protection Regulation (GDPR), where ensuring fairness and justifiability of automated decisions is paramount (Mirza et al., 2019).

The significance of counterfactual explanations extends beyond regulatory compliance. Over time, this method has witnessed widespread adoption across diverse domains, including but not limited to finance, healthcare, and criminal justice. Researchers and practitioners alike recognize its potential to not only uncover and mitigate biases within models but also to ensure that the decision-making processes align with broader societal values (Yang et al., 2021).

11.2.6 Rule-based Explanations

Rule-based explanations, a prominent technique in XAI, revolve around employing interpretable models, particularly decision trees and rule-based systems. These models play a pivotal role in augmenting the transparency of machine learning processes by furnishing explicit rules that establish a precise mapping between input features and predictions. The explicitness of these rules facilitates human understanding, a critical factor in cultivating trust and acceptance of AI-driven decision-making.

The foundational work of Breiman (2017), serves as the cornerstone of decision tree–based explanations. Breiman's comprehensive exploration encompasses the construction of decision trees and their versatile application in both classification and regression tasks.

The hierarchical structure of decision trees, characterized by a series of binary decisions, renders them inherently interpretable. This seminal work laid the groundwork for various rule-based systems, establishing decision trees as a fundamental tool in the realm of explainable AI. Caruana et al. (2015) advocate for the use of interpretable models in healthcare predictive analytics.

11.2.7 Layer-wise Relevance Propagation (LRP)

LRP is a technique like the GradCAM, with one major difference. GradCAM is directly applied on the output of the CNN model. However, in the LPR model, we start from the last layer and move backward to compute the relevance score for each neuron of the neural network model. Finally, by having all the scores for all the neurons in model, we can compute the importance score of each feature in the model. In the following paragraphs, we summarize the works carried out using LRP model.

Binder et al. (2021) present a sophisticated machine learning method that combines different aspects of breast cancer, such as shape and molecular makeup. It effectively identifies and locates cancer cells and immune cells within tissue images using LRP model. It also predicts molecular details like gene activity and protein amounts accurately. This method helps understand how cancer's appearance relates to its molecular properties (Ripoll et al., 2021). This approach not only enhances the interpretability of machine learning models in precision but also is compatible with clinical knowledge.

11.2.8 Fuzzy Classifier

Fuzzy classifier is a technique which works based on the fuzzy logic. In this logic, there is no absolute truth, but we are dealing with partial truth in fuzzy classifier. In the following paragraphs, we summarize the carried-out works using fuzzy classifier model.

Sabol et al. (2020) propose a cumulative fuzzy class membership criterion (CFCMC)–based classifier for colorectal cancer detection from histopathological images. This fuzzy classifier improves decision-making by providing a semantical explanation of the diagnosis, visualizing the most influential training samples for a given prediction, and showing samples from conflicting classes (Mothilal et al., 2020). The classifier is not fully automated but designed as a support system for medical experts while blending high accuracy with human-friendly explainability. Therefore, it enhances the reliability and accountability of medical diagnoses.

Bahani et al. (2021) explore the development of a fuzzy rule-based classification system (FRBCS) to diagnose heart disease using medical datasets. This system leverages fuzzy logic to interpret complex medical data which provide a more nuanced analysis than traditional binary classifiers. The FRBCS achieves high accuracy in heart disease prediction, making it a valuable tool for medical professionals in diagnosing and understanding the nuances of heart disease.

11.3 Conclusion

This study presents an overview of the papers in the domain of XAI methods and their utilization in the interpretability of tasks such as image classification and segmentation in the realm of healthcare and medical science. As we see in the previous studies, the integration of Explainable AI with deep neural network models has the potential to contribute to both disease detection and diagnosis by offering supplementary insights to healthcare professionals. It is also essential to create algorithms that enhance reasoning and explanatory capabilities, considering all relevant clinical parameters and the factors contributing to specific findings. Moreover, by applying the decision-making models, there are also opportunities to gain insights, enhance, and advance the development of more effective AI algorithms.

Furthermore, we classified some papers that applied various types of XAI methods, such as LIME, SHAP, Grade-CAM, and more, along with the diseases for which these methods can provide explanations. As a result, we can say that rising prevalence of health and legal regulations underscores the necessity for approval and compliance with deep learning techniques, a requirement that can be facilitated through the application of XAI methods. Successfully addressing challenges in the clinical adoption of XAI is necessary for the field's expansion, leading to enhanced health and safety measures. Results show that trust in the XAI model's predictions contributes to improved patient outcomes.

References

Abdulaziz Alorf. The practicality of deep learning algorithms in COVID-19 detection: Application to chest X-ray images. *Algorithms*, 14(6), 183, 2021.

Anna Markella Antoniadi, Yuhan Du, Yasmine Guendouz, Lan Wei, Claudia Mazo, Brett A Becker, and Catherine Mooney. Current challenges and future opportunities for XAI in machine learning–based clinical decision support systems: A systematic review. *Applied Sciences*, 11(11), 5088, 2021.

Linta Antony, Sami Azam, Eva Ignatious, Ryana Quadir, Abhijith Reddy Beeravolu, Mirjam Jonkman, and Friso De Boer. A comprehensive unsupervised framework for chronic kidney disease prediction. *IEEE Access*, 9, 126481–126501, 2021.

Mina Bahadori, Masoumeh Soleimani, Morteza Soltani, and Mehdi Davari. Application of IoT in drug supply chain management (SCM) during Covid-19 outbreak. In *Advanced IoT Technologies and Applications in the Industry 4.0 Digital Economy*, pp. 224–237. CRC Press, 2024.

Khalid Bahani, Mohammed Moujabbir, and Mohammed Ramdani. An accurate fuzzy rule-based classification systems for heart disease diagnosis. *Scientific African*, 14, e01019, 2021.

Shahab S. Band, Atefeh Yarahmadi, Chung-Chian Hsu, Meghdad Biyari, Mehdi Sookhak, Rasoul Ameri, Iman Dehzangi, Anthony Theodore Chronopoulos, and Huey-Wen Liang. Application of explainable artificial intelligence in medical health: A systematic review of interpretability methods. *Informatics in Medicine Unlocked*, 101286, 2023.

G Octo Barnett, James J Cimino, Jon A Hupp, and Edward P Hoffer. DXplain: An evolving diagnostic decision-support system. *JAMA*, 258(1), 67–74, 1987.

Nicasia Beebe-Wang, Alex Okeson, Tim Althoff, and Su-In Lee. Efficient and explainable risk assessments for imminent dementia in an aging cohort study. *IEEE Journal of Biomedical and Health Informatics*, 25(7), 2409–2420, 2021.

Alexander Binder, Michael Bockmayr, Miriam Häagele, Stephan Wienert, Daniel Heim, Katharina Hellweg, Masaru Ishii, Albrecht Stenzinger, Andreas Hocke, Carsten Denkert, et al. Morphological and molecular breast cancer profiling through explainable machine learning. *Nature Machine Intelligence*, 3(4), 355–366, 2021.

Leo Breiman. *Classification and Regression Trees*. Routledge, 2017.

Ross J Burton, Mahableshwar Albur, Matthias Eberl, and Simone M Cuff. Using artificial intelligence to reduce diagnostic workload without compromising detection of urinary tract infections. *BMC Medical Informatics and Decision Making*, 19(1), 1–11, 2019.

Rich Caruana, Yin Lou, Johannes Gehrke, Paul Koch, Marc Sturm, and Noemie Elhadad. Intelligible models for healthcare: Predicting pneumonia risk and hospital 30-day readmission. In *Proceedings of the 21th ACM SIGKDD International Conference on Knowledge Discovery and Data Mining*, 1721–1730, 2015.

Hugh Chen, Scott M Lundberg, Gabriel Erion, Jerry H Kim, and Su-In Lee. Forecasting adverse surgical events using self-supervised transfer learning for physiological signals. *NPJ Digital Medicine*, 4(1), 167, 2021.

Mohamed Chetoui, Moulay A Akhloufi, Bardia Yousefi, and El Mostafa Bouattane. Explainable COVID-19 detection on chest X-rays using an end-to-end deep convolutional neural network architecture. *Big Data and Cognitive Computing*, 5(4), 73, 2021.

FT De Dombal, DJ Leaper, John R Staniland, AP McCann, and Jane C Horrocks. Computeraided diagnosis of acute abdominal pain. *British Medical Journal*, 2(5804), 9–13, 1972.

Theekshana Dissanayake, Tharindu Fernando, Simon Denman, Sridha Sridharan, Houman Ghaem-maghami, and Clinton Fookes. A robust interpretable deep learning classifier for heart anomaly detection without segmentation. *IEEE Journal of Biomedical and Health Informatics*, 25(6), 2162–2171, 2020.

Christopher Duckworth, Francis P Chmiel, Dan K Burns, Zlatko D Zlatev, Neil M White, Thomas WV Daniels, Michael Kiuber, and Michael J Boniface. Using explainable machine learning to characterise data drift and detect emergent health risks for emergency department admissions during COVID-19. *Scientific Reports*, 11(1), 23017, 2021.

Kevin Chew Figueroa, Bofan Song, Sumsum Sunny, Shaobai Li, Keerthi Gurushanth, Pramila Mendonca, Nirza Mukhia, Sanjana Patrick, Shubha Gurudath, Subhashini Raghavan, et al. Interpretable deep learning approach for oral cancer classification using guided attention inference network. *Journal of Biomedical Optics*, 27(1), 015001–015001, 2022.

Pavel Hamet and Johanne Tremblay. Artificial intelligence in medicine. *Metabolism*, 69, S36–S40, 2017.

Intisar Rizwan I Haque and Jeremiah Neubert. Deep learning approaches to biomedical image segmentation. *Informatics in Medicine Unlocked*, 18, 100297, 2020.

Majid Harouni, Mohsen Karimi, Afrooz Nasr, Helia Mahmoudi, and Zakieh Arab Najafabadi. Health monitoring methods in heart diseases based on data mining approach: A directional review. In Tanzila Saba, Amjad Rehman, & Sudipta Roy (Eds.), *Prognostic Models in Healthcare: AI and Statistical Approaches*, pp. 115–159. Springer, 2022.

Mohammad Hesam Hesamian, Wenjing Jia, Xiangjian He, and Paul Kennedy. Deep learning techniques for medical image segmentation: Achievements and challenges. *Journal of Digital Imaging*, 32, 582–596, 2019.

Zhengyu Jiang, Lulong Bo, Zhenhua Xu, Yubing Song, Jiafeng Wang, Pingshan Wen, Xiaojian Wan, Tao Yang, Xiaoming Deng, and Jinjun Bian. An explainable machine learning algorithm for risk factor analysis of in-hospital mortality in sepsis survivors with ICU readmission. *Computer Methods and Programs in Biomedicine*, 204, 106040, 2021.

Md Sarwar Kamal, Aden Northcote, Linkon Chowdhury, Nilanjan Dey, Rubén González Crespo, and Enrique Herrera-Viedma. Alzheimer's patient analysis using image and gene expression data and explainable-AI to present associated genes. *IEEE Transactions on Instrumentation and Measurement*, 70, 1–7, 2021.

Amjad Rehman Khan, Majid Harouni, Sepideh Sharifi, Saeed Ali Bahaj, and Tanzila Saba. Face detection in close-up shot video events using video mining. *Journal of Advances in Information Technology*, 14(2), 2023.

Chew-Teng Kor, Yi-Rong Li, Pei-Ru Lin, Sheng-Hao Lin, Bing-Yen Wang, and Ching-Hsiung Lin. Explainable machine learning model for predicting first-time acute exacerbation in patients with chronic obstructive pulmonary disease. *Journal of Personalized Medicine*, 12(2), 228, 2022.

Mahantapas Kundu, Mita Nasipuri, and Dipak Kumar Basu. Knowledge-based ECG interpretation: A critical review. *Pattern Recognition*, 33(3), 351–373, 2000.

Eunsaem Lee, Se Young Jung, Hyung Ju Hwang, Jaewoo Jung, et al. Patient-level cancer prediction models from a nationwide patient cohort: Model development and validation. *JMIR Medical Informatics*, 9(8), e29807, 2021.

Shu-Cheng Liu, Jesyin Lai, Jhao-Yu Huang, Chia-Fong Cho, Pei Hua Lee, Min-Hsuan Lu, Chun- Chieh Yeh, Jiaxin Yu, and Wei-Ching Lin. Predicting microvascular invasion in hepatocellular carcinoma: A deep learning model validated across hospitals. *Cancer Imaging*, 21, 1–16, 2021.

Hui Wen Loh, Wanrong Hong, Chui Ping Ooi, Subrata Chakraborty, Prabal Datta Barua, Ravinesh C Deo, Jeffrey Soar, Elizabeth E Palmer, and U Rajendra Acharya. Application of deep learning models for automated identification of Parkinson's disease: A review (2011–2021). *Sensors*, 21(21), 7034, 2021.

Pavan Rajkumar Magesh, Richard Delwin Myloth, and Rijo Jackson Tom. An explainable machine learning model for early detection of Parkinson's disease using LIME on daTSCAN Imagery. *Computers in Biology and Medicine*, 126, 104041, 2020.

Andreas Maier, Christopher Syben, Tobias Lasser, and Christian Riess. A gentle introduction to deep learning in medical image processing. *Zeitschrift für Medizinische Physik*, 29(2), 86–101, 2019.

Mehdi Marani, Morteza Soltani, Mina Bahadori, Masoumeh Soleimani, and Atajahangir Moshayedi. The role of biometric in banking: A review. *EAI Endorsed Transactions on AI and Robotics*, 2(1), 2023.

Randolph A Miller, Harry E Pople Jr, and Jack D Myers. Internist-I, an experimental computer-based diagnostic consultant for general internal medicine. In James A. Reggia, & Stanley Tuhrim (Eds.), *Computer-assisted Medical Decision Making*, pp. 139–158. Springer, 1985.

Bilal Mirza, Wei Wang, Jie Wang, Howard Choi, Neo Christopher Chung, and Peipei Ping. Machine learning and integrative analysis of biomedical big data. *Genes*, 10(2), 87, 2019.

Richard F Mollica and Gregory L Fricchione. Mental and physical exhaustion of health-care practitioners. *The Lancet*, 398(10318), 2243–2244, 2021.

Ramaravind K Mothilal, Amit Sharma, and Chenhao Tan. Explaining machine learning classifiers through diverse counterfactual explanations. In *Proceedings of the 2020 Conference on Fairness, Accountability, and Transparency*, pp. 607–617, 2020.

Mobeen Nazar, Muhammad Mansoor Alam, Eiad Yafi, and Mazliham Mohd Su'ud. A systematic review of human–computer interaction and explainable artificial intelligence in healthcare with artificial intelligence techniques. *IEEE Access*, 9, 153316–153348, 2021.

Bernard Nordlinger, Cédric Villani, and Daniela Rus. *Healthcare and Artificial Intelligence.* Springer, 2020.

Iam Palatnik de Sousa, Marley Maria Bernardes Rebuzzi Vellasco, and Eduardo Costa da Silva. Local interpretable model-agnostic explanations for classification of lymph node metastases. *Sensors*, 19(13), 2969, 2019.

Atul Rawal, James McCoy, Adrienne Raglin, and Danda B Rawat. A quantitative comparison of causality and feature relevance via explainable AI (XAI) for robust, and trustworthy artificial reasoning systems. In *International Conference on Human–Computer Interaction*, pp. 274–285. Springer, 2023.

Daniel R Ripoll, Sidhartha Chaudhury, and Anders Wallqvist. Using the antibody–antigen binding interface to train image-based deep neural networks for antibody-epitope classification. *PLoS Computational Biology*, 17(3), e1008864, 2021.

Patrik Sabol, Peter Sinčák, Pitoyo Hartono, Pavel Kočan, Zuzana Benetinová, Alžbeta Blichárová, Ľudmila Verbóová, Erika Štammová, Antónia Sabolová-Fabianová, and Anna Jašková. Explainable classifier for improving the accountability in decision-making for colorectal cancer diagnosis from histopathological images. *Journal of Biomedical Informatics*, 109, 103523, 2020.

Hui Shi, Dong Yang, Kaichen Tang, Chunmei Hu, Lijuan Li, Linfang Zhang, Ting Gong, and Yanqin Cui. Explainable machine learning model for predicting the occurrence of postoperative malnutrition in children with congenital heart disease. *Clinical Nutrition*, 41(1), 202–210, 2022.

Edward Shortliffe. *Computer-based Medical Consultations: MYCIN*, volume 2. Elsevier, 2012.

Nima Tajbakhsh, Laura Jeyaseelan, Qian Li, Jeffrey N Chiang, Zhihao Wu, and Xiaowei Ding. Embracing imperfect datasets: A review of deep learning solutions for medical image segmentation. *Medical Image Analysis*, 63, 101693, 2020.

Erico Tjoa and Cuntai Guan. A survey on explainable artificial intelligence (XAI): Toward medical XAI. *IEEE Transactions on Neural Networks and Learning Systems*, 32(11), 4793–4813, 2020.

Sandra Wachter, Brent Mittelstadt, and Chris Russell. Counterfactual explanations without opening the black box: Automated decisions and the GDPR. *Harvard Journal of Law & Technology*, 31, 841, 2017.

Xing Wang, Xiaofang You, Li Zhang, Dayu Huang, Beatrice Aramini, Leonid Shabaturov, Gening Jiang, and Jiang Fan. A radiomics model combined with XGBoost may improve the accuracy of distinguishing between mediastinal cysts and tumors: A multicenter validation analysis. *Annals of Translational Medicine*, 9(23), 1737, 2021.

Sholom M Weiss, Casimir A Kulikowski, Saul Amarel, and Aran Safir. A model-based method for computer-aided medical decision-making. *Artificial Intelligence*, 11(1–2), 145–172, 1978.

Wikipedia. History of Artificial Intelligence. https://en.wikipedia.org/wiki/. 2023.

Fan Xu, Li Jiang, Wenjing He, Guangyi Huang, Yiyi Hong, Fen Tang, Jian Lv, Yunru Lin, Yikun Qin, Rushi Lan, et al. The clinical value of explainable deep learning for diagnosing fungal keratitis using in vivo confocal microscopy images. *Frontiers in Medicine*, 8, 797616, 2021.

Rui Yang, Fengkai Ke, Huanping Liu, Mingcheng Zhou, and Hui-Min Cao. Exploring sMRI biomarkers for diagnosis of autism spectrum disorders based on multi class activation mapping models. *IEEE Access*, 9, 124122–124131, 2021.

Xian Zeng, Yaoqin Hu, Liqi Shu, Jianhua Li, Huilong Duan, Qiang Shu, and Haomin Li. Explainable machine-learning predictions for complications after pediatric congenital heart surgery. *Scientific Reports*, 11(1), 17244, 2021.

Yiming Zhang, Ying Weng, and Jonathan Lund. Applications of explainable artificial intelligence in diagnosis and surgery. *Diagnostics*, 12(2), 237, 2022.

Jianpeng Zhang, Yutong Xie, Qi Wu, and Yong Xia. Medical image classification using synergic deep learning. *Medical Image Analysis*, 54, 10–19, 2019.

Chapter 12

Revolutionizing Prostate Cancer Diagnosis: Vision Transformers with Explainable Artificial Intelligence to Accurate and Interpretable Prostate Cancer Identification

Krunal Maheriya[1], Mrugendrasinh Rahevar[1], Martin Parmar[1], Deep Kothadiya[1], Atul Patel[1], and Amit Ganatra[2]

[1]*Chandubhai S. Patel Institute of Technology, Charotar University of Science and Technology, Anand, Gujarat, India*
[2]*Parul University, Vadodara, Gujarat, India*

12.1 Introduction

The diagnosis and treatment of cancer hold significant importance due to the pervasive occurrence of the disease, a high mortality rate, and the potential for recurrence following treatment. According to data from the National Vital Statistics

DOI: 10.1201/9781032626345-12

Reports, the incidence rate of cancer (per 100,000 persons) in the United States varied across racial groups from 2002 to 2006. For White individuals, the rate was 470.6, for Black individuals 493.6, for Asians 311.1, and for Hispanics 350.6. This indicates that cancer affects people of all races extensively. In the United States, lung cancer, breast cancer, and prostate cancer emerged as the top three causes of death, collectively claiming the lives of over 227,900 individuals in 2007, as reported by the National Cancer Institute.

Machine learning and deep learning hold a pivotal role in the automated identification, segmentation (Sevak et al., 2017), and computer-assisted diagnosis of malignant lesions. One of the most common medical conditions in males is prostate cancer (PCa). Each year, 300,000 men worldwide die of clinically significant PCa (csPCa), which is classified as cancer with an ISUP 2 score. The 2019 European Association of Urology (EAU) guidelines and the 2019 UK National Institute for Health and Care Excellence (NICE) guidelines both recommend using multiparametric magnetic resonance imaging (mpMRI) instead of biopsies in the early diagnosis of prostate cancer. However, the most recent recommendations for interpreting prostate mpMRI (PI-RADS v2.1) follow a semiquantitative assessment that necessitates a high level of knowledge for use. Additionally, MRI results for prostate cancer can show a wide range of clinical behavior and extremely variable morphology (The PI-CAI Challenge – Grand Challenge, n.d.).

Prostate cancer is the most common cancer among men, and while some types of prostate cancer grow slowly and require minimal or no treatment, others are aggressive and can spread rapidly (Santos et al., 2015). Detecting prostate cancer at an early stage is crucial for successful treatment, but it remains challenging. The current diagnostic tools include digital rectal examination, serum prostate-specific antigen (PSA) blood test, and transrectal ultrasound (TRUS)-guided biopsy, but they have limitations, leading to efforts to improve their accuracy (De Rooij et al., 2014). Figure 12.1 depicts the different types of cancer cases occurred in males worldwide.

The majority of PSA (prostate-specific antigen) (Smith & Catalona, 1994) in the bloodstream is bound to protease inhibitors, leaving only a small portion unbound. Men with prostate cancer often have lower free-to-total PSA ratios (also known as percent-free PSA) than men with noncancerous conditions in men with increased total PSA levels. Previous research has shown that calculating the percent-free PSA might be useful in separating prostate cancer from benign conditions. Based on the variations in percent-free PSA distribution between the cancer and benign groups, researchers have discovered possible biopsy thresholds. These limits have the ability to retain a sensitivity of over 90% while reducing needless biopsies by up to 50% (Partin et al., 1996).

The effectiveness of PSA in the identification of prostate cancer has also been found to be influenced by a number of variables, such as the size of the prostate and tumor, age, total PSA levels, and the history of prior biopsies (Parekh et al., 2007). This study aimed to determine the extent to which percent-free PSA could enhance the specificity of PSA in detecting prostate cancer among men with

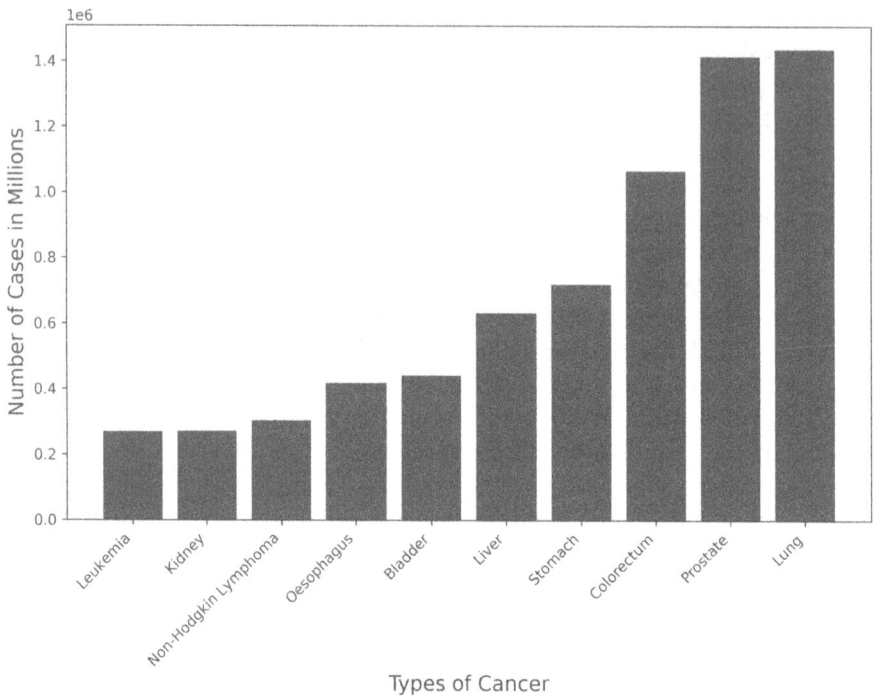

Figure 12.1   Different types of cancer cases occurred in males worldwide.

total PSA concentrations ranging from 4.0 ng/mL to 10.0 ng/mL. Additionally, it sought to assess the influence of population characteristics such as total PSA levels, prostate volume, and patient age on the measurement of percent-free PSA (Partin et al., 1996).

Prostate cancer diagnosis mostly targets urologists. In the United States, early detection primarily relies on prostate-specific antigen (PSA)-based screening, followed by prostate biopsy for confirmation of diagnosis. However, this guideline does not cover the detection of prostate cancer in symptomatic men who may exhibit symptoms associated with locally advanced or metastatic prostate cancer (such as new-onset bone pain or neurological symptoms affecting the lower extremities, among others) (Carter et al., 2013).

Explainable artificial intelligence (XAI) is a branch of artificial intelligence (AI) dedicated to enhancing the transparency, comprehensibility, and interpretability of AI models. Its significance lies in the increasing complexity of AI systems and their involvement in critical decision-making processes. Understanding how these systems function and the rationale behind their decisions is vital (Armato et al., 2011).

XAI endeavors to tackle the opaque nature prevalent in numerous AI models, often challenging to decipher due to intricate algorithms and extensive data utilization. Employing XAI methods involves dissecting these models to offer insights into their decision-making processes. This approach fosters trust in AI systems, ensures their fairness and impartiality, and enhances their overall performance.

Deep learning models showcase exceptional performance in critical domains such as medical science, national defense, sign language (Kothadiya, Bhatt, Saba, et al., 2023; Kothadiya et al., 2022; Kothadiya et al., 2024), automated driving (Kothadiya et al., 2021), finance, facial emotion recognition (Chaudhari et al., 2023), fingerprint liveness detection (Kothadiya, Bhatt, Soni, et al., 2023), and the COVID-19 detection (Patel et al., 2023), among others. However, these applications necessitate addressing trust-related issues. A system that delivers promising results alongside a comprehensible interpretation is more readily trusted (Afza et al., 2021). The remarkable performance of computer vision tasks leads to the generation of an extensive array of parameters and associations with the physical environment, rendering explanations exceedingly challenging. This intricate learning framework is often perceived as a "Black-Box" (Linardatos et al., 2020). With the advancement of deep learning, particularly in sensitive sectors like computer vision, the need for transparency and interpretability is paramount. The integration of explainability, commonly referred to as explainable artificial intelligence, becomes imperative (Giotis et al., 2015). Figure 12.2 illustrates the entire architectural overview of AI and XAI methodologies.

XAI, a swiftly evolving discipline, emerges as a crucial facet of AI (Dudekula et al., 2023; Kothadiya, Bhatt, Rehman, et al., 2023). Research endeavors in XAI within the realm of computer vision strive to unveil or decipher the inner workings of the black-box. Moreover, it furnishes trust and interpretability to aid in unbiased troubleshooting across various computer vision applications such as object detection, classification, and more. Insights derived from XAI models shed light on potential design flaws or structures (Calisto & Lai-Yuen, 2020).

Advancements in AI, notably employing transformers model (Chaudhari et al., 2022; Dosovitskiy et al., 2010; Kothadiya, Rehman, Abbas, et al., 2023) models,

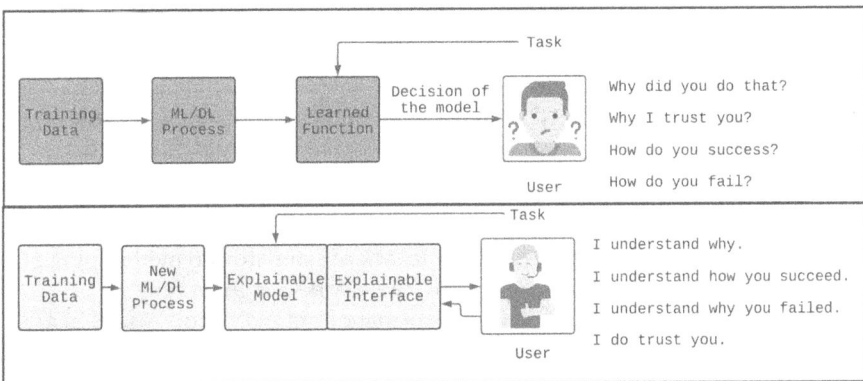

Figure 12.2 A comprehensive overview architecture of AI and XAI techniques.

show promise in refining the accuracy of prostate cancer detection. ViT models, originally intended for image classification, display remarkable proficiency across diverse computer vision applications. Within the realm of prostate cancer detection, researchers are exploring ViT models' potential to scrutinize multiparametric MRI scans and pinpoint tumor regions. Leveraging ViT models' sophisticated pattern recognition capabilities aims to heighten the precision and efficiency of detection, ultimately improving patient outcomes in managing prostate cancer.

In the field of medicine, such as brain cancer (Khan et al., 2019; Rehman et al., 2021), skin cancer (Saba et al., 2012), and prostate cancer, detection is crucial to clarify and understand how the internal learning process functions. Accurate internal learning patterns enhance confidence in prostate cancer detection models (Malaviya et al., 2023). However, this clarification can also reveal misclassification errors, prompting enhancements in the model or input methods. In tasks like sign language recognition, trustworthiness plays a critical role in predicting how the model learns specific gesture-based signs (Chen et al., 2017). The ability to interpret significantly enhances the approach to accurately forecast the intended label. Given the potential variability in detecting prostate cancer, there is a likelihood of identifying a different label. Using XAI for prostate cancer detection aids in refining the detection model to meet diverse expectations and assists end users in comprehending the deep learning model's learning process for detecting prostate cancer (Ganesan et al., 2022; Tahir et al., 2019). Table 12.1 presents an overview of the key challenges faced in achieving explainable AI.

Table 12.1 Overview of Challenges in Achieving Explainable AI

Challenges of Explainable AI	*Description*
The complexity of AI models	The complex architecture of advanced AI models, like deep neural networks, makes it difficult to decipher and explain their decision-making processes, posing a significant challenge in their widespread adoption
Balancing accuracy and interpretability	The pursuit of simultaneously achieving highly accurate AI predictions and readily understandable explanations is a persistent endeavor
Lack of standardization	The lack of standardized methodologies or frameworks for generating explanations in AI systems results in a lack of uniformity and consistency in explanation techniques

(Continued)

Table 12.1 (Continued)

Challenges of Explainable AI	Description
Scalability and performance impact	Integrating explainability methods into AI models might necessitate compromises in terms of their computational efficiency and scalability
Trade-offs between transparency and performance	While striving for greater interpretability in AI models, it is crucial to carefully balance the need for simplicity with the potential impact on model performance
Handling high-dimensional data	Unraveling the mechanisms underlying AI model decisions for high-dimensional data, like images or genomic data, poses a significant challenge in interpreting their outputs
Ethical and legal implications	Ethical considerations, including privacy, bias, and accountability, must be carefully addressed when developing AI explanation mechanisms

Moreover, integrating XAI into our vision transformers–based prostate cancer detection model augments doctors' understanding of the AI's decision-making process. This integration fosters trust in the AI's results by offering enhanced transparency, allowing medical professionals to discern specific features within prostate images contributing to the AI's cancer detection. Such transparency provides invaluable insights into the AI's reasoning, empowering clinicians to comprehend the basis of the AI's detections and further solidifying trust in the model's outcomes.

12.2 Related Work

In the realm of prostate cancer detection, extensive research has been conducted to enhance the accuracy and efficiency of diagnostic methods. Previous studies have explored various approaches, including traditional techniques such as digital rectal examination (Soronen et al., 2021), serum prostate-specific antigen (PSA) blood tests (Catalona et al., 1991), and transrectal ultrasound (TRUS)-guided biopsies (Harvey et al., 2012).

Early detection of prostate cancer is crucial for reducing mortality rates. The complexity of prostate cancer MRIs necessitates advanced diagnostic systems and tools. Researchers have developed computer-aided diagnosis (CAD) systems to help radiologists identify abnormalities. Hussain et al. (2018) utilized novel machine learning techniques (Chaudhari et al., 2023), including the Bayesian approach,

SVM kernels (polynomial, RBF, and Gaussian), and decision trees, for prostate cancer detection. They also proposed various feature extraction strategies based on texture, morphological, SIFT, and EFDs features to improve detection accuracy. The performance was evaluated using both single and combined features and machine learning classification techniques (Fahad et al., 2018; Meethongjan et al., 2013). Cross-validation was employed, and the results were assessed using ROC curves, specificity, sensitivity, PPV, NPV, and FPR. Among single-feature extraction strategies, the SVM Gaussian kernel achieved the highest accuracy of 98.34% with an AUC of 0.999. Combining feature extraction strategies, SVM Gaussian kernel with texture + morphological features and EFDs + morphological features yielded the highest accuracy of 99.71% and an AUC of 1.00.

A comprehensive review of the literature was conducted to identify and assess the potential of existing and emerging biomarkers for prostate cancer detection (Parekh et al., 2007). Recently proposed guidelines by the Early Detection Research Network for biomarker study phases were adapted for prostate cancer, and the current state of biomarker research was evaluated against these study phases. Additionally, current and potential biomarkers for prostate cancer detection were examined. Recent advancements in high-throughput bench research, such as high-dimensional genomic, proteomic, and autoantibody signatures, hold promise for enhancing the performance of prostate-specific antigens, but these techniques are still undergoing reproducibility and multicenter validation studies. Iftikhar et al. (2017) discussed the current evidence and research questions surrounding prostate cancer prevention, early detection, and the management of men at high risk of prostate cancer or diagnosed with low-grade prostate cancer.

Schröder et al. (2000) analyzed the diagnostic accuracy of prostate-specific antigen (PSA), digital rectal examination (DRE), transrectal ultrasonography (TRUS), and tumor characteristics in men with low PSA levels (0–4.0 ng/mL). Radical prostatectomy was performed on approximately half of the 478 men diagnosed with prostate cancer. Tumor characteristics, including pT category, Gleason score, and cancer volume, were evaluated in 166 processed radical prostatectomy specimens. Fifty of these specimens had PSA levels between 0 and 4.0 ng/mL. Our findings confirm and expand upon recent evidence suggesting that DRE has low predictive value and that many significant cancers may be missed at this PSA range.

Iqbal et al. (2021) investigated the effectiveness of deep learning and non-deep learning approaches for prostate cancer detection. They employed fine-tuned deep learning models (LSTM and ResNet-101) that operate directly on raw image data, without the need for hand-crafted features. Their performance was compared to non-deep learning classifiers trained on hand-crafted features extracted from carcinoma images, such as texture, morphology, and GLCM. They used a jackknife tenfold cross-validation method to evaluate the models and assessed their performance using sensitivity, specificity, PPV, NPV, accuracy, MCC, and AUC. The best results were obtained using the non-deep learning method with GLCM features and KNN-Cosine, achieving sensitivity (98.00%), specificity (99.25%), PPV (98.99%), NPV (99.11%), accuracy (99.07%), and AUC (0.998). The LSTM deep learning method also achieved impressive results, with sensitivity (98.33%), specificity (100%), PPV (100%), NPV (99.26%), accuracy (99.48%), MCC (0.9879), and AUC (0.9999). Notably, the ResNet-101 deep learning method outperformed both non-deep learning methods and LSTM, achieving perfect accuracy (100%) and AUC (1) for kernel naive Bayes, SVM Gaussian, and RUSBoost tree. These findings suggest that the ResNet-101 deep learning method holds promise as a more accurate and reliable tool for prostate cancer detection.

Yoo et al. (2019) employed deep convolutional networks (CNNs), which have shown remarkable success in computer vision tasks like object detection and segmentation. The medical imaging research community has increasingly explored different CNN architectures as promising solutions to develop more accurate CAD tools for cancer detection. Using axial diffusion-weighted imaging (DWI) of specific patients, Yoo et al. developed and put into practice an automated CNN-based workflow for the diagnosis of clinically relevant prostate cancer (PCa). The collection included DWI pictures from 427 individuals, including 175 with PCa and 252 without, totaling 427 cases. A second test set of 108 patients (out of a total of 427) was reserved and not used during training in order to assess the performance of the pipeline. With an area under the receiver operating characteristic curve (AUC) of 0.87 (95% confidence interval [CI]: 0.84–0.90) at the slice level and an AUC of 0.84 (95% CI: 0.76–0.91) at the patient level, the results showed encouraging performance. Figure 12.3 illustrates the proposed framework that integrates deep

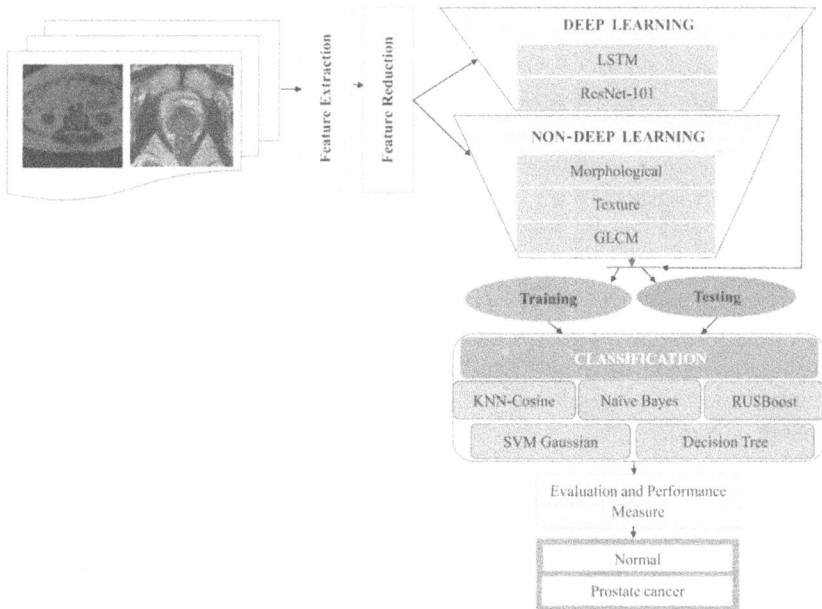

Figure 12.3 Proposed framework that combines deep learning methodologies with conventional techniques for prostate cancer detection by Iqbal et al. (2021).

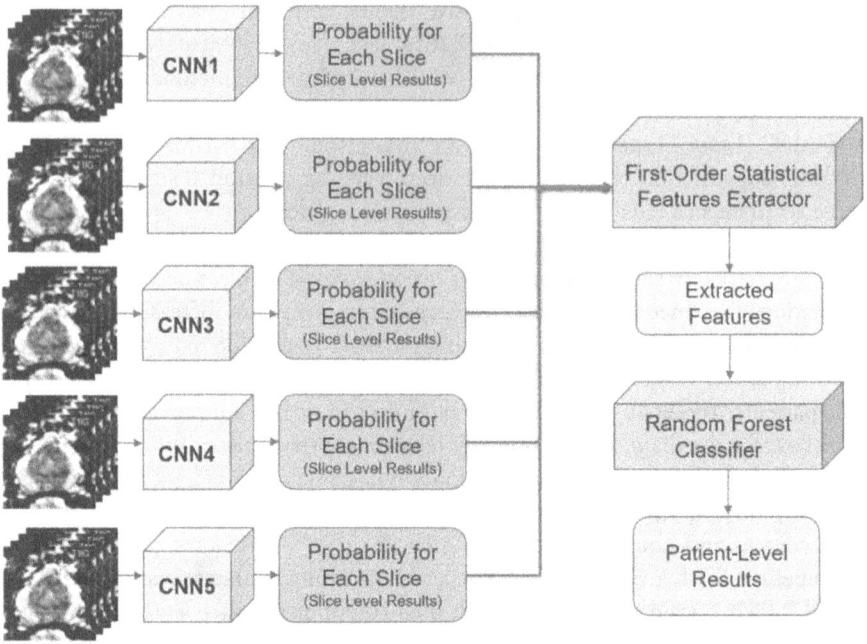

Figure 12.4   The proposed structural components outlined by Yoo et al. (2019).

learning methodologies with conventional techniques for the detection of prostate cancer. Figure 12.4 depicts the proposed structural components.

De Vente et al. (2020) proposed a strategy that, in comparison to conventional classification and detection approaches, is more therapeutically useful. They worked on creating a neural network that can evaluate cancer tissue holistically while simultaneously detecting it. They used a particular dataset for both training and testing. In their approach, they employed a 2D U-Net architecture, which takes MRI slices as input and generates lesion segmentation maps that encode the Gleason Grade Group (GGG), an indicator of cancer aggressiveness. The authors proposed a technique for encoding the GGG in the model target, leveraging the fact that the GGG classes have an inherent ordinal relationship. Additionally, they explored various methods for incorporating prior information such as prostate zone segmentation and employed assembling techniques.

Saha et al. (2021) introduced a multistage 3D computer-aided detection and diagnosis (CAD) model designed to automatically locate clinically significant prostate cancer (csPCa) in bi-parametric MR imaging (bpMRI). They utilized a substantial dataset consisting of 1,950 prostate bpMRI scans paired with radiologically estimated annotations. The authors proposed the idea or theory that CNN-based models, when trained using appropriate techniques, have the potential to accurately detect and identify cancerous abnormalities that have been confirmed through

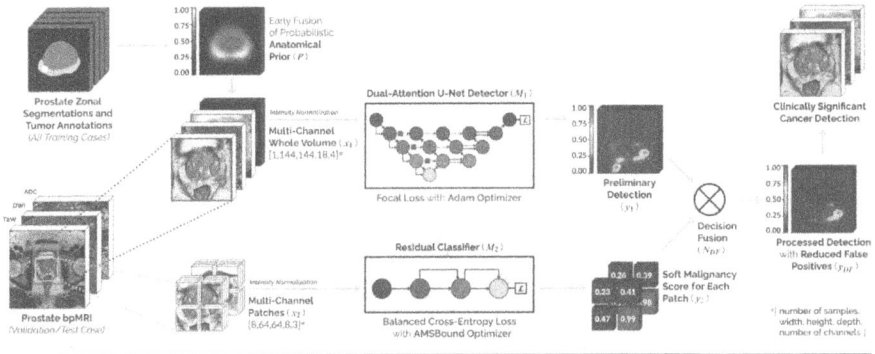

Figure 12.5   The proposed comprehensive framework for computing voxel-level detections of clinically significant prostate cancer, as proposed by Saha et al. (2021).

biopsy in a different group or population of individuals. Figure 12.5 presents the proposed comprehensive framework for computing voxel-level detections of clinically significant prostate cancer.

Chui et al. (2022) introduced a multiscale denoising convolutional neural network (MSDCNN) model specifically designed for prostate cancer detection (PCD). The model focuses on reducing noise in the images to enhance the accuracy of detection. Additionally, the model was optimized using transfer learning, a technique that leverages domain knowledge from a different but related dataset. In this case, the source datasets were artificially contaminated with Gaussian noise before transferring the acquired knowledge to the target dataset. Figure 12.6 illustrates

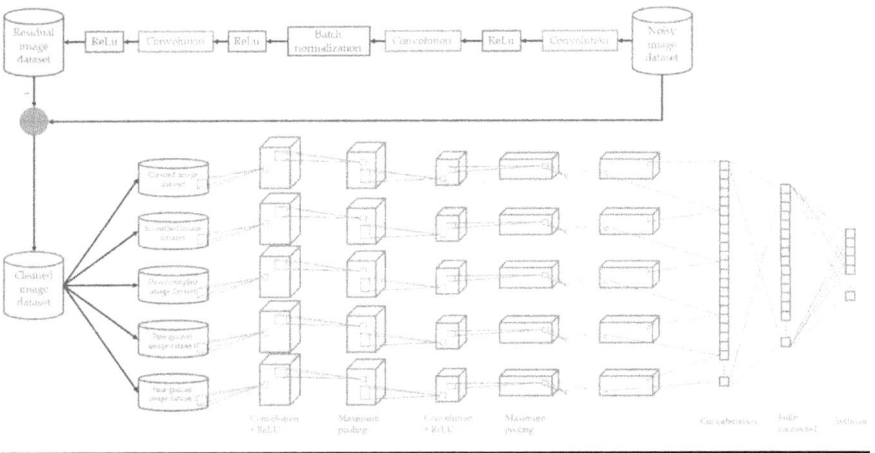

Figure 12.6   The proposed structure of MSDCNN developed by Chui et al. (2022).

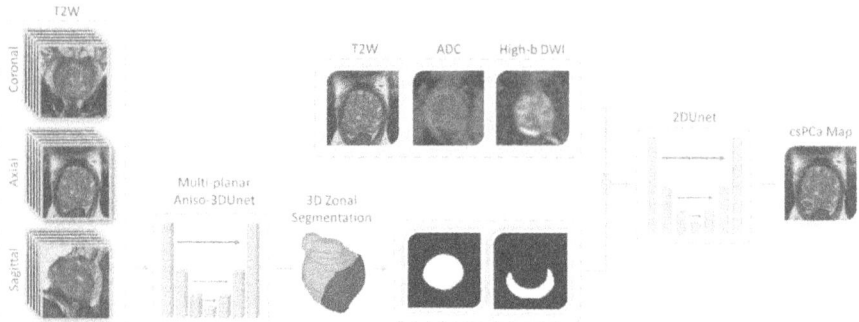

Figure 12.7   The proposed design of DL-CAD presented by Hosseinzadeh et al. (2022).

the proposed structure of the MSDCNN (Multi-Scale Deep Convolutional Neural Network).

Hosseinzadeh et al. (2022) introduced a fully automated deep learning–based system for the detection of prostate cancer in prostate MRI scans. The algorithm was trained, validated, and tested using MRI scans from two different institutions. An experienced radiologist delineated the boundaries of MRI-visible lesions, and all these lesions underwent biopsy using MRI TRUS guidance. The lesion masks and histopathological results served as ground truth labels to train the UNet and AH-Net architectures for detecting and segmenting prostate cancer lesions. The algorithm was trained to identify any prostate cancer lesion with an ISUP grade of 1 or higher. Performance metrics such as detection sensitivity, positive predictive values, and the average number of false positive lesions per patient were used to evaluate the algorithm's performance. Figure 12.7 presents the proposed design of the DL-CAD (Deep Learning Computer-Aided Detection) system.

However, these methods have limitations, leading researchers to explore innovative technologies and methodologies studies on ViT and GNN (Malaviya, 2023; Raisinghani et al., 2021) for lung cancer detection and HIV molecular prediction respectively. Du et al. (2023) introduced the first multi-domain vision transformer (MDViT) architecture, which incorporates domain adapters to address data scarcity and nontransferable knowledge (NKT) by adaptively leveraging knowledge from multiple small data sources (domains). To further enhance cross-domain representation learning, they integrated a mutual knowledge distillation framework that transfers knowledge between a universal network (encompassing all domains) and auxiliary domain-specific network branches. Experiments conducted on four skin lesion segmentation datasets confirm MDViT's efficacy in improving performance and generalizability. Inspired by this research, we did prostate detection using ViT (Figure 12.8). Table 12.2 provides an overview of publicly available datasets for various types of cancer.

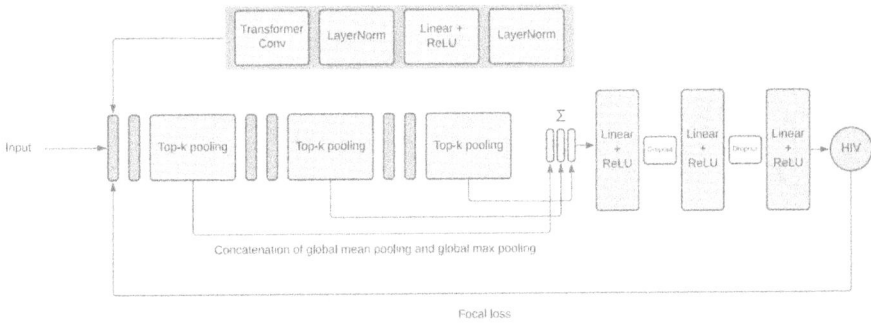

Figure 12.8 **The proposed structure for HIV molecular prediction utilizing stacked graph transformer, as outlined by Raisinghani et al. (2021).**

Table 12.2 **Overview of Publicly Available Datasets for Various Types of Cancer**

Sr. No.	Dataset	Type of Image	Cancer	No. of Images	Reference
1	IBSR	MRI	Brain	Total 38 scans	NITRC (n.d.)
	OASIS	Multi-model		MRI: 2168 and in PET: 1608	Marcus et al. (2007)
	BRATS (2012–2019)	MRI		65	CBICA, (n.d.)
	FIGSHARECJDATA	MRI		3,064	Cheng (2017)
2	INbrest	Mammograms	Breast	410	Moreira et al. (2012)
	BreaKHis	Microscopic image		7,909	Spanhol et al. (2017)
	MIAS/miniMIAS	Mammograms		330	Suckling (1994)
	DDSM	Mammograms		10,480	Heath et al. (2001)
	ICPR2014MITOSIS	Histopathology slides		1,420	Santos et al. (2015)
3	Kvasir	Endoscopic	Colon	8,000	Pogorelov, Randel, Griwodz, et al. (2017)
	Kvasir-SEG	Endoscopic		1,000	Jha et al. (2020)
	NerthusData-set	Endoscopic video		5,525 frames in 21 videos	Pogorelov, Randel, De Lange, et al. (2017)
	ASU-Mayo clinical database	Colonoscopy video		38 Videos	Tajbakhsh et al. (2015)
	EndoTech2020	Colonoscopy frames		1,000	EndoTect 2020 (n.d.)
	Hyper-kvasir	Binary mask images		1,000	Borgli et al. (2020)

(Continued)

Table 12.2   (Continued)

Sr. No.	Dataset	Type of Image	Cancer	No. of Images	Reference
4	LICD-IDRI	CT	Lung	224,527	Armato III et al., (2011)
	DLCST	CT		4,101	Danish Lung Cancer Group (2007)
	JSRT	X-ray		647	Japanese Society of Radiological Technology (n.d.)
	ACDC-LungHP	Histopathology		200	ACDC-LungHP – Grand Challenge (n.d.)
	ELCAP	CT		50 Scans	Reeves et al. (2009)
	NSCLC	CT		52,073	Aerts et al. (2019)
5	MICCSISliver	CT	Liver	30 patients' data	SLIVER07 – Grand Challenge (n.d.)
	PAIP	WSI		100	PAIP 2019 – Grand Challenge (n.d.)
6	PROSTATE-MRITCIA	MRI	Prostate	22,036	Choyke et al. (2016)
	ProstateEx Challenge	MRI		538	SPIE-AAPM-NCI PROSTATEx Challenges – The Cancer Imaging Archive (TCIA) Public Access - Cancer Imaging Archive Wiki (n.d.)
	ProstateEx-2 Challange	MRI		162	PROSTATEx-2 Challenge (n.d.)
7	DermIS	Dermoscopic	Skin	206	DermIS (n.d.)
	ISBI-2016	Dermoscopic		1,279	Rotemberg et al. (2021)
	Med-Node	Macroscopic		170	Giotis (2015)

12.3 Proposed Method

Figure 12.9 illustrates the process of our suggested approach. Initially, the method transforms image frames into various patches, which are then converted into vectors to facilitate input processing. To maintain the correct sequence of vectors, positional encoding is incorporated into the input vectors. Ultimately, the input vector undergoes processing through the encoder layer, yielding classification probabilities as the output.

(a)

(a)

| X1 | X2 | X3 | Xn |

CLS

Dens Layer

Z_0

$Z_n = MX_n + b$

P0 P1 P2 P3 $\cdots$ Pn

Z_0

Final Z Vector (Input)

Transformers Model (Encoder)

MHA (Multi-Head Algorithm)

Dense (FFNN)

Co C1 C2 C3 $\cdots$ Cn

Classification (Softmax)

Probabilities

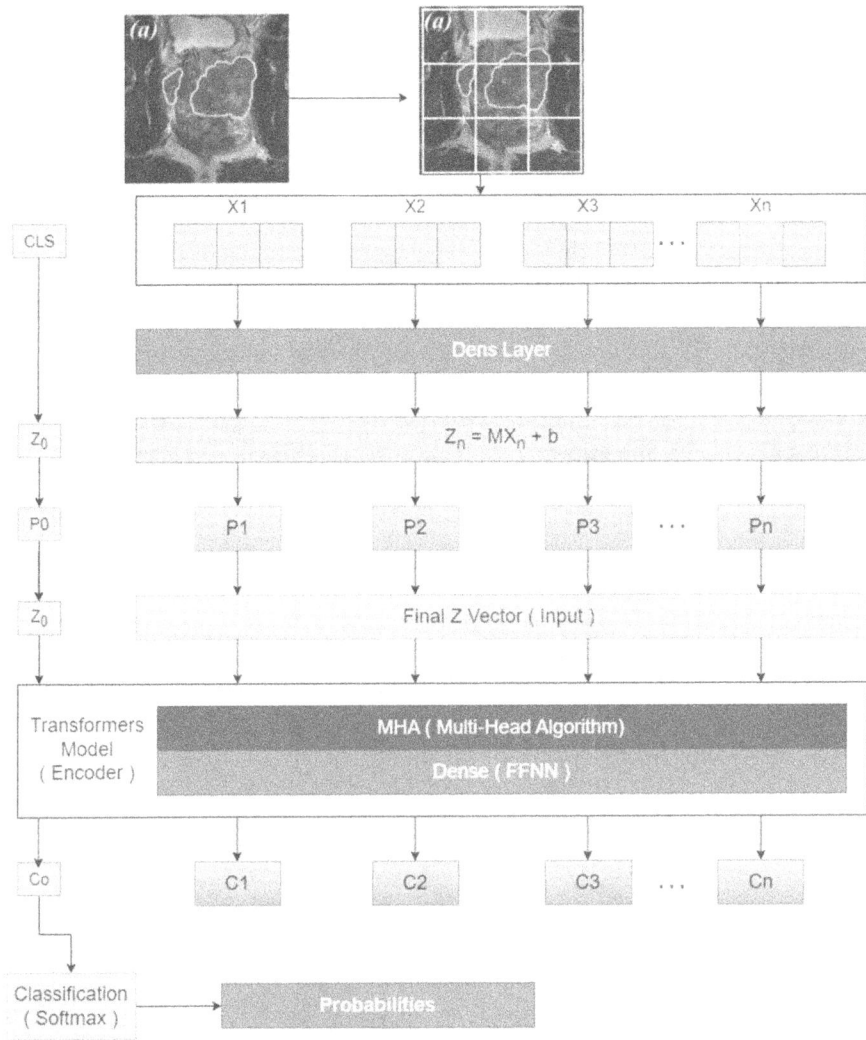

Figure 12.9 Proposed architecture to detect prostate cancer.

12.3.1 Input Embedding Layer

In the context of detecting prostate cancer, the vision transformer operates by processing an input image of the prostate area fragmented into separate patches. These patches then undergo an essential transformation called linear projection, converting each patch into an embedding. These embeddings act as concise representations of localized sections within the prostate image, condensed into smaller, lower-dimensional vectors. This layer establishes a significant link between specific patches within the prostate image and their corresponding embeddings, bridging the gap between the original visual data of the prostate and its more simplified representations. This step significantly rearranges the complex information within the prostate image, ultimately supporting subsequent analysis and processing to enhance accurate cancer detection within the vision transformer framework.

12.3.2 Positional Encoding

A critical element contributing to the model's understanding of the spatial layout within the prostate image is positional encoding. Vision transformers rely on positional encodings to explicitly provide spatial information, addressing the inherent limitation of transformers in processing sequential input devoid of positional or spatial awareness. To analyze the prostate image, vision transformers fragment it into patches arranged in a grid-like structure. These patches are considered as tokens or segments of a sequence, with each patch's visual characteristics encapsulated within an embedding vector representing it. However, these embeddings lack inherent spatial information regarding the positions of the patches within the image. To rectify this, positional encoding is integrated into the input embeddings. Positional encoding, sharing the same dimensions as the embeddings, incorporates positional details into the embeddings, enabling the model to discern the relative positions of the patches within the prostate image. This encoding mechanism plays a crucial role in assisting the model to understand and encode the spatial relationships among different regions within the prostate image, contributing significantly to accurate cancer detection (Figures 12.10 and 12.11).

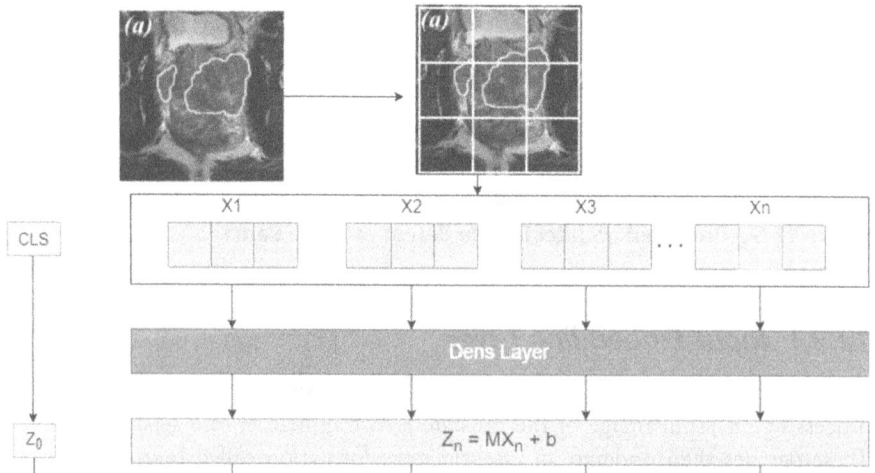

Figure 12.10 **Architectural representation of working of input embedding for the proposed approach.**

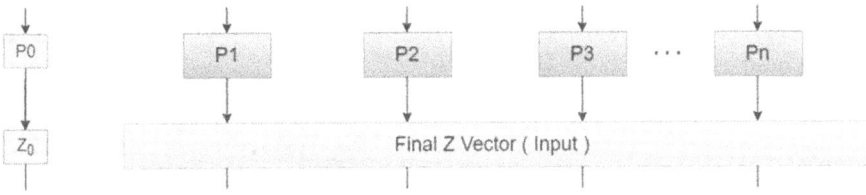

Figure 12.11 **Architectural representation of positional encoding for the proposed approach.**

$$p(k, 2i) = \sin\left(\frac{k}{n^{\frac{2i}{d}}}\right)$$ (12.1)

$$p(k, 2i+1) = \cos\left(\frac{k}{n^{\frac{2i}{d}}}\right)$$ (12.2)

The variable k signifies the position of a specific segment or patch within the input sequence of the prostate image. Meanwhile, d denotes the dimension of the output embedding space, representing the features extracted from these segments. The function $p(k, j)$ serves as the mapping function, associating the position k in the input sequence to the index (k, j) within the positional matrix. In this encoding process, n signifies a user-defined scalar, typically set to 10,000, impacting the encoding granularity. The variable i is employed to map column indices ranging from 0 to $(d/2 + 1)$. For each i value, both the sine and cosine functions play a significant role in generating the positional encoding, contributing distinct encoding patterns for different positions within the prostate image. This encoding technique aids the model in understanding the spatial relationships among various segments, enhancing the accurate identification of cancerous regions within the prostate image.

12.3.3 Transformers Encoder Layer

The fundamental structure of the vision transformer model consists of multiple transformer encoder layers, playing a vital role in its functioning for prostate cancer detection. Within each of these encoder layers, there are typically two primary sublayers that significantly impact the model's effectiveness and ability to analyze prostate images for cancer detection and localization. These sublayers serve a pivotal role in handling the input data, extracting intricate patterns, and fostering improved learning of distinctive features within the prostate image. This layered arrangement empowers the model to progressively understand and interpret visual information within the prostate image, resulting in more precise and accurate identification of cancerous areas within the prostate. This capability holds immense importance in the effective diagnosis and management of prostate cancer (Figure 12.12).

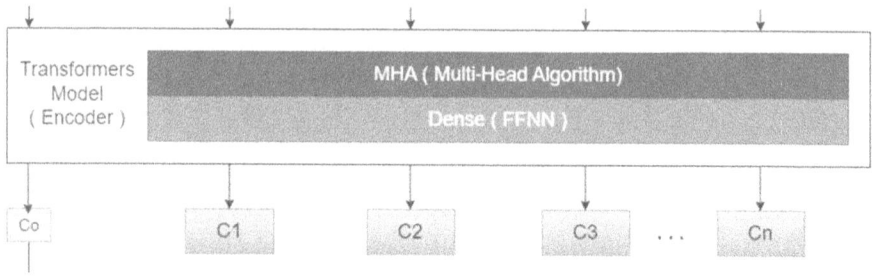

Figure 12.12 **Architectural representation of encoder layer of the proposed method.**

12.3.4 Multi-head Self-attention (MHA) Layer

This specific layer plays a pivotal role in directing the model's focus toward specific segments within the input sequence, which, in this scenario, corresponds to the embedded patches within the prostate image. Its function involves computing attention scores, essentially evaluating the significance or relevance of each patch concerning all others. Consequently, it consolidates essential information from pertinent patches, allowing the model to center its attention on critical regions within the prostate image that might indicate areas affected by cancer. This mechanism of attention is key to the model's capacity to comprehend relationships among various sections of the prostate image and generate meaningful representations. Ultimately, this process assists in capturing intricate connections among diverse regions of the prostate image, thereby enhancing the model's ability to accurately identify potential cancerous areas.

$$MHA = Z1 + Z2 + Z3 + \cdots + Zn \tag{12.3}$$

where

$$Z = \text{Attention}(Q, K, V) = \text{softmax}\left(\frac{QK^T}{\sqrt{d_k}}\right)V \tag{12.4}$$

12.3.5 Feed-Forward Neural Network (FFN) Layer

Following the MHA layer in the vision transformer model, the resulting output progresses into a feed-forward neural network. This network is responsible for implementing nonlinear transformations to the characteristics of each patch independently. By doing so, it enhances the model's capacity to model intricate relationships inherent within the patches of the prostate image (Larabi-Marie-Sainte et al., 2019; Mughal et al., 2018a,b). These nonlinear transformations introduce a heightened level of sophistication in understanding the complex interconnections between the different sections of the prostate image. Consequently, this expanded modeling capacity significantly contributes to the model's proficiency in comprehending and delineating nuanced patterns associated with potential cancerous regions within the prostate, facilitating more accurate detection and localization of malignancies.

$$FFN = wx + b \qquad (12.5)$$

12.3.6 Layer Normalization

Layer normalization serves as a fundamental technique embedded within vision transformers to augment stability and enhance the model's performance during both training and inference stages, crucial in the context of prostate cancer detection. Implemented after each sublayer within the transformer encoder layers, this normalization technique plays a pivotal role in standardizing inputs at every layer of the model. Specifically, it operates on a per-patch or per-token basis, effectively normalizing values across the dimensions of the embeddings. This normalization process is instrumental in mitigating the challenges posed by internal covariate shift within the model during training. Internal covariate shift refers to the fluctuations in the distribution of intermediate activations encountered throughout the training process. By leveraging layer normalization, the vision transformer model gains robustness, ensuring more consistent and reliable learning patterns, thereby aiding in the precise identification and characterization of cancerous regions within prostate images.

12.3.7 Output Layer

The final stage of the vision transformer model deals with a binary classification task aimed at determining if an input image depicts signs of prostate cancer. In the context of prostate cancer detection, the primary objective is to predict whether a given prostate image contains indications of the disease or not. During the training phase, the model is fine-tuned to minimize the binary cross-entropy loss, aligning the predicted probabilities with the actual ground truth labels. This loss function serves as a guide for the model to learn and make accurate classifications based on the visual information extracted from the input images. By optimizing the model through this process, the vision transformer becomes adept at distinguishing between cancerous and noncancerous regions within prostate images, significantly contributing to the accuracy and reliability of prostate cancer identification (Figure 12.13).

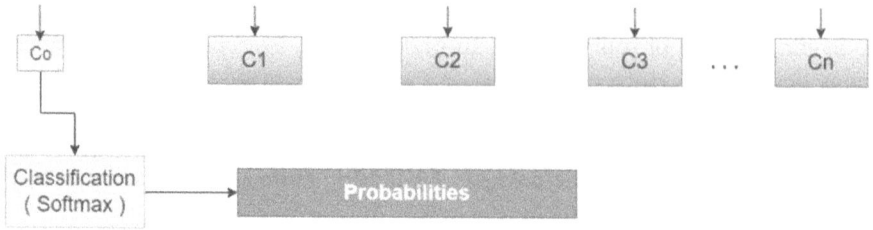

Figure 12.13 **Architecture of the proposed model to understand the output calculation of prostate cancer detection probabilities.**

12.4 Experiment

12.4.1 Training Details

For our experimental setup, we harnessed the computational prowess of the DGX100 system, a purpose-built computing platform tailored explicitly for handling deep learning tasks with optimal efficiency. The DGX100 infrastructure furnished an array of cutting-edge resources, encompassing a suite of multiple GPUs (Graphics Processing Units), substantially accelerating both training and inference phases. To execute the experiment seamlessly and effectively, we utilized the Jupyter Notebook environment. This interactive interface afforded us the flexibility to not only script and execute complex code, but also visualize and document every facet of the experimental workflow with ease.

To derive meaningful insights from the input images, we employed the ResNet50 model, a robust CNN, to extract pertinent features. Leveraging pre-trained weights from the imagenet dataset, we conducted feature extraction, meticulously capturing intrinsic characteristics and patterns encoded within the images. These extracted features, representing high-level visual attributes, were meticulously preserved in the. npy file format, a versatile and efficient file structure conducive for subsequent analyses. The extracted features, encapsulating essential information from the ResNet50 model, served as fundamental inputs for our subsequent vision transformer model. By employing this data as inputs, we facilitated the detection and localization of potential malignant regions within prostate images. This strategic integration of pre-extracted features seamlessly augmented the efficiency and accuracy of our vision transformer model in identifying nuanced patterns indicative of prostate cancer. This meticulous methodology in feature extraction and integration of preprocessed data forms a critical foundation in our approach toward the accurate detection of prostate cancer using the vision transformer architecture.

12.4.2 *Dataset*

Our dataset comprised mpMRI (multi-parametric magnetic resonance imaging) scans of the prostate obtained from the Radboud University Medical Center, originating from a previous comprehensive CAD investigation. Each mpMRI scan within the dataset underwent meticulous evaluation and assessment by a highly skilled radiologist boasting over two decades of experience in the field. This seasoned professional meticulously scrutinized the scans, meticulously identifying suspicious anomalies or areas of concern, and subsequently assigned a Prostate Imaging Reporting and Data System (PI-RADS) score to each identified region based on specific criteria. The PI-RADS scoring system, a standardized method for interpreting mpMRI results, is utilized to assess and stratify the probability of prostate cancer within the identified lesions. Specifically, findings with a PI-RADS score of 3 or higher were subjected to further clinical intervention, typically necessitating a subsequent biopsy procedure for confirmation and accurate diagnosis. Notably, all biopsies performed were precisely guided by MRI imaging, ensuring precise and targeted tissue sampling.

Following the biopsy procedure, an esteemed pathologist, holding an extensive track record of over two decades in the domain, meticulously examined and graded the biopsy specimens. These histopathological assessments served as the gold standard benchmark for subsequent analyses and formed the foundation for the PROSTATEx challenges, contributing invaluable insights into the diagnostic accuracy and performance of various prostate cancer detection methodologies. The inclusion of this meticulously curated dataset, spanning a range of PI-RADS scores and histopathological grades, represents a critical resource for benchmarking and evaluating novel detection algorithms and approaches for accurate prostate cancer detection and localization.

The dataset encompassed multiple imaging sequences in each mpMRI scan, encompassing a combination of T2-weighted, dynamic contrast-enhanced (DCE), and DWI sequences. These scans were conducted utilizing cutting-edge MRI equipment, particularly the 3T MAGNETOM Trio and Skyra systems developed by Siemens Medical Systems, ensuring high-quality and detailed imaging outcomes. The T2-weighted images were acquired utilizing a turbo spin echo sequence, producing images with a remarkable spatial resolution of approximately 0.5 mm in a 2D format and a slice thickness of 3.6 mm. These images provide detailed anatomical information of the prostate gland, enabling the visualization of structural abnormalities and lesions with remarkable clarity. The DCE sequences, essential for assessing the perfusion of tissues, were captured using a 3D turbo flash gradient echo sequence. This sequence produced images with a spatial resolution of $1.5 \times 1.5 \times 4$ mm^3 and a temporal resolution of 3.5 seconds, allowing for the visualization of contrast enhancement dynamics over time, particularly useful in identifying areas of abnormal vascularity.

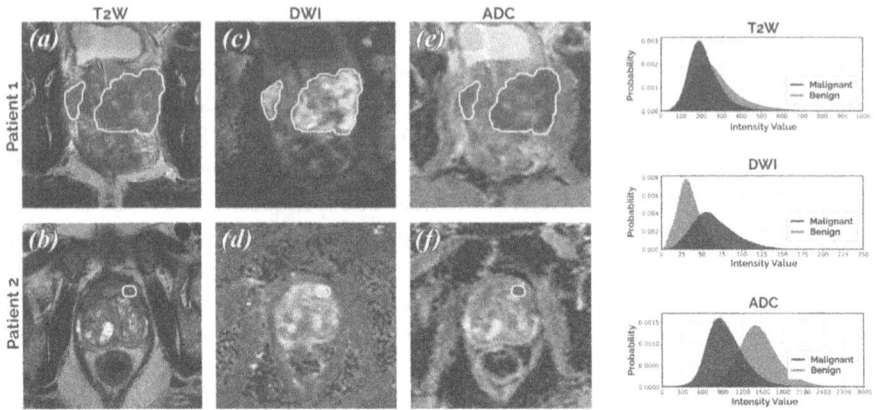

Figure 12.14 **Sample of the dataset used in the proposed algorithm.**

Furthermore, the DWI series, crucial for evaluating tissue microstructure, utilized a single-shot echo-planar imaging sequence. This sequence captured images with a resolution of $2 \times 2 \times 3.6$ mm³, incorporating diffusion-encoding gradients in three directions and employing three distinct b-values (50 s/mm², 400 s/mm², and 800 s/mm²). Additionally, a computed apparent diffusion coefficient map, an essential tool for assessing tissue cellularity and detecting abnormalities, was derived from the DWI series. Moreover, the study encompassed Ktrans images, derived from the DCE imaging, in mhd format. These Ktrans images, representing the volume transfer constant of contrast agent between blood plasma and the extravascular extracellular space, offered critical insights into tissue perfusion dynamics, aiding in the identification and characterization of suspicious lesions within the prostate. Each identified lesion within the dataset was meticulously documented, accompanied by detailed location information and a reference thumbnail image, providing a comprehensive resource for subsequent analyses. Furthermore, the pathology-defined Gleason Grade Group, a pivotal metric for characterizing prostate cancer aggressiveness, was meticulously documented for each identified lesion, ensuring a robust dataset for evaluating and validating detection methodologies and algorithms (Figure 12.14).

12.5 Results

Table 12.3 presents a comparison of different models based on their Test AUC (%), which is a measure of classification performance. Among the models listed, the ViT (vision transformer) stands out with the highest Test AUC of 95%, indicating superior performance in the classification task. The DeepCNN and CNN models

Table 12.3   Comparison of the Different Architecture with the Proposed Model

Model	Test AUC (%)
DeepCNN (Yoo et al., 2019)	87
2D U-Net (De Vente et al., 2020)	44.6
CNN (Saha et al., 2021)	86.69
U-Net + AH-Net (Hosseinzadeh et al., 2022)	70
ML (SVM, DT) (Hussain et al., 2018)	98
Resnet-101 (Iqbal et al., 2021)	100
EVT (Proposed)	100

also demonstrate good performance with Test AUC values of 87% and 86.69%, respectively. The U-Net + AH-Net model achieves a Test AUC of 70%, while the 2D U-Net lags behind with a Test AUC of 44.6%. Overall, the ViT model shows promising results, suggesting its effectiveness for the given classification task compared to the other models (Figures 12.15–12.17).

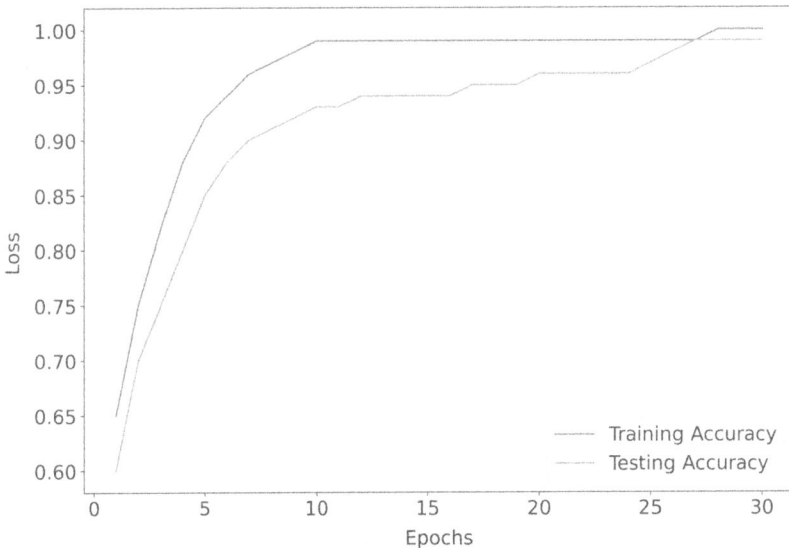

Figure 12.15   Training and testing accuracy curve for the proposed approach.

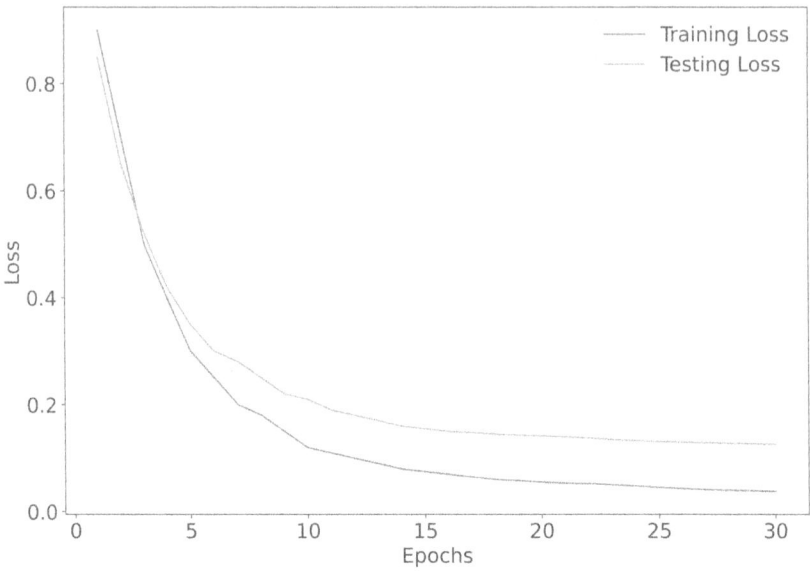

Figure 12.16   Training and testing loss curve for the proposed approach.

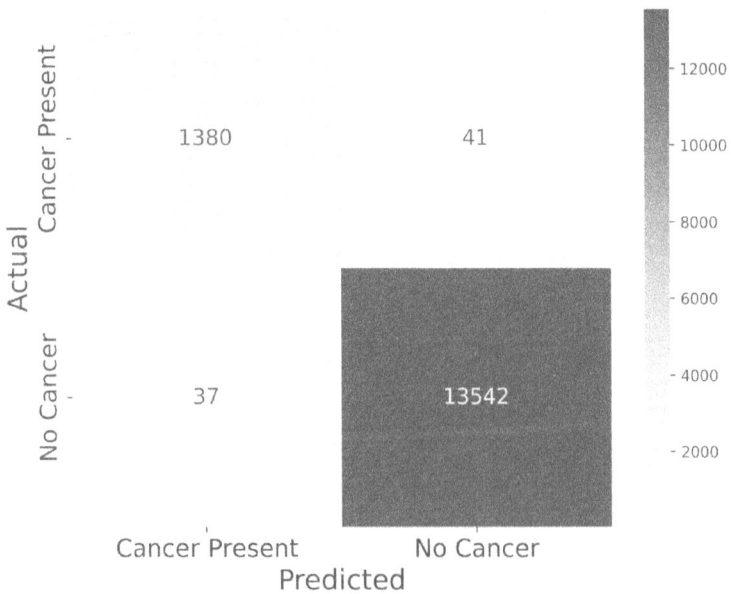

Figure 12.17   Diagnostic performance illustrated through a heatmap for prostate cancer detection.

12.6 Conclusion

The application of vision transformers in the context of prostate cancer detection emerges as a promising avenue in modern medical diagnostics. Through extensive analysis and rigorous experimentation, this study effectively showcased the superior efficacy and potential of vision transformers in augmenting the precision and accuracy of prostate cancer diagnosis. Leveraging the inherent capabilities of vision transformers, particularly their adeptness in capturing intricate relationships and discerning nuanced patterns within prostate images through self-attention mechanisms, has distinctly enhanced the diagnostic precision for prostate cancer. The experimental outcomes vividly underscored the considerable advantages of the proposed deep learning–based approach over conventional methodologies. Vision transformers exhibited exceptional performance metrics, boasting significantly heightened precision, recall, and overall accuracy in the identification of prostate cancer cases. This groundbreaking discovery offers a beacon of hope to the medical community by presenting a cutting-edge tool for the early and precise detection of prostate cancer, thereby potentially enhancing patient outcomes and bolstering survival rates.

Furthermore, this research spotlighted the remarkable adaptability of vision transformers in managing diverse and extensive medical datasets, encompassing multi-modal imaging alongside clinical information. By amalgamating various data sources, the suggested methodology holds tremendous promise in improving overall diagnostic capabilities. Additionally, the integration of XAI into the vision transformers–based model empowers medical practitioners by providing a transparent view into the decision-making process of the AI system. This heightened transparency instills greater trust in the AI's results and equips doctors with valuable insights into the specific features within prostate images contributing to the AI's cancer detection. As a forward-looking perspective, the future scope of this research entails further refinements and validations in real-world clinical settings, potentially paving the way for the seamless integration of vision transformers and XAI methodologies into routine prostate cancer diagnostic protocols. This amalgamation holds the potential to revolutionize the landscape of prostate cancer diagnosis, enabling comprehensive, individualized, and highly accurate evaluations by harnessing the synergistic power of cutting-edge deep learning techniques and XAI in clinical practice.

References

ACDC-LungHP - Grand Challenge. (n.d.). Grand-Challenge.Org. Retrieved November 29, 2023, from https://acdc-lunghp.grand-challenge.org/DATA/

Aerts, H. J. W. L., Wee, L., Rios Velazquez, E., Leijenaar, R. T. H., Parmar, C., Grossmann, P., Carvalho, S., Bussink, J., Monshouwer, R., Haibe-Kains, B., Rietveld, D., Hoebers, F., Rietbergen, M. M., Leemans, C. R., Dekker, A., Quackenbush, J., Gillies, R. J., & Lambin, P. (2019). *Data from NSCLC-radiomics* (Version 4) [dataset]. *The Cancer Imaging Archive.* https://doi.org/10.7937/K9/TCIA.2015.PF0M9REI

Afza, F., Khan, M. A., Sharif, M., Kadry, S., Manogaran, G., Saba, T., Ashraf, I., & Damaševičius, R. (2021). A framework of human action recognition using length control features fusion and weighted entropy-variances based feature selection. *Image and Vision Computing, 106*, 104090.

Armato III, S. G., McLennan, G., Bidaut, L., McNitt-Gray, M. F., Meyer, C. R., Reeves, A. P., ..., & Clarke, L. P. (2011). The lung image database consortium (LIDC) and image database resource initiative (IDRI): A completed reference database of lung nodules on CT scans. *Medical Physics, 38*(2), 915–931.

Borgli, H., Thambawita, V., Smedsrud, P. H., Hicks, S., & Jha, D., et al. (2020). HyperKvasir, a comprehensive multi-class image and video dataset for gastrointestinal endoscopy. *Scientific Data, 7*(1), 283. https://doi.org/10.1038/s41597-020-00622-y

Calisto, M. B., & Lai-Yuen, S. K. (2020). AdaEn-Net: An ensemble of adaptive 2D–3D fully convolutional networks for medical image segmentation. *Neural Networks, 126*, 76–94.

Carter, H. B., Albertsen, P. C., Barry, M. J., Etzioni, R., Freedland, S. J., Greene, K. L., Holmberg, L., Kantoff, P., Konety, B. R., & Murad, M. H. (2013). Early detection of prostate cancer: AUA guideline. *The Journal of Urology, 190*(2), 419–426.

Catalona, W. J., Smith, D. S., Ratliff, T. L., Dodds, K. M., Coplen, D. E., Yuan, J. J. J., Petros, J. A., & Andriole, G. L. (1991). Measurement of prostate-specific antigen in serum as a screening test for prostate cancer. *New England Journal of Medicine, 324*(17), 1156–1161. https://doi.org/10.1056/NEJM199104253241702

CBICA. (n.d.). Brain Tumor Segmentation (BraTS) Challenge 2020: Scope. Perelman School of Medicine at the University of Pennsylvania. Retrieved November 29, 2023, from https://www.med.upenn.edu/cbica/brats2020/

Chaudhari, A., Bhatt, C., Krishna, A., & Mazzeo, P. L. (2022). ViTFER: Facial emotion recognition with vision transformers. *Applied System Innovation, 5*(4), 80.

Chaudhari, A., Bhatt, C., Nguyen, T. T., Patel, N., Chavda, K., & Sarda, K. (2023). Emotion recognition system via facial expressions and speech using machine learning and deep learning techniques. *SN Computer Science, 4*(4), 363. https://doi.org/10.1007/s42979-022-01633-9

Chen, L.-C., Papandreou, G., Kokkinos, I., Murphy, K., & Yuille, A. L. (2017). Deeplab: Semantic image segmentation with deep convolutional nets, atrous convolution, and fully connected CRFs. *IEEE Transactions on Pattern Analysis and Machine Intelligence, 40*(4), 834–848.

Cheng, J. (2017). Brain tumor dataset. figshare. https://doi.org/10.6084/m9.figshare.1512427.v5

Choyke, P., Turkbey, B., Pinto, P., Merino, M., & Wood, B. (2016). *Data from PROSTATE-MRI* (Version 1). *The Cancer Imaging Archive*. https://doi.org/10.7937/K9/TCIA.2016.6046GUDV

Chui, K. T., Gupta, B. B., Chi, H. R., Arya, V., Alhalabi, W., Ruiz, M. T., & Shen, C.-W. (2022). Transfer learning-based multi-scale denoising convolutional neural network for prostate cancer detection. *Cancers, 14*(15), 3687.

Danish Lung Cancer Group. (2007). *Screening for Lung Cancer. A Randomised Controlled Trial of Low-Dose CT-Scanning*. (Clinical Trial Registration NCT00496977). clinicaltrials.gov. https://clinicaltrials.gov/study/NCT00496977

De Rooij, M., Hamoen, E. H., Fütterer, J. J., Barentsz, J. O., & Rovers, M. M. (2014). Accuracy of multiparametric MRI for prostate cancer detection: A meta-analysis. *American Journal of Roentgenology, 202*(2), 343–351.

De Vente, C., Vos, P., Hosseinzadeh, M., Pluim, J., & Veta, M. (2020). Deep learning regression for prostate cancer detection and grading in bi-parametric MRI. *IEEE Transactions on Biomedical Engineering, 68*(2), 374–383.

DermIS. (n.d.). DermIS.Net. Retrieved November 29, 2023, from https://dermis.net/dermisroot/en/home/index.htm

Dosovitskiy, A., Beyer, L., Kolesnikov, A., Weissenborn, D., Zhai, X., Unterthiner, T., Dehghani, M., Minderer, M., Heigold, G., & Gelly, S. (2010). An image is worth 16 × 16 words: Transformers for image recognition at scale. *arXiv:2010.11929*.

Du, S., Bayasi, N., Hamarneh, G., & Garbi, R. (2023). MDViT: Multi-domain Vision Transformer for Small. In: Greenspan, H., et al. Medical Image Computing and Computer Assisted Intervention – MICCAI 2023. Lecture Notes in Computer Science, vol. 14223. Springer, Cham. https://doi.org/10.1007/978-3-031-43901-8_43

Dudekula, K. V., Syed, H., Basha, M. I. M., Swamykan, S. I., Kasaraneni, P. P., Kumar, Y. V. P., Flah, A., & Azar, A. T. (2023). Convolutional neural network-based personalized program recommendation system for smart television users. *Sustainability, 15*(3), 2206.

EndoTect 2020. (n.d.). Retrieved November 29, 2023, from https://endotect.com/

Fahad, H. M., Ghani Khan, M. U., Saba, T., Rehman, A., & Iqbal, S. (2018). Microscopic abnormality classification of cardiac murmurs using ANFIS and HMM. *Microscopy Research and Technique, 81*(5), 449–457.

Ganesan, J., Azar, A. T., Alsenan, S., Kamal, N. A., Qureshi, B., & Hassanien, A. E. (2022). Deep learning reader for visually impaired. *Electronics, 11*(20), 3335.

Giotis, I., Molders, N., Land, S., Biehl, M., Jonkman M. F., & Petkov, N. (2015). MEDNODE: A computer-assisted melanoma diagnosis system using non-dermoscopic images. *Expert Systems with Applications, 42*, 6578–6585.

Harvey, C. J., Pilcher, J., Richenberg, J., Patel, U., & Frauscher, F. (2012). Applications of transrectal ultrasound in prostate cancer. *The British Journal of Radiology, 85*(special_issue_1), S3–S17. https://doi.org/10.1259/bjr/56357549

Heath, M., Bowyer, K., Kopans, D., Moore, R., & Kegelmeyer, P. (2001). The digital database for screening mammography, IWDM-2000. In *Fifth International Workshop on Digital Mammography*. Medical Physics Publishing (pp. 212–218).

Hosseinzadeh, M., Saha, A., Brand, P., Slootweg, I., de Rooij, M., & Huisman, H. (2022). Deep learning–assisted prostate cancer detection on bi-parametric MRI: Minimum training data size requirements and effect of prior knowledge. *European Radiology, 32*, 2224–2234.

Hussain, L., Ahmed, A., Saeed, S., Rathore, S., Awan, I. A., Shah, S. A., Majid, A., Idris, A., & Awan, A. A. (2018). Prostate cancer detection using machine learning techniques by employing combination of features extracting strategies. *Cancer Biomarkers, 21*(2), 393–413.

Iftikhar, S., Fatima, K., Rehman, A., Almazyad, A. S., & Saba, T. (2017). An evolution based hybrid approach for heart diseases classification and associated risk factors identification. *Biomedical Research, 28*(8), 3451–3455.

Iqbal, S., Siddiqui, G. F., Rehman, A., Hussain, L., Saba, T., Tariq, U., & Abbasi, A. A. (2021). Prostate cancer detection using deep learning and traditional techniques. *IEEE Access, 9*, 27085–27100.

Japanese Society of Radiological Technology. (n.d.). JSRT Database. Retrieved November 29, 2023, from http://db.jsrt.or.jp/eng.php

Jha, D., Smedsrud, P. H., Riegler, M. A., Halvorsen, P., de Lange, T., Johansen, D., & Johansen, H. D. (2020). Kvasir-SEG: A Segmented Polyp Dataset. In Y. M. Ro, W.-H. Cheng, J. Kim, W.-T. Chu, P. Cui, J.-W. Choi, M.-C. Hu, & W. De Neve (Eds.), *MultiMedia Modeling* (pp. 451–462). Springer International Publishing. https://doi.org/10.1007/978-3-030-37734-2_37

Khan, M. A., Lali, I. U., Rehman, A., Ishaq, M., Sharif, M., Saba, T., Zahoor, S., & Akram, T. (2019). Brain tumor detection and classification: A framework of marker-based watershed algorithm and multilevel priority features selection. *Microscopy Research and Technique*, *82*(6), 909–922, *11*, 47410–47419. https://doi.org/10.1002/jemt.23238

Kothadiya, D. R., Bhatt, C. M., Rehman, A., Alamri, F. S., & Saba, T. (2023). SignExplainer: An explainable AI-enabled framework for sign language recognition with ensemble learning. *IEEE Access*. https://ieeexplore.ieee.org/abstract/document/10122570/

Kothadiya, D. R., Bhatt, C. M., & Rida, I. (2024). Simsiam Network Based Self-Supervised Model for Sign Language Recognition. In A. Bennour, A. Bouridane, & L. Chaari (Eds.), *Intelligent Systems and Pattern Recognition* (Vol. 1941, pp. 3–13). Springer Nature Switzerland. https://doi.org/10.1007/978-3-031-46338-9_1

Kothadiya, D., Bhatt, C., Sapariya, K., Patel, K., Gil-González, A.-B., & Corchado, J. M. (2022). Deepsign: Sign language detection and recognition using deep learning. *Electronics*, *11*(11), 1780.

Kothadiya, D., Bhatt, C., Soni, D., Gadhe, K., Patel, S., Bruno, A., & Mazzeo, P. L. (2023). Enhancing fingerprint liveness detection accuracy using deep learning: A comprehensive study and novel approach. *Journal of Imaging*, *9*(8), 158.

Kothadiya, D., Chaudhari, A., Macwan, R., Patel, K., & Bhatt, C. (2021). The convergence of deep learning and computer vision: Smart city applications and research Challenges. *3rd International Conference on Integrated Intelligent Computing Communication & Security (ICIIC 2021)*, 14–22. https://www.atlantis-press.com/proceedings/iciic-21/125960870

Kothadiya, D., Rehman, A., Abbas, S., Alamri, F. S., & Saba, T. (2023). Attention-based deep learning framework to recognize diabetes disease from cellular retinal images. *Biochemistry and Cell Biology*, *101*(6), 550–561. https://doi.org/10.1139/bcb-2023-0151

Kothadiya, D. R., Bhatt, C. M., Saba, T., Rehman, A., & Bahaj, S. A. (2023). SignFORMER: DeepVision transformer for sign language recognition. *IEEE Access*, *11*, 4730–4739.

Larabi-Marie-Sainte, S., Aburahmah, L., Almohaini, R., & Saba, T. (2019). Current techniques for diabetes prediction: Review and case study. *Applied Sciences*, *9*(21), 4604.

Linardatos, P., Papastefanopoulos, V., & Kotsiantis, S. (2020). Explainable AI: A review of machine learning interpretability methods. *Entropy*, *23*(1), 18.

Malaviya, N., Rahevar, M., Virani, A., Ganatra, A., & Bhuva, K. (2023). LViT: Vision Transformer for Lung Cancer Detection. *2023 International Conference on Artificial Intelligence and Smart Communication (AISC)*, Greater Noida, India, pp. 93–98, doi: 10.1109/AISC56616.2023.10085230.

Marcus, D. S., Wang, T. H., Parker, J., Csernansky, J. G., Morris, J. C., & Buckner, R. L. (2007). Open access series of imaging studies (OASIS): Cross-sectional MRI data in young, middle aged, nondemented, and demented older adults. *Journal of Cognitive Neuroscience*, *19*(9), 1498–1507. https://doi.org/10.1162/jocn.2007.19.9.1498

Meethongjan, K., Dzulkifli, M., Rehman, A., Altameem, A., & Saba, T. (2013). An intelligent fused approach for face recognition. *Journal of Intelligent Systems*, *22*(2), 197–212.

Moreira, I. C., Amaral, I., Domingues, I., Cardoso, A., Cardoso, M. J., & Cardoso, J. S. (2012). Inbreast: Toward a full-field digital mammographic database. *Academic Radiology*, *19*(2), 236–248.

Mughal, B., Muhammad, N., Sharif, M., Rehman, A., & Saba, T. (2018a). Removal of pectoral muscle based on topographic map and shape-shifting silhouette. *BMC Cancer*, *18*(1), 1–14.

Mughal, B., Sharif, M., Muhammad, N., & Saba, T. (2018b). A novel classification scheme to decline the mortality rate among women due to breast tumor. *Microscopy Research and Technique*, *81*(2), 171–180.

NITRC. (n.d.). IBSR: Tool/Resource Info. Retrieved November 29, 2023, from https://www.nitrc.org/projects/ibsr

PAIP 2019—Grand Challenge. (n.d.). Grand-Challenge.Org. Retrieved November 29, 2023, from https://paip2019.grand-challenge.org/

Parekh, D. J., Ankerst, D. P., Troyer, D., Srivastava, S., & Thompson, I. M. (2007). Biomarkers for prostate cancer detection. *The Journal of Urology*, *178*(6), 2252–2259.

Partin, A. W., Catalona, W. J., Southwick, P. C., Subong, E. N., Gasior, G. H., & Chan, D. W. (1996). Analysis of percent free prostate-specific antigen (PSA) for prostate cancer detection: Influence of total PSA, prostate volume, and age. *Urology*, *48*(6), 55–61.

Patel, B., Kothadiya, D., & Patel, R. (2023). COVID-19 detection on chest X-ray image using YOLO based architecture. *2023 International Conference on Artificial Intelligence and Smart Communication (AISC)*, 27–30. https://ieeexplore.ieee.org/abstract/document/10085498/

Pogorelov, K., Randel, K. R., De Lange, T., Eskeland, S. L., Griwodz, C., Johansen, D., Spampinato, C., Taschwer, M., Lux, M., Schmidt, P. T., Riegler, M., & Halvorsen, P. (2017). Nerthus: A bowel preparation quality video dataset. *Proceedings of the 8th ACM on Multimedia Systems Conference*, 170–174. https://doi.org/10.1145/3083187.3083216

Pogorelov, K., Randel, K. R., Griwodz, C., Eskeland, S. L., De Lange, T., Johansen, D., Spampinato, C., Dang-Nguyen, D.-T., Lux, M., Schmidt, P. T., Riegler, M., & Halvorsen, P. (2017). KVASIR: A multi-class image dataset for computer aided gastrointestinal disease detection. *Proceedings of the 8th ACM on Multimedia Systems Conference*, 164–169. https://doi.org/10.1145/3083187.3083212

PROSTATEx-2 Challenge. (n.d.). Retrieved November 29, 2023, from https://www.aapm.org/GrandChallenge/PROSTATEx-2/default.asp

Raisinghani, Y., Shah, A., & Rahevar, M. (2021). Stacked graph transformer for HIV molecular prediction. *2021 2nd International Conference on Communication, Computing and Industry 4.0 (C2I4)*, 1–6. https://doi.org/10.1109/C2I454156.2021.9689399

Reeves, A. P., Biancardi, A. M., Yankelevitz, D., Fotin, S., Keller, B. M., Jirapatnakul, A., & Lee, J. (2009). A public image database to support research in computer aided diagnosis. *2009 Annual International Conference of the IEEE Engineering in Medicine and Biology Society*, 3715–3718. https://ieeexplore.ieee.org/abstract/document/5334807/

Rehman, A., Khan, M. A., Saba, T., Mehmood, Z., Tariq, U., & Ayesha, N. (2021). Microscopic brain tumor detection and classification using 3D CNN and feature selection architecture. *Microscopy Research and Technique*, *84*(1), 133–149. https://doi.org/10.1002/jemt.23597

Rotemberg, V., Kurtansky, N., Betz-Stablein, B., Caffery, L., Chousakos, E., Codella, N., Combalia, M., Dusza, S., Guitera, P., Gutman, D., Halpern, A., Helba, B., Kittler, H., Kose, K., Langer, S., Lioprys, K., Malvehy, J., Musthaq, S., Nanda, J., …, Soyer,

H. P. (2021). A patient-centric dataset of images and metadata for identifying melanomas using clinical context. *Scientific Data, 8*(1), 34. https://doi.org/10.1038/s41597-021-00815-z

Saba, T., Al-Zahrani, S., & Rehman, A. (2012). Expert system for offline clinical guidelines and treatment. *Life Science Journal, 9*(4), 2639–2658.

Saha, A., Hosseinzadeh, M., & Huisman, H. (2021). End-to-end prostate cancer detection in bpMRI via 3D CNNs: Effects of attention mechanisms, clinical priori and decoupled false positive reduction. *Medical Image Analysis, 73*, 102155.

Santos, A., Wernersson, R., & Jensen, L. J. (2015). Cyclebase 3.0: A multi-organism database on cell-cycle regulation and phenotypes. *Nucleic Acids Research, 43*(D1), D1140–D1144.

Schröder, F. H., Van Der Cruijsen-Koeter, I., De Koning, H. J., Vis, A. N., Hoedemaeker, R. F., & Kranse, R. (2000). Prostate cancer detection at low prostate specific antigen. *The Journal of Urology, 163*(3), 806–812.

Sevak, J. S., Kapadia, A. D., Chavda, J. B., Shah, A., & Rahevar, M. (2017). Survey on semantic image segmentation techniques. *2017 International Conference on Intelligent Sustainable Systems (ICISS)*, 306–313. https://doi.org/10.1109/ISS1.2017.8389420

SLIVER07 – Grand Challenge. (n.d.). Grand-Challenge.Org. Retrieved November 29, 2023, from https://sliver07.grand-challenge.org/

Smith, D. S., & Catalona, W. J. (1994). Rate of change in serum prostate specific antigen levels as a method for prostate cancer detection. *The Journal of Urology, 152*(4), 1163–1167.

Soronen, V., Talala, K., Raitanen, J., Taari, K., Tammela, T., & Auvinen, A. (2021). Digital rectal examination in prostate cancer screening at PSA level 3.0-3.9 ng/ml: Long-term results from a randomized trial. *Scandinavian Journal of Urology, 55*(5), 348–353. https://doi.org/10.1080/21681805.2021.1966095

Spanhol, F., Oliveira, L. S., Petitjean, C. and Heutte, L. (2017, June 20). Breast Cancer Histopathological Database. BreakHis—Laboratório Visão Robótica e Imagem. https://web.inf.ufpr.br/vri/databases/breast-cancer-histopathological-database-breakhis/

SPIE-AAPM-NCI PROSTATEx Challenges: The Cancer Imaging Archive (TCIA) Public Access (n.d.). Retrieved November 29, 2023, from https://wiki.cancerimagingarchive.net/display/Public/SPIE-AAPM-NCI+PROSTATEx+Challenges

Suckling, J., et al (1994). The mini-MIAS database of mammograms. Retrieved November 29, 2023, from http://peipa.essex.ac.uk/info/mias.html

Tahir, B., Iqbal, S., Usman Ghani Khan, M., Saba, T., Mehmood, Z., Anjum, A., & Mahmood, T. (2019). Feature enhancement framework for brain tumor segmentation and classification. *Microscopy Research and Technique, 82*(6), 803–811.

Tajbakhsh, N., Gurudu, S. R., & Liang, J. (2015). Automated polyp detection in colonoscopy videos using shape and context information. *IEEE Transactions on Medical Imaging, 35*(2), 630–644.

The PI-CAI Challenge – Grand Challenge. (n.d.). Grand-Challenge.Org. Retrieved May 29, 2023, from https://pi-cai.grand-challenge.org/

Yoo, S., Gujrathi, I., Haider, M. A., & Khalvati, F. (2019). Prostate cancer detection using deep convolutional neural networks. *Scientific Reports, 9*(1), 1–10.

Index

For Product Safety Concerns and Information please contact our EU
representative GPSR@taylorandfrancis.com
Taylor & Francis Verlag GmbH, Kaufingerstraße 24, 80331 München, Germany

www.ingramcontent.com/pod-product-compliance
Lightning Source LLC
Chambersburg PA
CBHW060351220326
41598CB00023B/2880